ACCESSIBILITY AND ACTIVE OFFER

ACCESSIBILITY AND ACTIVE OFFER

HEALTH CARE AND SOCIAL SERVICES IN LINGUISTIC MINORITY COMMUNITIES

Edited by Marie Drolet, Pier Bouchard
and Jacinthe Savard

With the collaboration of Josée Benoît
and Solange van Kemenade

University of Ottawa Press
2017

uOttawa

The University of Ottawa Press (UOP) is proud to be the oldest of the francophone university presses in Canada and the only bilingual university publisher in North America. Since 1936, UOP has been "enriching intellectual and cultural discourse" by producing peer-reviewed and award-winning books in the humanities and social sciences, in French or in English.

Copy Editing: Robert Ferguson
Proofreading: Lesley Mann
Typesetting: Interscript & Édiscript enr.
Cover Design: Édiscript enr.
Cover Image: Shutterstock

Library and Archives Canada Cataloguing in Publication
Accessibilité et offre active. English
Accessibility and active offer: health care and social services in linguistic minority communities / edited by Marie Drolet, Pier Bouchard and Jacinthe Savard with the collaboration of Josée Benoît and Solange van Kemenade.

(Health and society)
Translation and adaptation of: Accessibilité et offre active.

Includes bibliographical references.
Issued in print and electronic formats.
ISBN 978-0-7766-2563-8 (softcover)
ISBN 978-0-7766-2564-5 (PDF)
ISBN 978-0-7766-2565-2 (EPUB)
ISBN 978-0-7766-2566-9 (Kindle)

1. Health services accessibility—Canada. 2. Human services—Canada. 3. Linguistic minorities—Services for—Canada. 4. Canadians, French-speaking—Services for. 5. Canadians, English-speaking—Services for—Québec (Province). I. Drolet, Marie, 1957-, editor II. Bouchard, Pier, 1956-, editor III. Savard, Jacinthe, 1961-, editor IV. Title. V. Title: Accessibilité et offre active. English.

RA450.4.F74A3313 2017   362.84'114071   C2017-907036-3
                                                        C2017-907037-1

Legal Deposit:
Library and Archives Canada

The editors gratefully acknowledge the financial support of Health Canada for the translation and adaptation of this work (Original: *Accessibilité et offre active: Santé et services sociaux en contexte linguistique minoritaire*, Presses de l'Université d'Ottawa, 2017) and the close collaboration of the CNFS—Secrétariat national. The views expressed herein do not necessarily represent the views of Health Canada.

The University of Ottawa Press gratefully acknowledges the support extended to its publishing list by the Government of Canada, the Canada Council for the Arts, the Ontario Arts Council, and the Federation for the Humanities and Social Sciences through the Awards to Scholarly Publications Program and by the University of Ottawa.

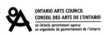
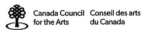

Contents

Introduction: Social Services and Health Services in Minority-Language Communities: Towards an Understanding of the Actors, the System, and the Levers of Action

Marie Drolet, Pier Bouchard,

PART I. ENGAGING ACTORS: PUTTING THE STRATEGIC ANALYSIS TO THE TEST

PART II. POLICY LEVERS AND LEGAL MEASURES: THE INTERPLAY OF ACTORS

PART III. ACCESSIBILITY AND THE ACTIVE OFFER OF FRENCH-LANGUAGE SERVICES

List of Figures and Tables

Chapter 9

Chapter 10

Chapter 11

Chapter 12

Appendix

Chapter 13

Chapter 14

Conclusion

Abbreviations

AFMO	Association française des municipalités de l'Ontario/ Association of Francophone Municipalities of Ontario
AJEFO	Association des juristes d'expression française de l'Ontario (Association of French-language legal professionals in Ontario)
ALEQ	Alberta Language Environment Questionnaire
ANB/ANB	Ambulance Nouveau Brunswick/Ambulance New Brunswick
AOcVF	Action ontarienne contre la violence faite aux femmes (Ontario Francophone action network for violence against women)
AVC/CVA	Accident vasculaire cérébral/cerebral vascular accident or cerebrovascular accident
BACLO/OLCDB	Bureau d'appui aux communautés de langue officielle/Official Language Community Development Bureau
CA/Board	Conseil d'administration/Board of Directors
CALACS	Centres d'aide et de lutte contre les agressions à caractère sexuel (rape crisis and sexual assault centres offering French-language services; most provinces have their own networks offering services in one or both official languages, such as the Ontario Network of Rape Crisis Centres)
CASC/CCAC	Centre d'accès aux soins communautaires/Community Care Access Centre
CCCFSM	Comité consultatif des communautés francophones en situation minoritaire/Consultative Committee for French-Speaking Minority Communities
CCM	Chronic Care Model
CFMNB	Centre de formation médicale du Nouveau-Brunswick (Francophone medical training centre located in Moncton, NB)

CFSM/FMC Communautés francophones en situation minoritaire/ Francophone minority communities

CHSSN Community Health and Social Services Network

CLOSM/OLMC Communautés de langues officielles en situation minoritaire/official language minority communities

CNFS Consortium national de formation en santé (National consortium of health education; association for Francophone post-secondary health science programs)

CSF Commissariat aux services en français/Office of the French Language Services Commissioner

DEAAC Direction de l'éducation des adultes et de l'action communautaire (Adult education and community action bureau)

DEP Diplôme d'études professionnelles (Professional studies diploma; received on completion of one year in a vocational stream in a CÉGEP or college in Quebec)

ECCM Expanded Chronic Care Model

ÉMNO École de médecine du Nord de l'Ontario/Northern Ontario School of Medicine

ESCC/CCHS Enquête sur la santé dans les collectivités canadiennes/ Canadian Community Health Survey

FARFO Fédération des aînés et retraités francophones de l'Ontario (Ontario federation of Francophone seniors and retired people)

FCFA Fédération des communautés francophones et acadiennes (Federation of Acadian and Francophone communities)

FESFO Fédération de la jeunesse franco-ontarienne (Federation of Franco-Ontarian youth)

GRC/RCMP Gendarmerie Royale du Canada/Royal Canadian Mounted Police

GReFoPS Groupe de recherche sur la formation professionnelle en santé et en service social en contexte francophone minoritaire (Group for research on professional education in social service and health care disciplines)

GRIOSS	Groupe de recherche et d'innovation sur l'organisation des services de santé (Group for research and innovation on the organization of health services)
HINT	Hearing In Noise Test
ICRML/CIRLM	Institut canadien de recherche sur les minorités linguistiques/Canadian Institute for Research on Linguistic Minorities
ICS	Intelligibility in Context Scale
LEAP-Q	Language Experience and Proficiency Questionnaire
LLO/OLA	Loi sur les langues officielles du Canada/Official Languages Act, Canada
LLON/OLAN	Loi sur les langues officielles du Nunavut /Official Languages Act, Nunavut
LLONB/OLANB	Loi sur les langues officielles du Nouveau-Brunswick/Official Languages Act, New Brunswick
LSF	Loi sur les services en français
NB	Nouveau-Brunswick/New Brunswick
OA/AO	Offre active/Active Offer
OAF/OFA	Office des affaires francophones/Office of Francophone Affairs
OHIP	Ontario Health Insurance Plan
OMS/WHO	Organisation mondiale de la Santé/World Health Organization
OPP	Police provincial de l'Ontario/Ontario Provincial Police
OPS	Ontario Public Service
QCGN	Quebec Community Groups Network
RLISS/LHIN	Réseaux locaux d'intégration des services de santé/ Local Health Integration Network
SEF/FLS	Services en français/French-language services
SSF	Société santé en français (Association to promote health services in French)
SSI-ICM	Synthetic Sentence Identification and Ipsilateral Competing Message

TCS/CHT	Transfert canadien en matière de santé/Canada Health Transfer
TMB	Test de Mots dans le Bruit (Word recognition in noise test)
TNO/NWT	Territoires-du-Nord-Ouest/Northwest Territories

Social Services and Health Services in Minority-Language Communities: Towards an Understanding of the Actors, the System, and the Levers of Action

Marie Drolet, *University of Ottawa*, Pier Bouchard, *Université de Moncton*,
Jacinthe Savard, *University of Ottawa*,
and Solange van Kemenade, *University of Ottawa*

Have you ever imagined what it would be like to communicate with a doctor or other health care or social services professional in a language you cannot speak or only speak occasionally? That is the everyday experience of many Francophones living in Francophone minority communities (FMCs) and many Anglophones living in Quebec, especially in areas outside Montréal. It is very common for people in these situations, particularly among seniors and young children, to be unable to access comparable social services and health care in both official languages even though many do not speak the language of the majority—English in FMCs and French in Quebec.

The first multidisciplinary volume of its kind, this collective work presents current research on language issues in the area of health and social services in Canadian official language minority communities. The chapters in the collection, covering major topics in the field, are anchored in the notion of active offer. From an operational perspective, "[a]ctive offer can be defined as a verbal or written invitation to users to express themselves in the official language of their choice. The active offer to speak their language must precede the request for such services" (Bouchard, Beaulieu, & Desmeules, 2012, p. 46). Moreover, the results of several studies to date reveal that the active offer of health and social services in both official languages in minority situations is a matter of quality and safety (Drolet, Dubouloz, & Benoît, 2014; Lapierre *et al.*, 2014; Roberts & Burton, 2013); humanization of care and services; professional ethics; rights and equity (Bouchard, Beaulieu, & Desmeules, 2012; Vézina & Dupuis-Blanchard, 2015); and satisfaction on the part of users and their caregivers (Drolet *et al.*, 2014; Éthier & Belzile, 2012; Roberts & Burton, 2013).

It is interesting, too, that active offer practices are also part of other minority language situations, such as among Welsh speakers in Wales. Active offer is part of an approach that involves developing best practices in the planning and organization of health and social services and fostering the emergence of a social service and health care system that is linguistically appropriate (Roberts & Burton, 2013). Along the same lines the United States adopted the National Standards on Culturally and Linguistically Appropriate Services (CLAS) in 2001. The objectives of these standards are to improve the social services and health care provided to minority populations through (1) better access to services in the user's language; (2) culturally sensitive care; and (3) organizational support (U.S. Department of Health and Human Services, 2001).

All these studies and analyses suggest that efforts must continue to enhance the education offered in post-secondary institutions, thereby enabling future health and social services professionals to better understand the issues they will face in the workplace: accessibility and the active offer of services in official language minority communities. It is essential that students be equipped to become leaders who are able to intervene effectively in this regard and to support changes in the organizations for which they will work.

The Importance of Health and Social Services in the Official Language of One's Choice

Before turning to the specific content of the chapters in this volume, it would be beneficial to offer some reflections on the importance of access to health and social services in the official language of the user's choice, and the reasons that lie behind such active offer. These thoughts can be framed by international research work on the vulnerability of people with limited language and literacy skills, which introduced the concepts of health literacy and Limited English Proficiency (LEP) (Andrulis & Brach, 2007; Derose, Escarce, & Lurie, 2007).

If we examine the rates of bilingualism in Canada, it is Francophones living in minority language communities (i.e., outside Quebec) who have the highest rate: 87% speak both official languages. In Quebec, which at 42.6% has the highest overall rate of bilingualism in Canada, 61% of Anglophones and 38% of Francophones speak both languages fluently (Lepage & Corbeil, 2013). On the other hand, New Brunswick, Canada's only officially bilingual province, has an overall rate of bilingualism of 33.2%; 72% of Francophones are bilingual, representing two thirds (67.4%) of bilingual residents in the province (Pépin-Filion & Guignard Noël, 2014). Furthermore, immigrants, who constitute the primary factor of demographic growth in Canada, represent 20% of the Canadian population, and approximately 20% of these newcomers speak a language other than French or English as their mother tongue. The result is that a large proportion (82.5%) of Canadians cannot speak both official languages (Lepage & Corbeil, 2013). Finally, more than 86% of bilingual people live in Quebec, Ontario, and New Brunswick, while they make up only 63% of the overall Canadian population (ibid.).

Despite the high rate of bilingualism among Francophones in official language minority communities, they prefer to receive social services and health care in French (Gagnon-Arpin *et al.*, 2014). The same is true for English-speaking Quebeckers, who prefer to receive these services in English. Indeed, language plays a fundamental role in the ability of the user and/or the user's caregiver or family members to build a relationship of trust with the health or social service professional. In terms of safety, when the professional and user share a common language, verbal communication is clearer and more efficient. As a result, the professional's treatments and interventions are better able to respond to the needs expressed by the people concerned and the experiences and conditions they describe (Snowden, Masland, Peng, Wei-Mein Lou, & Wallace, 2011).

This observation also holds true for bilingual people seeking services; they are generally more comfortable and have a higher language proficiency in one of the two languages they speak (Boudreault & Dubois, 2008). It is wrong to assume that a bilingual person who can converse in a second language can express him/herself at the same level in this language as a person for whom it is the first language. For example, in a study by Manson (1988, cited by Ferguson & Candib, 2002), Spanish-speaking people in the United States ask more questions when a physician from the same language group is present.

Furthermore, various factors can affect the language in which people who have learned several languages are best able to express themselves on a given subject. Among the factors are the order and the context in which they learned the language, and how often they use each of the languages in different contexts (Köpke & Schmid, 2011; Pavlenko, 2012). People who speak an official language in a minority context may switch regularly between the language of the minority and that of the majority. For example, they may prefer to use the language of the majority to find a specific element in their environment (Santiago-Rivera *et al.*, 2009). These authors emphasize the tendency for the language of the minority, or of the majority, to adapt to the way people speak and the terms they use in their everyday speech (ibid.). An individual may rely predominantly on one language to express ideas that are work-related and another to express emotions, or share a situation in the language in which it occurred.

Finally, words spoken by an individual in their first language seem to be more emotionally charged or have a higher affective value and be more complex and spontaneous (Santiago-Rivera *et al.*, 2009). This is even more apparent when the person is distressed or suffering, expressing emotions, or analyzing events in depth and interpreting their meaning (Castaño, Biever, González, & Anderson, 2007; Madoc-Jones, 2004). Understanding this is vital for helping the relationship or problem-solving when a health or social issue arises, and for empowering people to overcome their situation.

A number of studies from Canada, Wales, the U.S. and other countries also have demonstrated the consequences of not receiving care and services in the language of one's choice. In terms of access, people in official language minority communities are less likely to consult health professionals who provide examinations and primary care, and to receive preventive care. They have a weaker understanding of the care and services they receive (Bonacruz Kazzi & Cooper, 2003) and are, therefore, less likely to follow the recommendations of a health professional compared to people in the majority language group (Jacobs, Chen, Karliner, Agger-Gutpa, & Mutha, 2006; Qualité de services de santé Ontario, 2015). Mainly because of this context, people in the minority language group are at greater risk of being admitted to the hospital (Drouin & Rivet, 2003) and, once there, tend to remain there longer (Jacobs *et al.*, 2006).

The safety and quality of care are also affected: users have a greater tendency to experience diagnostic errors and negative repercussions from their treatments (Bowen, 2015; Drouin & Rivet, 2003; Ferguson & Candib, 2002; Irvine *et al.*, 2006; Flores *et al.*, 2003). For example, they may have an adverse reaction to their medication if they do not completely understand the instructions, at least in part because of the complexity of the medical and professional language used (Drouin & Rivet, 2003). When dialogue becomes difficult, language barriers, trust, and confidence in the health or social service professional can be diminished (Anderson *et al.*, 2003), the user's confidentiality can be violated, especially if there is an interpreter or if has been hard to obtain informed consent (Flores *et al.*, 2003), and the user is less satisfied with the care and services received (Bowen, 2015; Drolet *et al.*, 2014; Irvine *et al.*, 2006; Mead & Roland, 2009; Meyers *et al.*, 2009).

For seniors, proficiency in the second language has often deteriorated because of age-related conditions such as loss of hearing or neurological damage (Alzheimer's disease, related dementia, cardiovascular accident, etc.) (Madoc-Jones, 2004). In this case, research has found that the first language learned is connected to procedural memory, as it has been learned implicitly; the second or even third languages are more often learned explicitly and draw instead on the declarative memory (Paradis, 2000; Köpke & Schmid, 2011). These different types of memory are associated with different brain structures. Thus, in the case of a brain injury, the first and second languages learned can be affected in similar or distinct ways and recovery can follow various paths: parallel, differential, selective, etc. (Paradis, 2000; Köpke & Prod'homme, 2009).

When they are in need of social service and health care procedures in which communication is of paramount importance, people in an official language minority community are less likely to consult professionals; their weak skills in the language of the majority are among the reasons (Kirmayer *et al.*, 2007). Difficulties finding a general practitioner able to refer them to a specialist, long wait times, the inability to find relevant and reliable information on mental health (especially in the minority language), and the differences in perspective in this area cause additional limitations and significantly decrease the use of mental health services by immigrant, refugee, and cultural minority citizens (Fenta *et al.*, 2006; Reitmanova & Gustafson, 2009; Lachance *et al.*, 2014). Moreover, immigrants are often unfamiliar with the Canadian health and social service system in general (Zanchetta & Poureslami, 2006). Combined with migratory and social integration issues, these challenges make newcomers and cultural minority citizens even more vulnerable and put them at increased risk for further health disparities compared to the overall population.

In addition to all these issues, Francophones who live in official language minority contexts face specific challenges. They are not necessarily comfortable nor confident enough to ask for services in French (Forgues & Landry, 2014) for such reasons as: (1) linguistic insecurity (Deveau, Landry, & Allard, 2009); (2) fear of not receiving services as quickly (Drolet *et al.*, 2014); (3) the conviction that it is impossible to receive these services (Société santé en français, 2007); (4) internalization of the minority identity (Tajfel, 1978; Tajfel & Turner, 1986), which can lead to two consequences: difficulty asking for or insisting on services in their language, and the belief that services in French may be of inferior quality (Drolet *et al.*, 2015); (5) ease of agreeing to speak English rather than listening to a service provider who has trouble speaking French (Deveau *et al.*, 2009); and (6) lack of French vocabulary for medical issues or health care, which may make the person wonder if it would be harder to understand verbal or written information in French than in English (Bouchard, Vézina, & Savoie, 2010; Deveau *et al.*, 2009). Likewise, some Francophones attended English schools, even though they spoke French more often at home. In some cases, this was their choice, and in others it was because of rules in the past that prevented the use of French in the schools or access to French-language schools. Francophones educated in English may find it easier to read and write in English, although they prefer to converse in French.

Towards an Understanding of Actors, the System, and Levers of Action

The idea of publishing this particular volume, a collaborative work issued in both official languages, has its roots in the research of two teams, both of which had been working for several years in the area of French-language health care and social services within Francophone minority communities throughout Canada. The *Groupe de recherche de l'innovation sur l'organisation des services de santé* (GRIOSS) at the Université de Moncton, which took the initiative for this book, and the *Groupe de recherche sur la formation professionnelle en santé et en service social en contexte francophone minoritaire* (GReFoPS) at the

University of Ottawa, collaborated closely to bring the project to fruition. In the interest of presenting a rich variety of analytical perspectives and further developing multiple collaborations in the field, members of the two groups also invited contributions from other Canadian researchers in the fields of health care, social work, political science, law, public administration, psychology, and education, all recognized for their expertise in the area.

It is useful to review the legal context. In 1969, the Parliament of Canada adopted the first *Official Languages Act*, making English and French the two official languages of Canada and guaranteeing access to federal government services in both languages. The amendments made to the *Act* in 1988 (the addition of Part VII) affirmed the Government of Canada's commitment to enhancing the vitality of the English and French linguistic minority communities (OLMCs) in Canada and supporting and assisting their development. Moreover, Parliament inserted a section protecting the rights of the English and French linguistic minority populations into the *Canadian Charter of Rights and Freedoms* in 1981 (Allaire, 2001). Although the *Canadian Constitution* gives provinces and territories the responsibility for social services and health care, Parliament adopted the *Canada Health Act* in 1984, stating: "The primary objective of Canadian health care policy is to protect, promote and restore the physical and mental well-being of residents of Canada, and to facilitate reasonable access to health services without financial or other barriers" (Bowen, 2001, p. 18).

Table 1. Timeline of Important Canadian Events

EVENTS	DATES
The first *Official Languages Act* recognizes the equal status of English and French in all institutions of the Government of Canada	1969
Amendment of the *Constitution Act* and introduction of the *Canadian Charter of Rights and Freedoms*	1982
Canadian Health Act	1984
Amendment of the *Official Languages Act* adding, among other items, Part VII: Advancement of English and French (enhancing the vitality of the English and French linguistic minority communities in Canada and supporting and assisting their development)	1988
The Government of Canada's *Action Plan for Official Languages* policy statement is released; $2 million per year is allocated for creating networks and organizing activities.	March 2003
Creation of the *Consortium national de formation en santé*, the successor of the *Centre national de formation en santé*	2003
Part X of the *Official Languages Act* (Court Remedy) makes it possible to enforce Part VII of the *Act* (Advancement of English and French)	2005
Roadmap for Canada's Linguistic Duality 2008–2013	June 2008
Roadmap for Canada's Official Languages 2013–2018	March 2013
Statement of commitment to education on the active offer of French language health services is signed by the leaders of *Consortium national de formation en santé* (CNFS) member institutions; launch of the *Tool Box for the Active Offer*	2013

In this volume, the researchers we invited to contribute have highlighted the diversity of the provinces in applying this legal framework, as well as the socio-demographic complexity of the Canadian context in the area of official languages. While certain constitutional and legal measures facilitate access to social services and health care in linguistic minority contexts (Chapter 3), the demographic weight of official language minority communities (OLMCs) and their vitality can also be a lever to establish policies and practices that have a positive impact on the active offer of services in the official language of the minority (Chapters 3, 4 and 14).

Federal and provincial jurisdiction and unwritten constitutional principles are also discussed: these authors present an illuminating and nuanced view of the complexity and diversity of the situations and issues they've encountered. In their chapters we learn, for instance, that New Brunswick has the most highly developed legal framework to govern the provision of social services and health care in the minority official language as it is the only officially bilingual Canadian province. Ontario follows, with its system for designated French-language services in designated regions. Finally, a law passed in 2016 created a legal framework that fosters French-language services in the province of Manitoba. Balancing these provisions is Quebec, with a population that is 78.9% Francophone (Verreault, Fortin, & Gravel, 2017). It is the only province that has adopted French as its official language, prompting the Anglophone minority to assert its language rights. Despite its attention to the Canadian context as a whole and in all its complexity, this volume focuses more on these four provinces and on Nova Scotia. However, research on regions with smaller concentrations of Francophone minorities and on Anglophones outside Montreal is becoming more prevalent.

In order to enhance the quality of our reflections on the subject, we decided to adopt a theoretical framework based on the strategic analysis first developed by Crozier and Friedberg (1977), and presented in Chapter 1. The sociology of organizations provided an overall framework to analyze the relationship between the actor and the system. This framework allowed us to examine the issues and challenges of access to and the active offer of social services and health care in official language minority communities in greater depth, as well as to investigate the strategies and levers of action implemented by actors in linguistic minority contexts.

Thus each contribution on the challenges of active offer contained in this book is a source of information on the *actors* (their role, their behaviours, their actions, their strategies, their interactions, etc.); on the *system* (the organization of services, measures promoting active offer, limitations, etc.); and/or the *relationship* between the actors and the system. We believe this is an original and unique contribution to research on the practices and challenges related to active offer. Indeed, when we are confronted with one of the issues raised by active offer, all of us, researchers as well as practitioners and community members, have to address the following question: Is the problem, strategy for action, or solution primarily a matter of actors (e.g., an insufficient number of health or social service professionals who are aware and equipped to actively offer services), or does it lie within the system (lack of policies, procedures, or measures favourable to active offer within organizations; inadequate networking opportunities among professionals; or a lack of directories of bilingual, Francophone, or Francophile professionals outside Quebec or Anglophone professionals in Quebec)? The fact that the two are interrelated makes the question even harder to answer.

We should specify that the authors do not use the model of strategic analysis as the only framework to guide the analysis and reflection in each of their chapters. In the interest of the wealth and diversity of expertise, the contributors to this book hope, instead, to improve our understanding of the role of the actor and the system by offering current perspectives on the principles of active offer. Each of them in their own way contributes to the study of the dynamics of the actors, system, and relationships involved in the active offer of services in the minority official language.

In the following fourteen chapters (grouped into five sections), our colleagues pursue their examination of the issues, challenges, and possible solutions related to promoting the active offer of services in the official languages in minority settings, as well as its challenges in terms of human resources (recruitment and retention) and elements to consider for education and training in this area. The authors share the results of their studies as well as their understanding of the different dimensions that come into play in an analysis of the active offer of social services and health care to linguistic minority populations across Canada.

While some authors discuss theoretical foundations, others present findings from their empirical studies. Some of them make recommendations for improving access to services and the active offer of services in the minority language. The authors raise issues that do not appear to be insurmountable and which organizations, service providers, individuals, and communities as well as decision-makers could address.

The following paragraphs briefly outline each of the chapters.

Part I — Engaging Actors: Putting the Strategic Analysis to the Test

Chapter 1 lays the foundations for a theoretical framework designed to give a general readership interested in the subject a better idea of the active offer of social services and health care services in official language minority communities. Sylvain Vézina and Sébastien Savard explain how the sociology of organizations, and more specifi-cally strategic analysis, can help us better understand the relation-ships of conflict and cooperation between actors and the system. The authors believe this is a major contribution to both research on and the practice of active offer. Strategic analysis enables us to determine how to articulate the research problem and how to develop a strategy for action. Is the answer to be found among the actors, or in the poli-cies and procedures? The appropriate response will be found in the complexity of the interactions between and among them, which are set out in the theoretical model. These divergent and sometimes contradictory interests, as well as the power relationships founded on resources and assets (among other elements), play out in different ways in the interactions. In the chapters that follow, other researchers will explore the question of active offer in the same theoretical per-spective. Some give us a better understanding of the role of the actor, and others focus on the system or the interaction between the two. All help to shed light on the subject.

Based on research on the provision of French-language services and the results of a national dialogue, Pier Bouchard *et al.* examine the education and training of health and social service professionals in **Chapter 2**, as well as the competencies these professionals need to develop to better serve Francophone minority communities. This is a line of research and reflection that threads through other chapters in the book and is of great significance. The authors offer new insights about the active offer of French-language services in relation to future graduates in post-secondary health and social service programs, notably those that are part of the *Consortium national de formation en santé* (CNFS). Among the essential elements to be included in these professional programs, the authors stress the importance of information on language as a health determinant, on living conditions in minority language communities, and on working in minority language settings. Competencies associated with skills and attitudes for working with Francophones in minority contexts are also considered important components of education and training.

Part II — Policy Levers and Legal Measures: The Interplay of Actors

Chapter 3 is distinct from the other chapters in that the author approaches the questions of language and access to health and social services from a legal standpoint. Is the state legally required to provide free universal access to health care? The answer, according to Pierre Foucher, author of this chapter, is "no." Access to the health system in Canada is not a "fundamental right;" instead, it is a political decision. The author then studies the legal aspects of language rights, examining two components: federalism and its impact on French-language health services, and fundamental rights protected by the *Canadian Charter of Rights and Freedoms*. This chapter allows readers to grasp an extremely important issue: although the Canadian approach is geared to cooperation and coordination of federal-provincial-territorial efforts and respects the division of powers, it does not provide for firm legal guarantees of the right to receive health care in one's own official language. Instead, Foucher suggests it is in provincial legislation that linguistic minority groups can find elements that protect certain rights to access health services.

    Chapter 4 provides a critical reflection on active offer in the justice sector in Ontario, with ideas that could be considered in the health and social services sector. Linda Cardinal *et al.* focus first on legislative and policy instruments and outline the evolution of French-language services (FLS) in the province. Based on a review of literature dating from the 1980s and continuing to the time the first strategic plan for developing the active offer of FLS was created, the authors consider the positive aspects of these instruments, which represent the outcome of dialogues between community actors and government actors. However, even though there is a process to co-construct the provision of FLS, and this co-construction is founded on dialogue, the authors feel that the process often relies on the willingness of various actors. This is inadequate for ensuring FLS will continue to be offered. The authors suggest that policies, directives, planning, and accountability should become the standard instruments for ensuring the active offer of French-language services. Results from a series of interviews support the authors' findings.

Part III — Accessibility and the Active Offer of French-Language Services

In **Chapter 5**, Louise Bouchard and Martin Desmeules look at the situation of Francophone seniors (65 years and over) in the linguistic minority population and draw a socio-sanitary portrait of their living conditions. The authors point out that the rate of aging is more rapid in this population than in the overall population of Canada. Moreover, Francophone seniors who live in minority settings are comparatively less well off, with fewer financial and cultural resources. Overall, these individuals are more vulnerable to health problems. The findings are based on the authors' analysis of data from the Canadian Community Health Survey (CCHS) in three large Canadian regions (Atlantic Canada, Ontario, and the West). The authors conclude the chapter with interesting suggestions for actions that could be undertaken to improve the situation. These include, for example, strengthening literacy programs for Francophone seniors who live in minority language communities, and enhancing the active offer of the areas of preventive health, health education, and programs that empower individuals to take ownership of their health care and social services.

Chapter 6 describes the experience of Francophone users in eastern Ontario accessing French health services. Based on qualitative research and an analysis of the actors and the system, Marie Drolet *et al.* reveal the paradoxes inherent in the complex identity construction processes of users in the health and social service network. These users must navigate through English and French services and settings, and at the same time maintain the quality of their mother tongue. For staff providing services, the fear of being marginalized and sometimes their own linguistic insecurity are among the feelings that are ever-present and prevent some professionals from serving users in French and practising active offer.

The authors' analysis is informed by tools such as the Chronic Care Model and the Expanded Chronic Care Model, which outline the conditions enabling users to take charge of their chronic health problems. In particular, these models describe the roles that users, their caregivers, and service providers play in care and services. Concepts such as "productive interaction," "proactive," and "better-informed and better-equipped caregivers" are introduced by the authors, in order to explain the paradoxes facing actors in a system that is not always positive towards the active offer of social services and health care in the minority language.

In **Chapter 7**, Éric Forgues *et al.* review the legal and political context as well as achievements made by Francophone minority communities, in particular following the conflict surrounding the Ontario Conservative government's plan to close Hôpital Montfort in 1997. This event was a milestone, the authors remind us, in the struggle of Francophone minority communities for the right to access social services and health care in their own language. Inequalities in health and social services were at the centre of their protests that, in the end, brought about improvements in FLS. This chapter illustrates the complexity of the barriers that prevent access to services. The barriers cannot be attributed solely to the lack or shortage of health professionals. In fact, in an empirical study to identify the factors that foster health and social services for Francophone users in four Canadian provinces, the author focuses on factors related to the social, political, and legal environments, as well as the organization of work. Compliance with policy decisions and the vigilance of actors ready to take the political and legal action necessary for change seem to constitute the basic conditions that guarantee access to health and social services in an official language minority community.

Part IV — Bilingualism and the Active Offer of French-Language Services

In **Chapter 8**, Danielle de Moissac *et al.* explore the point of view of Francophone and bilingual professionals on access to French-language health and social services by Francophone minority populations in Manitoba and eastern Ontario. Their research combines two qualitative studies underlining the challenges that professionals face in those two environments. Some of the challenges are not unique to Manitoba or Ontario, as other chapters show. Among the challenges identified are the shortage of bilingual, Francophone, and Francophile professionals; the difficulty of identifying bilingual clients and service providers; a lack of networks to support bilingual professionals; and often a lack of organizational support to make an active offer of services in bilingual health and social services facilities. The authors present options for improving access to services, suggesting, among other possibilities, that various organizational strategies may be adopted.

Along the same thematic lines, **Chapter 9**, by Sébastien Savard *et al.*, studies factors contributing to the recruitment and retention of bilingual health and social service professionals, again in a minority language setting. The qualitative research on which this chapter is based took place in the two Canadian cities of Winnipeg and Ottawa. The results demonstrate that the most significant factor in retaining these professionals is the quality of the work environment. The quality of the connections professionals make with their co-workers and with users is one of the primary sources of job satisfaction for them, contributing to the overall satisfaction and retention of employees. The authors conclude the chapter with several recommendations that could lead to a better use of resources, especially through the education and training of service providers working in the sector.

In **Chapter 10**, the author examines active offer under the lens of organizational culture, hoping to identify, through empirical research, the predominant language-related values operating in Anglophone and Francophone hospitals in New Brunswick. These values are fundamental to organizational culture and determine the importance of the active offer of French-language services in a given setting. Informed by a perspective drawing from the sociology of organizations as a starting point, Sylvain Vézina believes that actors may interpret the idea of bilingualism as a threat to the balance of power in the system, and that such an attitude may create resistance among members of the linguistic majority. This is the reason he suggests a discourse that promotes the value of a culture of active offer by emphasizing the goals of safety and quality of care and services in both official languages.

Part V — Issues and Strategies in Educating and Training Future Professionals

Chapter 11 turns to the question of educating educators, that is, the university professors offering education and training on active offer to future graduates. The authors found that most of them had not received training on the teaching and learning strategies best suited for students in professional programs who would be working with Francophone minority communities. This realization led Claire-Jehanne Dubouloz *et al.* to explore educational theory in the area of andragogy (adult education) and to propose a conceptual framework within which an educational component on active offer could be developed. Three types of knowledge can be distinguished in this framework: knowledge, skills, and people skills or attitudes. The authors also reflect on the particular issues of teaching active offer that they discovered while conducting a pilot project on the implementation of education on active offer.

Chapter 12 by Jacinthe Savard *et al.* discusses a research program whose objective was to design and validate measurement tools for active offer behaviours. Three tools were developed: the first was intended to measure the perception of service providers regarding their own behaviours to promote active offer; the second measured the perception of service providers with respect to the actions taken by their organization to support active offer behaviours (organizational support); the third investigated factors believed to determine the provision of an active offer of French-language services (e.g., the ethnolinguistic vitality of a person's community, a person's identity and acculturation, etc.). According to the author, these factors are determinants of active offer. The tools, which are robust, reliable, and constructed according to recognized theoretical models, fill a major gap in the field since no measurement tools existed before this research began. In a series of tables, the authors synthesize the contents of the measurement tools (questionnaires) as well as the results obtained through statistical tests. The findings reveal, among other facts, that the perceived organizational support and certain individual behaviours (notably the affirmation of identity, education in active offer, and proficiency in French) are positively associated with active offer. In this sense, the research offers concrete knowledge we can use to improve education on active offer in programs for future health and social service professionals.

In **Chapter 13**, Josée Lagacé and Pascal Lefebvre compile data from scholarly studies and present new research data. They show a gap between best practices and current practices in the use of normalized tests for audiology and speech-language pathology assessment of bilingual children. In Canada, most Francophone children who live in linguistic minority settings are bilingual. However, as the authors explain, audiologists and speech-language pathologists who assess clients for communication disorders do not have tests that have been normalized in this population. Better tests that can more accurately identify the difficulties found in official language minority communities are needed. Moreover, these tests should also account for the complexity and the value of learning two languages at the same time. For this reason, the authors make recommendations for university programs and professional development in audiology and speech-language pathology. Recommendations are also made for employers and parents.

Last but not least, **Chapter 14** is entirely dedicated to the English-speaking communities of Quebec. In it, Richard Bourhis presents a theoretical model that helps us to understand the relations between majority and minority groups. The author explains how the Interactive Acculturation Model (IAM) provides an intergroup approach to minority/majority group relations in multilingual settings. He points out the importance of the ethnolinguistic vitality as the first element of this model, which describes the relative strengths and weaknesses of linguistic communities in contact. Additionally, he examines the types of language policies that regulate the status of linguistic communities, which is the second element of the IAM. Thirdly, the acculturation orientations of minority and majority group speakers are described as they interact to yield harmonious, problematic, or conflictual intergroup relations. In the second part of his chapter, M. Bourhis analyses bilingual health care policies for official language minorities in Canada and in Quebec. Finally, the author presents in a detailed analysis the implications of the 2014 Quebec government health care Bill 10 for the vitality of the English-speaking communities of Quebec.

In the **Conclusion**, we present the contribution made by each author to a cohesive reflection on active offer, considering each of them in the light of strategic analysis. We then propose six strategies to promote active offer, locating them in an analytical framework that allows us to reconcile the largest possible number of perspectives possible and, thus, capture the object of study in its full complexity. Levers and options for action serve as different angles from which to look ahead to further explorations in the field. The framework is founded on theory and empirical data and, at the same time, oriented towards action. In this way, it encompasses the limitations of the system as well as the opportunities it offers to the various actors involved, who can then adapt their actions to their respective environment in which they operate.

References

Allaire, G. (2001). *La Francophonie canadienne: Portraits*. Québec: CIDEF-AFI, and Sudbury: Prise de parole.

Anderson, L. M., Scrimshaw, S. C., Fullilove, M. T., Fielding, J. E., & Normand, J. (2003). Culturally competent healthcare systems: A systematic review. *American Journal of Preventive Medicine*, 24(3, Supplement), 68–79. doi:10.1016/S0749-3797(02)00657-8

Andrulis, D. P. & Brach, C. (2007). Integrating literacy, culture, and language to improve health care quality for diverse populations. *American Journal of Health Behavior*, 31(Supplement 1), S122–S133. Retrieved from http://search.proquest.com.proxy.bib.uottawa.ca/docview/211891742?accountid=14701

Bonacruz Kazzi, G., & Cooper, C. (2003). Barriers to the use of interpreters in emergency room paediatric consultations. *Journal of Paediatrics and Child Health*, 39: 259–263.

Bouchard, L., Beaulieu, M., & Desmeules, M. (2012). L'offre active de services de santé en français en Ontario: Une mesure d'équité. *Reflets: Revue d'intervention sociale et communautaire*, 18(2), 38–65. http://doi.org/10.7202/1013173ar

Bouchard, P., Vézina, S., & Savoie, M. (2010). *Rapport du Dialogue sur l'engagement des étudiants et des futurs professionnels pour de meilleurs services de santé en français dans un contexte minoritaire: Formation et outillage, Recrutement et Rétention* (pp. 43–43). Ottawa, ON: Consortium national de formation en santé (CNFS). Retrieved from http://www.weebly.com/uploads/7/4/7/3/7473881/rapport_projet_de_loutillage.nov2010.pdf

Boudreau, A., & Dubois, L. (2008). Représentations, sécurité/insécurité linguistique. In S. Roy & P. Dalley (Eds.). *Francophonie, minorités et pédagogie*. Ottawa: Presses de l'Université d'Ottawa, 145–175.

Bowen, S. (2001). *Barrières linguistiques dans l'accès aux soins de santé*. Ottawa: Santé Canada. Retrieved from http://www.offreactive.com/wp-content/uploads/2013/08/1-barrieres-linguistiques-sarah-bowen-email1.pdf

Bowen, S. (2015). *Impact des barrières linguistiques sur la sécurité des patients et la qualité des soins* (p. 62). Retrieved from http://francosantesud.ca/wp-content/uploads/SSF-Bowen-S.-%C3%89tude-Barri%C3%A8res-linguistiques.pdf

Castaño, M. T., Biever, J. L., González, C. G., & Anderson, K. B. (2007). Challenges of providing mental health services in Spanish. *Professional Psychology: Research and Practice*, 38(6), 667–673. http://doi.org/10.1037/0735-7028.38.6.667

Crozier, M., & Friedberg, E. (1977). *L'acteur et le système*. Paris: Seuil.

Derose, K. P., Escarce, J., & Lurie, N. (2007). Immigrants and health care: Sources of vulnerability. *Health Affairs*, (26) 5, 1258–1268. Retrieved from http://content.healthaffairs.org/content/26/5/1258

Deveau, K., Landry, R., & Allard, R. (2009). Utilisation des services gouvernementaux de langue française. Une étude auprès des Acadiens et francophones de la Nouvelle-Écosse sur les facteurs associés à l'utilisation des services gouvernementaux en français (p. 195). *Institut canadien de recherche sur les minorités linguistiques (ICRML)*. Retrieved from http://www.weebly.com/uploads/7/4/7/3/7473881/rapport_deveau_utilisation_services_gouv.pdf

Drolet, M., Arcand, I., Benoît, J., Savard, J., Savard, S., et Lagacé, J. (2015). Agir pour avoir accès à des services sociaux et de santé en français: Des Francophones en situation minoritaire nous enseignent quoi faire! *Revue canadienne de service social*, 32(1–2), 5–26.

Drolet, M., Dubouloz, C.-J., & Benoît, J. (2014). L'accès aux services sociaux et de santé en français et la formation des professionnelles et des professionnels en situation francophone minoritaire canadienne. *Reflets: Revue d'intervention sociale et communautaire*, 20(2), 10–19. http://doi.org/10.7202/1027584ar

Drolet, M., Savard, J., Benoît, J., Arcand, I., Savard, S., Lagacé, J., ... Dubouloz, C-J. (2014). Health Services for Linguistic Minorities in a Bilingual Setting: Challenges for Bilingual Professionals. *Qualitative Health Research*, University of Ottawa, Ottawa, Ontario, Canada, 24(3), 295–305. https://doi.org/10.1177/1049732314523503

Drouin, J., & Rivet, C. (2003). Training Medical Students to Communicate with a Linguistic Minority Group. *Academic Medicine*, 78(6), 599–604. Retrieved from https://www.ncbi.nlm.nih.gov/pubmed/12805039

Éthier, S., & Belzile, L. (2012). *Améliorer l'accès des personnes âgées de Saint-Boniface et de Saint-Vital aux services de santé en français / Improving St. Boniface and St. Vital Seniors' Access to French-language Health Services.* Conseil communauté en santé du Manitoba. Université de Saint-Boniface. Retrieved from http://ustboniface.ca/file/documents-recherche/RAPPORT-Objectif-3-pratiques-exemplaires-version-finale-BILINGUE.pdf

Fenta, H., Hyman, I., & Noh, S. (2006). Mental health service utilization by Ethiopian immigrants and refugees in Toronto. *The Journal of Nervous and Mental Disease,* 194(12), 925–934.

Ferguson, W. J., & Candib, L. M. (2002). Culture, language, and the doctor-patient relationship. *Family Medicine,* 34(5), 353–361.

Flores, G., Laws, M. B., Mayo, S. J., Zuckerman, B., Abreu, M., Medina, L., & Hardt, E. J. (2003). Errors in Medical Interpretation and Their Potential Clinical Consequences in Pediatric Encounters. *Pediatrics,* 111(1), 6–14. http://doi.org/10.1542/peds.111.1.6

Forgues, É., & Landry, R. (2014). L'accès aux services de santé en français et leur utilisation en contexte francophone minoritaire (p. 158–159). Moncton, Nouveau-Brunswick: *Institut canadien de recherche sur les minorités linguistiques (ICRML).* Retrieved from http://www.icrml.ca/fr/recherches-et-publications/publications-de-l-icrml/item/8709-acces-aux-services-de-sante-en-francais-et-leur-utilisation-en-contexte-francophone-minoritaire

Gagnon-Arpin, I., Bouchard, L., Leis, A., et Bélanger, M. (2014). Accès et utilisation des services de santé en langue minoritaire. In R. Landry (Ed.), *La vie dans une langue officielle minoritaire au Canada.* Sainte-Foy, QC: Presses de l'Université Laval.

Irvine, F. E., Roberts, G. W., Jones, P., Spencer, L. H., Baker, C. R., & Williams, C. (2006). Communicative sensitivity in the bilingual healthcare setting: A qualitative study of language awareness. *Journal of Advanced Nursing,* 53(4), 422–434. http://doi.org/10.1111/j.1365-2648.2006.03733.x

Jacobs, E., Chen, A. H., Karliner, L. S., Agger-Gupta, N. & Mutha, S. (2006). The Need for More Research on Language Barriers in Health Care: A Proposed Research Agenda. *Milbank Quarterly,* 84: 111–133.

Kirmayer, L. J., Narasiah, L., Munoz, M., Rashid, M., Ryder, A. G., Guzder, J., & coll. (2011). Common mental health problems in immigrants and refugees: General approach in primary care. *CMAJ: Canadian Medical Association Journal,* 183(12), E959–67.

Köpke, B., & Prod'homme, K. (2009). L'évaluation de l'aphasie chez le bilingue: une étude de cas. *Glossa,* 107, 39–50. http://doi.org/http://glossa.fr/pdfs/107_2009 1204092949.pdf

Köpke, B., & Schmid, M. S. (2011). L'attrition de la première langue en tant que phénomène psycholinguistique. *Language, Interaction and Acquisition,* 2(2), 197–220. http://doi.org/10.1075/lia.2.2.02kop

Lachance, L., Martin, M., Kaduri, P., Godoy-Paiz, P., Ginieniewicz, J., Tarasuk, V., & McKenzie. K. (2014). Food insecurity, diet quality, and mental health in culturally diverse adolescents. *Ethnicity and Inequalities in Health and Social Care,* 7(1), 14–22. http://doi.org/10.1108/EIHSC-02-2013-0002

Lapierre, S., Coderre, C., Côté, I., Garceau, M-L., & Bourassa C. (2014). Quand le manque d'accès aux services en français revictimise les femmes victimes de violence conjugale et leurs enfants. *Reflets: Revue d'intervention sociale et communautaire,* 20(2), 22–51. http://dx.doi.org/10.7202/1027585ar

Lepage, J.-F., & Corbeil, J.-P. (May 2013). L'évolution du bilinguisme français-anglais au Canada de 1961 à 2011. *Regards sur la société canadienne.* Ottawa: Statistique Canada. No 75 006 X.

Madoc-Jones, I. (2004). Linguistic sensitivity, indigenous peoples and the mental health system in Wales. *International Journal of Mental Health Nursing,* 13: 216–224.

Mead, N., & Roland, M. (2009). Understanding why some ethnic minority patients evaluate medical care more negatively than white patients: A cross sectional analysis of a routine patient survey in English general practices. *BMJ,* 339, b3450–b3450. http://doi.org/10.1136/ bmj.b3450

Meyers, K., Tang, G., & Fernandez, A. (2009). Responding to the Language Challenge: Kaiser Permanente's Approach. *The Permanente Journal,* 13(3), 77.

Paradis, M. (2000). Generalizable Outcomes of Bilingual Aphasia Research. *Folia Phoniatrica et Logopaedica,* 52(1–3), 54–64. http://doi.org/10.1159/000021513

Pavlenko, A. (2012). Affective processing in bilingual speakers: Disembodied cognition? *International Journal of Psychology,* 47(6), 405–428. http:// dx.doi.org/10.1080/00207594.2012.743665

Pépin-Filion, D. (in collaboration with Guignard Noël, J.). (2014). *Évolution du bilinguisme au N.-B.* Rapport rédigé pour le Commissariat aux langues officielles du N.-B. Retrieved from http://www.droitslinguistiques.ca/ index.php?option=com_content&view=article&id=372%3Aevolution-du-bilinguisme-au-n-b&catid=1%3Aactualites&Itemid=1&lang=fr

Qualité de services de santé Ontario. (2015). *Les soins intégrés: point de vue des Ontariens concernant la communication et la coordination dans les soins de santé. Résultats de l'Enquête internationale de 2014 auprès des adultes âgés sur les politiques de santé du Fonds du Commonwealth.* Toronto: Qualité de services de santé Ontario.

Reitmanova, S., & Gustafson, D. L. (2009). Mental Health Needs of Visible Minority Immigrants in a Small Urban Center: Recommendations for Policy Makers and Service Providers. *Journal of Immigrant and Minority Health,* 11(1), 46–56. http://doi.org/10.1007/s10903-008-9122-x

Roberts, G. W., & Burton, C. R. (2013). Implementing the evidence for language-appropriate health care systems: The Welsh context. *Canadian Journal of Public Health*, 104(6), 88–90.

Santiago-Rivera, A. L., Altarriba, J., Poll, N., Gonzalez-Miller, N., & Cragun, C. (2009). Therapists' views on working with bilingual Spanish–English speaking clients: A qualitative investigation. *Professional Psychology: Research and Practice*, 40(5), 436–443. http://doi.org/10.1037/a0015933

Snowden, L.R, Masland, M.C, Peng, C.J, Wei-Mein Lou, C., & Wallace, N.T. (2011). Limited English proficient Asian Americans: Threshold language policy and access to mental health treatment. *Social Science & Medicine*, 72(2), 230–7.

Société santé en français. (2007). *Une offre active de services en santé pour une meilleure santé des francophones en situation minoritaire*. Ottawa, ON: Société santé en français (SSF). Retrieved from http://www.weebly.com/uploads/7/4/7/3/7473881/ssf_plans_directeurs _sommaire_2007-11-26.pdf

Tajfel, H. (1978). *The social psychology of minorities*. Sacramento: Minority Rights Group. Retrieved from http://books.google.ca/books?id=q7 ULAQAAIAAJ

Tajfel, H., & Turner, J. C. (1986). The social identity theory of intergroup behavior. In W. G. Austin & S. Worchel (Ed.). *Psychology of Intergroup Relations*, 7–24. Chicago, IL: Nelson-Hall.

United States (US) Department of Health and Human Services, O. of M. H. (2001). *National Standards for Culturally and Linguistically Appropriate Services*. Final Report.

Verreault, B., Fortin, J.F. & Gravel, P.L. (2017). Tableau statistique Canadien. *Institut de la statistique du Québec (ISQ)*. Retrieved from http://www.stat.gouv.qc.ca/statistiques/economie/comparaisons-economiques/interprovinciales/tableau-statistique-canadien.pdf

Vézina, S., Dupuis-Blanchard, S. (2015). La recherche au profit d'un meilleur accès aux services de santé en français / Research Benefiting Better Access to Health Care Services in French. *Linguistic Minorities and Society*, 6: 3–16.

Zanchetta, M. S., & Poureslami, I. M. (2006). Littératie en matière de santé dans la réalité des immigrants, sur le plan de la culture et de la langue. *Canadian Journal of Public Health / Revue Canadienne de Santé Publique*, 97, S28–S33. Retrieved from http://www.jstor.org/ stable/41995834

PART I

ENGAGING ACTORS: PUTTING THE STRATEGIC ANALYSIS TO THE TEST

Active Offer, Actors, and the Health and Social Service System: An Analytical Framework

Sylvain Vézina, *Université de Moncton*
and Sébastien Savard, *University of Ottawa*

Abstract

This chapter presents a theoretical framework inspired by strategic analysis, also called the sociology of organizations. By adopting this approach, researchers try to uncover the objectives and strategies used by the actors involved in order to better grasp the dynamics of the system of action, while at the same time taking into consideration the constraints arising from the formal structure. The concepts dealt with include the system of action, power, rules of the game, change, strategy, actor, issue, organization, and environment, all of which take into account the complexity of the challenges surrounding the practice of active offer in health and social services. One of the major contributions of this approach is that it provides an analytical framework making it possible to gain a better comprehension of the relationship between the actor and the system. These two components are essential not only for understanding the subject explored here, but also for identifying the strategies for action used by actors in a given community.

Key Words: active offer, social services and health, system of action, power, zone of uncertainty, strategic analysis, sociology of organizations, change, strategy, actor, issue, organization, environment.

Introduction

Access to health and social services that are safe and of comparable quality for official language minority communities (OLMCs) is a subject explored by a growing number of surveys, and, as a result, analyses (Vézina, 2015). Each one proceeds according to theoretical positions that are often conscious and acknowledged but are sometimes difficult to identify. Suggesting an analytical framework that makes it possible to amalgamate the greatest possible number of these perspectives in order to consider matters related to active offer is an onerous task. It is, nevertheless, what we propose to do in this chapter. We will argue that the organization is a construct in which we observe, among other things, relations of power and dependence, which rely on strategies developed around zones of uncertainty and give rise to the establishment of ever-evolving rules framing the cooperation of actors within as well as outside the organization. Although our choices are, by definition, subjective, we hope we are able to propose a way of theorizing the subject which will be of interest to many researchers and, especially, will enable us to address multiple aspects of active offer.

Thus, our first challenge is to identify an existing theoretical model that can integrate a wide variety of perspectives. Our second challenge is to establish, as clearly as possible, its potential, in view of the multiple dimensions of the subject of our research, active offer. Choosing a theoretical framework means adopting a series of general analytical tools developed by others before us through observations of reality and that allow us to explain the phenomena we are examining. Any theoretical model proposes a specific and consistent use of concepts that become analytical tools, in order to bring to light the logic underlying the phenomena observed, or even to predict these phenomena. In the following pages, we will suggest some tools we believe are most apt to help us understand active offer, its meaning, and the issues and challenges that come with it.

In concrete terms, we will refer to propositions and concepts drawn from the sociology of organizations.[1] These propositions seem useful to us in a number of ways. First, they offer a series of concepts to which researchers from different disciplines are able to relate, including the concepts of system of action, power, rules of the game, change, strategy, actor, issue, organization, and environment. Such concepts are able to take into account the complexity of challenges around the practice of active offer. We will consider them in more detail later on.

Next, the sociology of organizations provides an analytical framework that makes it possible to gain a better grasp of the relation between the actor (individual or group) and the system (hospital, social services, society…). From our perspective, this is a major contribution to the study of active offer. When considering the issues raised by active offer (either in research or in the offer of direct services to the population), we are faced with a significant challenge: we must decide if the problem, like the strategy of action, is first and foremost a matter of the actors involved; that is, the need for people working in health and social services who are conscious of the need for active offer and equipped to provide it. Or, on the other hand, is it a matter of the system; that is, the lack of up-to-date policies and procedures in the rules governing the employment of resources for the purpose of putting active offer into practice? The sociology of organizations addresses precisely the interaction between the two.

Finally, this theoretical model is intended to be concrete and move beyond the question of "why" to "how." Indeed, the primary interest to those who work with this approach understands how human beings (all of whom pursue their individual goals, which can be divergent, or even completely opposite, from those of others) manage to resolve the problem of their cooperation in an organization and what their cooperation costs them. In a way, we are trying to understand the mechanisms and conditions of integrating diverse rationalities[2] and divergent interests in the pursuit of common objectives that are basic to the organization and indispensable to its survival. Here is a simple illustration of the problem in the context of our subject. We need to specify from the outset that the particular challenge of active offer occurs in organizations where individuals working in a variety of professions must perform their duties in a minority setting. We could, then, state that the sociology of organizations examines how these actors, be they Anglophone or Francophone, unilingual or bilingual, manage to reconcile their often divergent interests when it comes to providing safe and quality social services and health services in the official language of the choice of the person requiring a service. It is the relation between conflict and cooperation that we are trying to better understand, here. Both are inherent in the dynamics of organized action (Friedberg, 1993).

Furthermore, the health care sector interests a large number of researchers in the field of sociology of organizations. During the second half of the 1980s, driven by the research of Michel Crozier (1987), researchers focused mainly on hospital organizations (Bélanger, 1988; Binst, 1994; De Pouvourville, 1994; Gonnet, 1994; Moisdon, 1994). Since then, they have diversified into other areas of health care, notably from the angle of public policy (Borraz, 2008; Bergeron, 2010), rationalization (Benamouzig, 2005), prevention (Crespin & Lascoumes, 2000), the practice of medicine (Castel & Merle, 2002; Castel, 2008) &, consequently, the place of expertise (Henry, Gilbert, Jouzel, & Marichalar, 2015). In the field of social services, Savard, Turcotte, and Beaudoin (2004) used the framework of strategic analysis to study the power relations between public facilities and community organizations serving children and families, both of which provide social services to this population. This shows that the framework can be used to study the dynamics of inter-organizational partnership.

Organization as a Construct

For those who take this approach, the organization is contingent, in the sense that no "best" way of organizing human activity exists. Instead, there are infinite possible variants, depending on the objective situation—and the intentions—of individuals for which it is comprised. When considered from a subjectivist viewpoint (Burrell & Morgan, 1979), the organization is seen as a construct formed from conflictual and cooperative relations between individuals and groups they call "actors." More precisely, the organization is recognized here according to the interactionist paradigm (Boudon, 1977); in other words, as the product of encounters between actors who are trying to define a framework to cooperate around common objectives. Starting from the idea that interactions between actors in a system are based on interests and objectives that may be concurrent or contradictory, the paradigm shows how power relations develop, as each person uses the resources in his or her own possession, and the zones of uncertainty under his or her own control, in order to force other actors to make concessions. This way, each person can achieve, at least in part, her or his own objectives. Conversely, however, this same actor, dependent on the resources possessed by others, cannot unilaterally impose rules and must instead negotiate and make compromises.

Physicians, managers, nursing staff, social workers, Francophones, Anglophones, men, and women, to name only a few, are connected in a variety of configurations according to the issues and the resources they have available to influence the dynamics of the system. Thereby, the system can respond as well as possible to their individual and collective interests when dealing with the issue at hand. In the perspective of the sociology of organizations, the active offer of social services and health care in the two official languages represents one issue among others. The way it is dealt with depends on both the performance of the actors and the recognition, by everyone involved, of its importance in achieving the objectives of the system. Starting from this idea, we would suggest that active offer cannot take place without an effective cooperation among actors, through their acknowledgement of their complementary roles and the clarification of the division of skills. Nonetheless, this cooperation will always be interrupted by conflict, whether on the level of values, interests, or objectives. A major part of the conflict is related to the competition among different actors for obtaining and using limited resources to achieve specific objectives. In short, cooperation cannot rely on a simple agreement around common values; it requires mechanisms such as learning and negotiation, or even bargaining (Castel & Carrère, 2007). Furthermore, cooperation will be impossible unless people consider the legitimate interests of the actors involved, be they interests of a professional, cultural, or labour condition, or of a different nature.

Power and Dependence: At the Heart of the Analysis

Power, a central notion of this model, is viewed from the angle of a transactional dynamics, where the logic of exchange, of negotiation, of giver-giving is predominant, rather than from the angle of oppression. The conception of power transmitted by this approach is also based on the principle that every power relationship is founded on a relationship of dependence that is fairly reciprocal between the actors in interaction. Thus, for exchanges or transactions to take place between actors, there must be interdependence between them. For example, one actor has one resource that I need. I negotiate with that actor so that either the resource is given to me or the resource does not infringe on my pursuit of my objectives. The other actor negotiates with me because I control one zone of uncertainty that is necessary for the actor to pursue his or her own objectives.

The notion of interdependence is therefore central to our understanding of how systems of action function. However, it is not to be confused with the notion of balance. Indeed, certain actors may possess more resources and control larger zones of uncertainty, giving them more negotiating power than other actors in the system. On the other hand, given that (according to this model) no actor possesses all the resources, the vision of power that is transmitted here is pluralist; that is to say, it introduces *a priori* the hypothesis that power is spread out among different actors. This conception is thus placed in opposition to the totalitarian vision of power, which postulates a relationship between dominant and dominated, where power is concentrated in the hands of dominant (often majority) groups. Crozier and Friedberg (1977) affirm that this vision of power ignores a fundamental aspect: that of exchange.

Even if the actor is constrained by the rules of the game and the strategies of other actors, this does not mean the actor is totally powerless: "Even in extreme situations, a man always retains a margin of liberty and cannot help but use it to beat the system." (Crozier & Friedberg, 1977: 42, our translation). Inspired by the work of Leavitt (1958), the authors affirm that even the most disadvantaged actor will always have the final choice to accept or refuse what the other asks so that the "changer," as well as the "changed," will experience tension in the power relationship. The idea presents itself as follows: there is no power without a relationship, no relationship without an exchange, no exchange without a negotiation. For these authors, then, although organizations are established around the necessary cooperation between individuals, they also involve an exercise of power because cooperation will never be totally balanced. To summarize, the exercise of power in our organizations seems to be a phenomenon every bit as normal as cooperation.

Concrete System of Action

These relations, characterized by negotiation, transaction, and compromise, take the form of games that regulate, we might say, the behaviour, decisions, and actions of people working within the system. Crozier and Friedberg (1977) suggest that these dynamics can be explained through the concept of "concrete system of action," or:

> A structured group of humans who coordinate the actions and participants by using relatively stable mechanisms that maintain its structure (that is, the stability of its games and relationships among them) by mechanisms of regulation that constitute other games. (286, our translation)

In accordance with this concept, these authors suggest that the behaviour of the actors cannot be explained solely by the rationality of the formal organization—its objectives, functions, and structures—as if it were a set of data and circumstances to which individuals would have no other choice than to adapt, and which they would, in the end, internalize in order to conform. Instead, they posit that actors' margins of liberty can never be completely restricted. The formal dimension of the organization—structure and rules—is exploited, interpreted, and modified by the actors in the course of confronting issues in their day-to-day relations. One of the key points of this concept to remember is that issues associated with active offer, such as access to safe and quality services and care, must be placed at the centre of the dynamics of the system of action in such a way as to ensure that, as a natural outcome, the formal dimension of the system incorporates the rules of the game. The actors from the minority—in our case, the linguistic minority—must take advantage of their margin of liberty in order to influence the system in this direction.

Strategies and Zones of Uncertainty
The capacity of actors to influence the dynamics of the system will depend on their ability to control any substantial and relevant resources available to them, as well as their ability to deal with the various constraints whether organizational, political, economic, or normative.

In the relational perspective of power transmitted by this theoretical approach, the zone of uncertainty is defined as an element not controlled by all, or at least not mastered by one of the actors involved. The more relevant resources an actor possesses, the more zones of uncertainty the actor controls—assuming that there are other actors with whom there is a power relationship and who depend on these zones—the greater the actor's margin of liberty and therefore capacity for action. Nevertheless, it often happens that the objectives pursued by an actor meet the resistance of another actor.

It is at this point that the objectives become issues around which alliances form (if the issues are convergent), or oppositions form (if the issues are divergent) between different actors in the system. It is in such oppositions that power relations appear.

Mastering relevant resources does not only determine the margin of liberty actors can have. It also determines, in part, the strategies that can be envisaged by the actors to achieve their objectives. Indeed, the more relevant resources an actor possesses—that is, resources that "the adversary" depends on or which correspond to a zone of uncertainty—the easier it will be to shift the power relation to the actor's favour. The importance of the resources owned, and the zones of uncertainty controlled, also have an influence on the ability of an actor to create alliances with other actors, thereby increasing opportunities to reach his or her objectives. In short, this approach invites us to demonstrate the capacity of actors and the strategies used to encourage actors to cooperate and provide active offer, or, inversely, to erect obstacles to doing both.

Rules and Collaboration

However, if a concrete system of action is, in reality, interrupted by power struggles, actors are just as concerned about reaching the objectives of the system, because they are aware that they depend, individually and collectively, on the survival of the system. This is why they will define and adjust, through their relationships, the formal rules and the structure of the system. This formal dimension of the organization can be considered as a crystallization of the state of relations among actors at a given time. It represents a form of compromise which will ultimately structure their relationships by defining, in a sense, the assets each person has and can use, and which limits the margin of liberty of the participants as a whole, so that all are encouraged to cooperate to achieve the objectives of the system.

The organizational structure and rules would serve to regulate the power relations among the actors in order to establish a minimum of consistency. Constructed around power relations, organizations are essentially trying to reduce the margin of manoeuvre and the leeway of its actors in an attempt to ensure their actions become predictable and their activities become controllable, and to force cooperation. Of interest here is the process by which standards, norms, and rules in an organization are produced (Castel, 2002, 2009). In the case of active offer, we might ask if the existence of certain standards of practice and procedure defining the individual's role in communicating with those concerned and in respecting the official languages would be favourable to establishing a dynamics of cooperation that benefits the whole. Would the implementation of standards and processes make it easier to control the activities and relationships among actors in terms of active offer, especially if it limits interpersonal contact, which is a source of conflict (Jacobsson, 2000)? This is an example of the kind of question explored in the sociology of organizations.

In addition, the approach we have been laying out here shows that structures, standards, and processes cannot regulate all aspects of action. There will always be remaining zones of uncertainty, issues, and sources of power for which there are no rules that will, therefore, continue to be sources of power struggles among actors. For example, while education has been ground for equality claims by Francophones in Canadian minority contexts for several decades, it is only in recent years—at the time of the crisis over the closure of Ottawa's Montfort hospital in 1997—that access to quality social services and health care for minority language groups has been recognized as a central issue that can inspire a community's advocacy and activism. This issue, long ignored by these communities, now influences the dynamics of our health and social service systems. Similarly, and despite the fact that it should have been addressed long ago, active offer only appeared as an issue in health and social services a few years ago. The rules of the game within our health and social service systems remain, in this regard, to be determined.

Relationship to the Environment

Furthermore, since the organization rarely functions outside a larger social system, and instead most often exists to respond to the needs and demands of people in a community, it must remain in contact with its environment. It is, in fact, dependent on its environment, and its environment will always be a zone of uncertainty threatening its internal balance. As a result, there will be a power relationship, notably in the exchange of information. Accordingly, the actors who make up the organization will constantly try to control their environment, all the while being dependent on it. The organization will attempt through various specialized services to structure its relations with the environment in such a way as to stabilize them. Inversely, it has to be recognized that the environment includes actors who are also, to a certain degree, dependent on the organization and trying to control it.

Crozier and Friedberg (1977) introduce here the concept of relays. Basically, this refers to actors who are present inside and outside the system who are vehicles for the exchange of information. Examples are information agents working within the organization and in the media, as well as actors in the community—Consortium national de formation en santé (CNFS), Société santé en français (SSF), Quebec Community Groups Network (QCGN), Community Health and Social Services Network (CHSSN), community associations, federal and provincial governments, professional associations, researchers, educational institutions, etc.—all of which become actors in the system of action and play a role influencing its dynamics.

Phenomenon of Change

All this leads us to the problem of change, viewed here along the same lines as the organization, as a construct. Thus, the reality is—from the point of view of the sociology of organizations—an ongoing collective creation that is always in a process of "becoming," and will evolve through, and be shaped by, conflicts, negotiations, bargaining, and relationships among individuals. Change is thus considered as a process of collective creation whereby members learn together. They invent and determine new ways of performing the social games of cooperation and conflict, giving rise to the establishment of new organizational structures. For people who work from this approach, change is related to the nature of individuals who are changing in their relations to each other and in the organization.

Beyond contradictory interests, strategies, and alliances, we find actors who seek to innovate, to develop new organizational tools and practices to encourage change oriented towards collective objectives. These "organizational champions" (Bloch & Hénaut, 2014) are positioned in a unique and tenuous space in the system as they embody change and, therefore, threaten the established order.

Conclusion

The sociology of organizations allows us to approach the active offer of health and social services in Canada's official languages according to a wide variety of perspectives including change, conflict, decision-making, public action, the mobilization of actors and their cooperation (Bergeron & Castel, 2014). It invites us to pay particular attention to the relations among actors, in order to see how they influence change toward active offer, and how they are, in turn, affected by this change. We might explore such questions as: To what extent does each of the strategies chosen lead (or not lead) to the implementation of practices favourable to active offer? Which of the strategies—radical change or incremental incentive—best enables leaders to convince the largest number of actors (Castel, 2002)? Which political measures, for example, could work in favour of active offer?

The sociology of organizations also provides us with tools to see how heavily professional issues (Borraz, 1998) weigh on strategies of change. This applies especially to those issues linked to the official languages in health care and social service organizations.

That is the presentation of the major ideas we have drawn from the sociology of organizations for this book. We have also described the use that can be made of the analytic framework of issues and challenges surrounding the implementation of active offer of services in minority official languages. Now we will see how the following analyses enable us to gain a better understanding of the role of the actor and the system, as well as their interactions, in advancing and updating principles of active offer.

Notes

1. Also called strategic analysis. The core propositions are contained in a seminal work (Crozier & Friedberg, 1977) and a title that revisits the model, responding to some of the criticisms levelled against it and specifying some of its ambiguities (Friedberg, 1993).
2. For more on the concept of rationality, see the work of Raymond Boudon (Boudon 1988, 1989, 1996).

References

Bélanger, P. R. (1988). Santé et services sociaux au Québec: un système en otage ou en crise? De l'analyse stratégique aux modes de régulation. *Revue internationale d'action communautaire*, 20(60), 145–156.

Benamouzig, D. (2005). *La santé au miroir de l'économie*. Paris : PUF.

Bergeron, H. (2010). Les politiques de santé publique. In O. Borraz, and V. Guiraudon (Ed.), *Politiques publiques 2: changer la société*. Paris: Presses de Sciences Po, pp. 79–111.

Bergeron, H., & Castel, P. (2014). *Sociologie politique de la santé*. Paris : PUF.

Binst, M. (1994). Vertus et limites de l'analyse stratégique pour l'intervention à l'hôpital. In F. Pavé, *L'analyse stratégique autour de Michel Crozier. Sa genèse, ses applications et ses problèmes actuels*. Paris: Seuil, pp. 369–372.

Bloch, M.-A., & Hénaut L. (2014). *Coordination et parcours: la dynamique du monde sanitaire, social et médico-social*. Paris: Dunod.

Borraz, O. (1998). *Les politiques locales de lutte contre le sida*. Paris: L'Harmattan.

Borraz, O. (2008). *Les politiques du risque*. Paris: Presses de Sciences Po.

Boudon, R. (1977). *Effets pervers et ordre social*. Paris: PUF.

Boudon, R. (1988). Rationalité et théorie de l'action sociale. In E. Guibert-Sledziewski and J.L. Vieillard-Baron (Eds.), *Penser le sujet aujourd'hui*. Paris: Méridiens Klincksieck, pp. 139–263.

Boudon, R. (1989). Subjective Rationality and the Explanation of Social Behavior, *Rationality and Society*, 1(2), 173–196.

Boudon, R. (1996). Au-delà de la rationalité limitée ? *Environnement et société*. 17: 85–111.

Burrell, G, & Morgan, G. (1979). *Sociological paradigms and organisational analysis*. London: Heinemann.

Castel, P. (2002). *Normaliser les pratiques, organiser les médecins: la qualité comme stratégie de changement* (Doctorat dissertation). IEP, Paris.

Castel, P. (2008). La gestion de l'incertitude médicale: approche collective et contrôle latéral en cancérologie. *Sciences sociales et santé*, 26(1), 9–32.

Castel, P. (2009). What's behind a Guideline? Authority, Competition and Collaboration in the French Oncology Sector. *Social Studies of Science*, 39(5), 743–764.

Castel, P., & Carrère, M.-O. (Eds.) (2007). *Soins en réseau: Pratiques, acteurs et régulation en cancérologie*. Montrouge: Éditions John Libbey Eurotext.

Castel, P., & Merle, I., (2002). Quand les normes de pratique deviennent une ressource pour les médecins. *Sociologie du travail*, 44(2), 337–355.

Crespin, R., & Lascoumes, P. (2000). Régulation de la carrière d'un instrument de santé: les parcours de l'usage du test du VIH dans l'emploi en France et aux États-Unis. *Sociologie du travail*, 42(1), 133–157.

Crozier, M. (1987). L'analyse stratégique en milieu hospitalier: pertinence et méthodologie. *Gestion hospitalière*, 261: 787–791.

Crozier, M., & Friedberg E. (1977). *L'acteur et le système*. Paris: Seuil.

De Pouvourville, G. (1994). La sociologie, l'ingénieur et l'hôpital. In F. Pavé, *L'analyse stratégique autour de Michel Crozier. Sa genèse, ses applications et ses problèmes actuels*. Paris: Seuil, pp. 357–361.

Friedberg, E. (1993). *Le pouvoir et la règle: dynamiques de l'action organisée*. Paris: Seuil.

Gonnet, F. (1994). Application du raisonnement stratégique et systémique aux hôpitaux publics. In F. Pavé, *L'analyse stratégique autour de Michel Crozier. Sa genèse, ses applications et ses problèmes actuels.* Paris: Seuil, pp. 337–344.

Henry, E., Gilbert, C., Jouzel, J.-N., & Marichalar, P. (Eds.) (2015). *Dictionnaire critique de l'expertise: santé, travail, environnement.* Paris: Presses de Sciences Po.

Jacobsson B. (2000). Standardization and expert knowledge. In Brunsson, N., & Jacobsson B., *A World of Standards,* Oxford: Oxford University Press, pp. 40–49.

Leavitt H. J. (1958). *Psychologie des fonctions de direction dans l'entreprise.* Paris: Ed. Hommes et Techniques.

Moisdon, J.-C. (1994). Hôpital, instrumentation de gestion et analyse stratégique. In F. Pavé, *L'analyse stratégique autour de Michel Crozier. Sa genèse, ses applications et ses problèmes actuels.* Paris: Seuil, pp. 350–356.

Savard, S., Turcotte, D., & Beaudoin, A. (2004). Le partenariat et les organisations sociosanitaires du secteur de l'enfance, de la famille et de la jeunesse: une analyse stratégique. *Nouvelles pratiques sociales,* 16(2), 160–177.

Vézina, S. (2015). Bilan de santé: une analyse descriptive de l'état de la recherche sur la santé et les communautés francophones en situation minoritaire. *Minorités linguistiques et société,* 6: pp. 202–223.

CHAPTER 2

Engaging Future Professionals in the Promotion of Active Offer for a Culturally and Linguistically Appropriate System[1]

Pier Bouchard, Sylvain Vézina, Manon Cormier, and
Marie-Josée Laforge, Groupe de recherche et d'innovation sur
l'organisation des services de santé (GRIOSS), *Université de Moncton*

"With their cultural competence reinforced by the awareness-raising efforts of the CNFS, these graduates are ready to become change makers, if not driving forces, to improve the health system wherever Francophones live, in every region of the country."

(LeBlanc, 2008, p. 42)

Abstract

In this chapter, the authors examine the approach of the *Consortium national de formation en santé* (CNFS) in the area of the active offer of health care and social services in French, in light of ideas from strategic analysis. We will look at the steps the CNFS has taken with regard to a consortium of Francophone post-secondary institutions offering programs in the area of health and social services, to design and share resources to prepare Francophone professionals to take up the challenge of improving access to French-language services in minority settings. In response to a recommendation made in an evaluation report in 2008, the CNFS has undertaken a process to prepare graduates of its post-secondary programs to become ambassadors who are prepared to improve access to safe, quality services for Francophone communities in minority settings.

Readers will learn about an actor-centred strategy enabling professionals to provide active offer of services in French. Readers will also learn about the series of challenges, issues, and ideas for action that occur as resources are developed. Because the process is dynamic we conclude by introducing some of the measures now being developed or implemented.

Key Words: language and health, issues and challenges of active offer, quality and safety of care, actor, strategy, commitment, education and training.

Introduction

Building the active offer capacity of Francophone professionals in health care and social services is a major undertaking, particularly in a setting where there is a very large majority of Anglophones. That is the subject of the current chapter. More specifically, we will be revisiting—in light of ideas proposed as part of a strategic analysis (Crozier & Friedberg, 1977; Friedberg, 1993)—the approach developed by the *Consortium national de formation en santé* (CNFS), with the support of the *Groupe de recherche et d'innovation sur l'organisation des services de santé* (GRIOSS),[2] to meet this challenge. Our goal is to give readers a better understanding of the foundations of the CNFS strategy in this area. The Consortium is an umbrella organization of several post-secondary educational institutions and regional partners across Canada whose purpose is to strengthen post-secondary French-language programs offered in the field of health care and social services. Therefore, the CNFS has a mission to better prepare future professionals in these disciplines to improve access to safe, quality health services[3] for Francophone minority communities. The CNFS was well positioned to initiate the reflection surrounding the means and materials available, and to select those best suited to preparing future health professionals—in particular, motivating them to take action to promote the active offer of health and social services. To carry out this project, the CNFS called on researchers affiliated with the GRIOSS, a group dedicated to research and innovation on the organization of health services, to collect information on the subject and to facilitate a dialogue with the primary actors involved, particularly researchers, educators, managers, health professionals, and students.

In our essay we present the results of an action research project[4] whose results are still being used to guide the active offer work of the CNFS. Through the perspective of the theoretical approaches of Crozier and Friedberg, we will consider how the CNFS articulated its plan to provide tools to actors, in particular health professionals, so they can act on the system (structures, procedures, conventions) in a way that promotes and improves access for Francophone minority communities (FMCs) to health services comparable to those available to the majority. This strategic orientation is closely aligned to the core mandate of the CFNS.

Background

To begin, we need to recall the decisive event that occurred in 1997, when the existence of the Hôpital Montfort, the only Francophone university hospital in Ontario, was in jeopardy. The plan proposed by the Government of Ontario resulted in an unprecedented protest against the idea, engaging the Canadian Francophone community to speak out and take action on the need for French-language health care (Lalonde, 2004). The crisis also led to the decision of the Ontario Court of Appeal, which concluded that the Hôpital Montfort was essential to the preservation and enhancement of the Franco-Ontarian community and contributed to the vitality of this minority linguistic community. Not only did the efforts of Montfort's advocates allow the hospital to survive, and even thrive, they also fostered the creation of networks of actors such as the *Société santé en français* (SSF), which has alliances in every province and territory, and the array of Francophone post-secondary health programs that make up the *Consortium national de formation en santé* (CNFS).

The initial mandate of the CNFS is to contribute to improving French-language services by educating and training a growing number of Francophone health care and social service professionals, and by developing research on the needs of Francophone minority communities in the area of health and wellness (CNFS n.d., para. 4). A proposal to adjust this mandate was made in a 2008 report evaluating the education and research orientation of the CNFS that was intended to better prepare future health and social service professionals to deal with the realities of working in minority settings (LeBlanc, 2008). In the report, the author raises the point that a large number of Francophone professionals will be asked not only to work in an environment where access to French-language services is limited, but one in which the workload of bilingual staff members is sometimes so demanding that there is a real risk of assimilating Francophone professionals. He describes workplaces where the organizational culture is not very favourable towards providing services in French: namely, medical records written in English, and the isolation of Francophone professionals surrounded by Anglophone team members. To counter these barriers and the spillover effect of a strongly Anglophone work environment on the linguistic behaviour of Francophone professionals, the author suggests that measures be taken to incorporate the concept and implications of working in Francophone minority communities into existing programs. Such measures would raise awareness and make future professionals more committed and better equipped to engage confidently in the work of offering quality services in the official language of the user's choice.

LeBlanc noted graduates felt poorly prepared, or even powerless, when they started to work in a minority context. This is why he felt it was time to improve their understanding of the issues and challenges of providing services in French by ensuring that their programs introduce them to some key ideas—for example, the link between language and quality of services, or the practice of actively offering social services and health services in French.

In other words, the evaluation established the premise that improving French-language services would necessarily involve motivating and engaging future health and social service professionals to become creative change makers. Guided by the belief actors have the capacity to influence the system, LeBlanc recommended that the CNFS pay particular attention to the issue of preparing and motivating students for action:

> We recommend that the CNFS analyze the problem of equipping students with the tools and resources they need to enable them to take up the challenge of actively offering health services in French in health facilities, and that it develop a teaching strategy designed to transmit an understanding of the issues and the aptitudes and abilities required to meet this challenge. (LeBlanc, 2008, p. 41)

According to LeBlanc, the arrival of a critical mass of better-equipped professionals in different health facilities should result in a tangible improvement in the provision of French-language services. Moreover, since some of these professionals would eventually rise into management positions, they could contribute to adapting the system to better respond to the linguistic needs of its users. This idea is perfectly aligned with the orientation suggested in 2001 by the Consultative Committee for French-Speaking Minority Communities / *Comité consultatif des communautés francophones en situation minoritaire* (CCCFSM). Its members believed it was vital that the community foster and develop organizations managed by and for Francophones and that these organizations be given adequate human and financial resources. In other words, progress in the area of service provision would, they thought, necessarily include governance and the participation of Francophones in decision-making:

> . . . the more Francophones are involved in the care delivery process, including managing health care institutions, the more French is respected and reflected in service delivery. This participation is also crucial if the population is to take real responsibility for health. (CCCFSM, 2001, p. 16)

This is the context in which GRIOSS researchers were asked to analyze the challenges of better preparing future professionals for the CNFS. The GRIOSS mandate was to compile more extensive information on this issue, and to develop a process to raise awareness and encourage the active engagement of stakeholders (researchers, professors, program directors, managers, practitioners, and students) in the design of resources and tools that could be integrated into programs preparing future professionals to actively offer social services and health care in French. In conjunction with the GRIOSS, the national secretariat of the CNFS also agreed to begin a dialogue with the actors involved with the aim of identifying content that should be included in post-secondary programs for professionals, as well as the tools and methods necessary to deliver this content. At the same time, it was a way of meeting the need for greater awareness and stronger motivation to act for change among the actors involved and to develop strategies to do so across Canada.

Methodological Considerations

Researchers used three methods of data collection to obtain a current picture of the situation. Nearly 40 interviews were conducted with experts and people familiar with issues related to education and training and the quality of French-language health services in minority settings (professors, researchers, managers, health professionals, CNFS coordinators). The participants interviewed included 15 men and 24 women; 3 were from Alberta, 3 from Manitoba, 4 from Nova Scotia, 10 from New Brunswick, and 19 from Ontario.

Drawing from the strategic analysis approach, the interview protocol was designed to elicit comments about the problems and challenges confronting Francophone minority communities in terms of the quality of services, on one hand, and on the other, the challenges that professionals must tackle if they wish to promote equal access to quality services in French.

Simultaneously, researchers conducted a survey of students and new health professionals to document their perception of the challenges to be met in the field of health care in minority settings and to assess their level of motivation to act. To participate, respondents had to be enrolled in one of the health programs supported by the CNFS and to have completed a minimum of 66% of the credits in their program, or to be new graduates from programs supported by the CNFS and be working in the health sector for at least three years.[5] The questionnaire included 48 statements on the following themes: perception of the link between language and health services; concerns about the work environment; avenues to explore to improve French-language services; and knowledge base to build and skills to develop in professional programs, so that health professionals will be better prepared to work effectively in a minority context.

The survey was delivered electronically.[6] Of the 898 potential participants, a total of 143 respondents followed up, including 127 (109 students and 18 new professionals) who completed the entire questionnaire, giving us a response rate of 16%. The profile of the respondents was as follows: 86% were students (70% in universities, 30% in colleges), 79% spoke French at home, 85% were women, and all age groups were represented, with a majority between 19 and 26 years of age.

The questionnaire was designed for students and professionals in all Canadian provinces and territories except Quebec. To identify the source of the responses, a question about the respondent's province of residence was included. Several people opted to answer that question by giving the province of their permanent residence; as a result, in the case of students listing the parental residence, the latter sometimes differed from the place where they studied. This resulted in a proportion of 10% of people who identified themselves as residents of Quebec. Given the small number of respondents from each province (with the exception of New Brunswick and Ontario), it became difficult to make comparisons according to province of residence. The researchers therefore agreed to combine the answers to certain questions from Alberta, British Columbia, Manitoba, and Nova Scotia, where Francophone minority communities are smaller. However, readers should not assume that the situations in these provinces are the same. We should also specify that the total number of respondents in these four provinces represents only 11% of the sample, so it is important to be cautious about the findings and to avoid any attempt to generalize.

The third method of data collection consisted of a national dialogue,[7] organized as part of a series of regional gatherings, which brought together a total of approximately 100 actors. The participants comprised students, new professionals, people familiar with the subject, researchers, coordinators, managers and representatives from educational programs and from organizations such as the SSF and the CNFS, and citizens. There were equal numbers from three regions of the country: from the East (these participants met in Moncton), the Centre (in Ottawa), and the West (in Winnipeg). The objectives of these discussions were to identify the educational content about active offer that should be included in training programs for professionals, and to determine the best way of delivering this content.

It was hoped that dialogue would make it possible to determine strategies for concrete action, thus enabling key actors in the system to work with new generations of professionals in a way that would foster their commitment to cooperative leadership for the benefit of safe and quality health and wellness services in French. The exercise was based on a model of mutual learning and the sustained commitment of actors in a strategy of cooperative action, for the purpose of influencing the system and of improving the policies, programs, and services for FMCs.

Issues Related to Access to French-Language Health Services: Perspective and Dynamics of Actors

The actors we interviewed emphasize the fact that quality French-language services should be delivered within a wait time comparable to services offered in the language of the majority, and should include direct access to communication in one's own language, both oral and written, when receiving these services.[8] When asked about health services in French, study participants indicated that communicating in the user's language is an essential condition if services are to be considered safe and of quality. Several studies have shown that users who face language barriers are exposed to a higher risk of errors, complications, and adverse incidents (including a lack of understanding of the diagnosis or treatment; delay or lack of follow-up in the treatment protocol; increase in hospitalizations; unnecessary or inappropriate diagnostic tests). (Bowen, 2000, 2001, 2015; CCCFSM, 2007; Munoz & Kapoor-Kohli, 2007).

Moreover, our interviews allowed us to learn about concrete situations that clearly illustrated the impact of language on the quality and safety of care. For example, the people we consulted spoke about the risk of diagnostic errors when a Francophone patient is considered to be "confused" by a unilingual Anglophone physician unable to understand what the patient is saying in French or in broken English. The same participants also pointed out gaps in treatment, sharing several examples of people who could not fully understand the instructions given by a health professional about prescribed treatment, and dealing with health complications that affected their recovery and may even have put their life in danger.

Thus, beyond the question of users' rights, the comments made by the professionals and researchers with whom we spoke clearly indicated that a lack of access to health services in the language of the user's choice raises fundamental safety issues. Linguistic and cultural barriers are seen to make a significant impact on the quality of communication between the health professional and the user, and thus on the effectiveness of care: "When cultural and linguistic barriers in the clinical encounter negatively affect communication and trust, this leads to patient dissatisfaction, poor adherence . . . and poorer health outcomes" (Betancourt, Green, Carrillo, & Ananeh-Firempong, 2003, p. 297). Another essential element that arose from the interviews was the need to take specific measures to offer services in the language chosen by the user in order to ensure adequate access to quality services and safe care. The safety of users is closely linked to the quality of the services they receive (Smith, Mossialos, & Papanicolas, 2008). As Bowen points out, "that official language proficiency is in itself a determinant of health, and may interact with ethnicity and socio-economic status. Future research should incorporate these broader dimensions" (2001, n.p.).

The data we collected also reveal a vicious circle: limited access to French-language services generally causes lengthy delays before a service is received. Because they are aware of these additional delays, users opt to be served in English. The comments of one of the study participants clearly illustrate the rational basis for this decision: [original: French] "Is someone going to wait for a service in French if it takes more time? Usually, we prefer to be looked after as soon as possible, especially if waiting might have consequences for our health."

Several of the people we met provided different examples of situations in which the user does not risk asking for service in French, out of a fear of being considered a troublemaker or being treated poorly by professionals. It is important to remember that users often feel vulnerable, stressed, and dependent on professionals, particularly when they are hospitalized. Sometimes they are intimidated by the status of medical professionals, and do not always have the confidence to ask questions, let alone insist on having explanations given in their own language.

All the same, we did notice different and even contradictory positions among managers regarding the matter of asking for services in French. Some are resistant to change and, claiming there is a low demand for them, question the need to arrange for French-language services. Others are more inclined to redefine the rules of the game; they believe being aware of the vicious circle should make everyone more eager to act in order to solve the problem. For those more receptive to change, the assumption seems to be that if supply improves, the demand will increase and the needs of Francophone minority communities in general will be better met.

Discussions also allowed us to expose the different realities of Francophone communities between one province—or even one region of a province—and others. In some regions where there is a high concentration of Francophones, people live their everyday life in French. In other regions the Francophone population is spread out and lacks the critical mass needed to guarantee access to quality health and wellness services in French. The Francophone community in New Brunswick is generally viewed as privileged because it represents one-third of the total population of the province, and also enjoys legal protections.

The situation from the point of view of bilingual professionals.
Throughout the entire study, bilingual professionals mentioned that
their employers and unilingual colleagues call on them daily for help
to meet the needs of Francophone users. This means their language
skills result in added work; sometimes these duties are not even
related to their profession: [original: French] "Since other professionals can't communicate with Francophone patients, I'm asked to play
several roles at the same time: interpreter, nurse, and social worker."
It seems that the workload of these makeshift interpreters is significantly heavier than others. Not only do bilingual professionals face
the possibility of an overload of work, they may also have to take on
responsibility outside of their area of competence.

Since these additional duties are generally not valued by the
employer, some Francophone professionals stated that they avoid
announcing or displaying too openly the fact that they are "bilingual." Consequently, people who do this are less inclined to make
an active offer of French-language services. Some professionals at
the dialogue mentioned they hesitated for a long time before "coming
out of the closet," for fear of having to deal with a heavier workload.
Other comments made by professionals also reveal some ambiguity
in the behaviour of employers towards their Francophone or bilingual
employees. Even though they had recruited the staff members
because of their language skills, managers seem to restrict their use
of French on the job. As well as requiring them to write medical
records in English, managers often supply information in English
only and ask staff to speak in English with their co-workers, even
when it is two Francophones who are talking.

> [original: French] My boss is an Anglophone and she doesn't
> want me to speak French to Francophone patients, because she
> doesn't understand French. So I have two options: either I can
> be assimilated into the Anglophone group, or I can quit and find
> a Francophone facility. Either way, I'm not helping Francophones
> who come to my facility. (A nurse)

It is as though some employers want to show off the bilingual nature
of the facility, without compromising the predominance of English.
It can be difficult for a bilingual professional, in these conditions, to
maintain both a high level of proficiency in French and a level of
commitment towards the Francophone cause.

Similarly, it seemed that unions sometimes slow the progress towards an active offer of French-language services. For example, we were told of a case in which the union brought a complaint forward, due to the hiring of what was considered an excessive number of bilingual staff. According to the union, too many French-speaking professionals could put the health of patients in danger. The real problem here seems to be the desire to limit the number of bilingual positions which, by definition, are closed to unilingual Anglophones from the majority community.

> [original: French] Imagine a young Francophone professional who is confronted with this reality. It's difficult for him to assert himself and work in French. He is told from the start: "You were hired because you're bilingual, but you have to speak English to your co-workers, patients, etc." When your union says this kind of thing, you can imagine what that does for a health professional's motivation to use French. (A manager)

The perspective of professionals starting their career. When we spoke about workplace issues to Francophone professionals who are at the beginning of their career, their responses made it clear that their commitment to providing services in the language of the minority represents a significant challenge. In the survey, for example, they were invited to indicate their level of concern about five issues: workload, career advancement, difficulty of working in French, relationships with service users, and the atmosphere in the workplace.

Figure 1. Concerns about the Work Environment

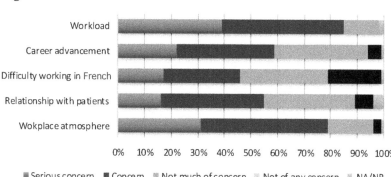

When the results were compiled, workload came first on the list, with 85.5% of respondents expressing concern about this issue. This is definitely a matter for concern, considering the link we established earlier between workload and commitment, on one hand, and the active offer of services in French, on the other. It is even more of a worry if active offer is not valued in the workplace.

Ranked next among their concerns, 79% of respondents noted the atmosphere in the workplace with co-workers. Once again, this situation could detract from a professional's commitment to active offer. As mentioned earlier, there is a tendency in a workplace with an Anglophone majority to discourage conversations in the language of the minority, whether the discouragement comes from managers or unions. When this happens, it does not take much pressure from peers or people in authority to make a new professional, eager to maintain a pleasant environment at work, decide to assimilate into the majority and, in so doing, neglect the role of promoting an active offer of services.

It is interesting to note that the concern ranked lowest by professionals was the difficulty of working in French; more than 52% of respondents said they were "not concerned" or "had little concern" about this issue. Given this result, there is no doubt about the crucial importance of the plan to better prepare students and new professionals by making them more aware of the issues in actively offering services in French.

While this profile of the situation might make us rather pessimistic, our study also revealed some promising avenues to explore. For example, the national dialogue allowed us to better understand the extent to which young people headed towards a career in health or social services are doing so because they want to "make a difference" and have a "meaningful career." Several young professionals stated that they seek out opportunities to get involved and would like to contribute, as Francophones, to their community.

We should also point out that a large number of young professionals state that they are in favour of bilingualism, and that they feel it is important for users to be able to access services in the language of their choice in order to be properly understood. More than 79% of respondents agreed it was either "important" or "very important" to receive French-language health services.

Figure 2. Importance of Offering French-Language Services

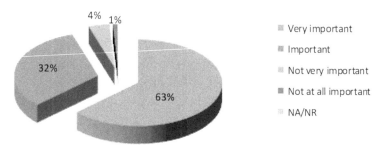

Regarding the working language, over 73% stated they would prefer to use French at work. However, this varies greatly depending on the place of residence. Respondents from New Brunswick are (second only to those from Quebec) the most likely to prefer French as their working language (84%), while residents of Ontario were more likely to state they have no preference (32%). Those in the other four provinces are more likely to express a preference for English (22%).

In spite of these numbers, respondents were very positive when asked how much importance they place on being able to offer French-language health services in a minority setting: more than 95% replied that it was either "important" or "very important."

Figure 3. Importance of Obtaining French-Language Services

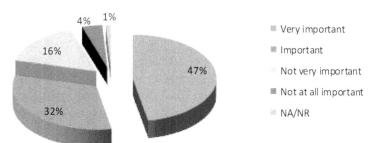

Moreover, young professionals starting careers want their organizations to make a statement in favour of diversity. Not only did they specify that the issue of equity was of great importance to them, they expressed their desire for the user to be at the centre of professionals' concerns. In other words, they want to work in an inclusive, client-centred environment where professionals are welcoming both to service users from official language minority communities *and* to those from other linguistic communities.

Project to Promote the Active Offer, Competency Profile, and Means for Action

According to the model of strategic analysis, information and expertise play an important role among the sources of recognized power (Crozier & Friedberg, 1977, p.71). We cannot help but recognize the almost complete absence in post-secondary programs of any content that could help future professionals take action for change, and specifically to contribute to creating a system in which services are more linguistically and culturally appropriate (in other words, sensitive and responsive to the challenges of the minority language community). Yet the future professionals we met during the study clearly wanted the issue of French-language health and wellness services to be examined more closely. They also wanted the curriculum and resources to be designed to make them more aware and better informed about the issues and challenges facing Francophone communities in a minority setting, and desired a greater emphasis to be placed on the cultural dimension of health during their studies.

Furthermore, a consensus rapidly emerged among the dialogue participants about the need to develop learning activities to help students gain a better understanding of the link between language and quality of care. They believed this would help professionals become more motivated to actively offering services in French. Thus, improving access to French-language services would rely on confident and engaged professionals, on one hand, and the access of educators to teaching and training tools on active offer on the other. Throughout their studies, for instance, future health professionals could discuss potential situations that could arise in a minority Francophone workplace so they would better understand the impact that speaking in French has on the quality and safety of care.

Finally, participants wished to have more opportunities for placements and internships in Francophone settings to acquire relevant experience as well as to strengthen their connections with people in the Francophone community.

Towards a competency profile. As part of this national conversation—intended to determine strategies for concrete action—participants acknowledged the necessity to develop a competency profile for health professionals working in minority contexts. Specifically, future professionals should have knowledge about the following themes: language as a determinant of health; conditions in which members of official language minority communities live; and characteristics of working in minority contexts. Professionals with this profile would be more inclined to adopt behaviours that promote the active offer of French-language services and be better prepared to take up the challenges they encounter while working in these settings.

Table 1. Competency Profile for Social Service and Health Professionals Working in Minority Contexts according to Dialogue Participants: "Knowledge"

Moncton	Ottawa	Winnipeg
– Language as a health determinant	– Language as a health determinant	– Language as a health determinant
– Characteristics of working in a minority context	– Realities and conditions in which members of official language minorities live	– Characteristics of work and profile of competency in a minority context
– Conditions in which members of official language minority communities live	– Practical examples of active offer	– Demographic information
	– Rights of minority language speakers	– Conditions in which members of official language minority communities live
– Identity construction		– Identity construction
		– Practical examples
		– Revitalizing language rights

Dialogue participants said the content included in the training of future professionals should promote the construction of meaning and pride in a Francophone identity, and commitment to the Francophone collectivity and bilingualism in particular. Comments from one of the participants are of particular interest: he said his experience in the dialogic exercise, in which different actors shared their perspectives, had enabled him to [original: French] "bathe in Francophone pride." Along the same lines, several participants in the dialogue verbalized their need for affirmation; this is clear in an example from one participant: [original: French] "We are often faced with the phenomenon of the 'Francophone in the closet.' People know they're in there, but they don't connect with them!" To summarize, participants feel action needs to be taken to develop a sense of pride and to encourage Francophones to "come out of the closet." This feeling of pride would, according to participants, allow health and social service professionals to show leadership in promoting access to safe, quality services in French: [original: French] "Leadership means being the voice of the family and the patient. It means accepting the idea of responding to questions that have nothing to do with our profession, and going beyond their common duties. We are the lifeline for our [Francophone] patients." (A nurse)

Table 2. Competency Profile for Social Service and Health Professionals Working in Minority Communities, according to Dialogue Participants: "Skills and Attitudes"

Moncton	Ottawa	Winnipeg
– Pride in Francophone identity	– Development of pride – attitudes (construction of meaning: logical / ideological)	– Commitment to Francophone community / bilingualism
		– Openness to diversity
– Leadership	– Leadership	– Leadership
– Self-knowledge and self-affirmation	– Networking	– Networking
		– Self-knowledge and self-affirmation
– Linguistic competencies	– Linguistic and cultural competencies	– Linguistic and cultural competencies
– Social and interpersonal relationship skills	– Social skills	– Social and interpersonal relationship skills
	– Importance of French	– Autonomy
		– Competencies linked to working in a minority context
		– Importance of going beyond the profile of competencies (global strategy for Francophones)

In this regard, there was discussion of applying theories of a pedagogy of conscientization (Landry & Roussel, 2003), which is designed to motivate students to take action as well as to contribute to the identity construction and development of future health professionals; that is

> . . . a pedagogy of conscientization and involvement, which develops the students' critical thinking and reflexive analysis, so that they become conscious of their Francophone minority reality and of the power relationships at work in society, and so that they become capable of imagining ways to take charge of their own destiny. . . . This pedagogy of conscientization and involvement cultivates their consciousness of sources of inequity and injustice, and is aimed at helping them develop a critical social consciousness and to take charge of transforming historical, social, political, and economic conditions. (p. 128–129)

Challenges integrating this content. During the dialogue, participants also identified best practices for transferring knowledge and helping students acquire competencies. A priority-setting exercise narrowed the criteria for evaluating the approach down to two: the potential of the delivery method and its feasibility. Five modes of delivery met the criteria: case studies, placements and internships, lectures and conferences, networking activities, and the use of technology (websites, social media, etc.). The use of case studies was recognized by participants from all three regions as an effective learning method; they felt it was dynamic and well suited to the content needed for future professionals to be well prepared for their work. In their opinion, case studies would also enable students in professional programs to understand the importance of placing the user at the centre of their practice, and to make them aware of the impact of language on the quality of health services and patient safety.

One of the most significant projects to emerge from dialogue was the design of a "toolbox" for people interested in learning more about the subject. It would include patient testimonies, exercises, and resources adapted to different audiences (academic, workplace, etc.). In the spirit of the strategic analysis, this toolbox is intended to raise awareness on the reality of the workplace by bringing into the classroom the perspectives of different actors: users, professionals, managers, researchers, leaders in Francophone organizations, etc. The contents of the toolbox would be geared to action and designed to move learners from theory to practice, in particular through their study of different avenues for action. Its purpose was to lead learners to reflection and analysis by inviting them to take ownership of the issues and to examine various themes related to the subject more deeply.

In response to this recommendation, members of the GRIOSS team were charged with creating the toolbox. They started by gathering existing information on the subject in the literature and then adding to the contents by creating various types of pedagogical resources. In November 2013, the www.offreactive.com website was launched; it is available to educators and members of the public.

Since its launch, the toolbox has attracted growing interest from the full range of actors who have taken advantage of its high-quality, ready-to-use materials, available in both English and French. As well as video capsules based on real experiences, the toolbox presents reading notes on key themes identified by the national dialogue participants, such as language and health, issues and challenges of active offer, characteristics of working in minority settings, etc. As well, users have access to case studies that can help stimulate discussion and explore the subject in more depth through descriptions of real or fictitious examples. The tool box also includes an observation sheet that can be used for internships, a tool to help future professionals become more critically conscious and better prepared for the experiences they will have in the field, and to imagine solutions that will improve access to French-language health services. Finally, the toolbox offers a guide for educators, with suggestions on teaching active offer using its contents.

The team that designed the toolbox hopes that it will make a growing number of professors and educators more aware of active offer, and make it easier for them to include content on active offer in their classes. This way, future professionals will be able to acquire new knowledge and develop new competencies that will serve them well when they enter the workforce and also be of great benefit to the OLMCs with which they work. At the same time, these competencies become an added value for these programs of study.

It is interesting to note that the toolbox is now recognized by the Commissioner of Official Languages as an exemplary resource that could potentially inspire federal institutions to improve their practice of active offer.[9] More precisely, the Commissioner encourages federal institutions to "take measures that take into account the human aspects of front-line service," from the point of view of employees as well as citizens.

Conclusion

Developing an action research project inspired by the ideas emerging from our strategic analysis gave us an opportunity to focus on the needs of the actors involved: a data collection to better grasp the actors' perspective and dynamics; a dialogue among actors; and the production of videos to present testimonials from users and different actors' perspectives. Initiatives such as dialogue and testimonials have yielded a variety of benefits contributing to the engagement and preparation of future health professionals. In January 2012, the CNFS published a reference framework for education and training on the active offer of French-language services. It presents the profile of competencies that emerged from the dialogue, continues with a series of learning components that begins with awareness and the development of a critical consciousness among future professionals, and finishes with the exercise of an ethical and engaged leadership (Lortie, Lalonde, & Bouchard, 2012).[10]

We would be remiss if we did not mention the new initiatives taken in recent years that are also part of the strategy to engage actors so they can influence change in the health system and improve the active offer of health services in both official languages. Here are some examples:

- Mobilization of professors who show leadership in teaching about active offer.
- Integration of content of learning on the active offer in health care programs (universities and colleges).
- Training of trainers (professors and teachers) in CNFS member institutions.
- Development of a national certification program on active offer.
- Design and production of tools to assess behaviours related to active offer.

Beyond describing some of the activities undertaken since 2008 by the CNFS in the area of active offer, we have also highlighted, in this chapter, the strategic orientation adopted by its members. Relying on the information and expertise available, the CNFS wants to make it possible for professionals to act for change and to improve the active offer of French-language services in the health system. Developing new studies enabling us to measure the impact of this type of strategy on the quality of health care offered to minority communities is vital. However, we have to wait until more ways have been found to apply this strategy to concrete action; tools to do so must be produced, applied to different situations, and refined. At this stage, there are numerous challenges in the implementation and evaluation of these actions. Here is one example: Despite all the efforts made to provide the health and social service sector with Francophone professionals who are prepared and equipped to ensure an active offer of services, the way services are organized still needs to be adapted in a way that optimizes the use of these resources. Perhaps we even have to ask ourselves if it is realistic to envisage transforming the system without first engaging the support of actors from the Anglophone majority communities. Since health and social service facilities are predominantly managed by actors speaking the language of the Anglophone majority, raising their awareness of the realities of the minority is necessary and must be taken into consideration when any strategy is being developed. Hence, new alliances have to be developed in order to support efforts to promote a linguistically and culturally appropriate health system. Because of this, should we not be just as concerned with finding ways to make actors from the majority aware, critically conscious, and well prepared? Is it not essential to engage them, as well, in our efforts to transform the system and to change the rules of the game so as to protect the safety of their patients from official language minority communities?

Despite concrete progress made towards access to French-language health care and social services, many roadblocks remain. Actors from the minority must, therefore, persevere in their efforts to deepen their understanding of the issues, in particular by collectively identifying the relevant zones of uncertainty that need to be monitored as well as the best strategies to adopt. These are promising opportunities for research and action.

Notes

1. The authors acknowledge the financial contribution of Health Canada to research on the commitment of future professionals, carried out in close cooperation with the national secretariat of the *Consortium national de formation en santé* (CNFS).

2. This cooperative project has already resulted in the submission of two research reports (Bouchard & Vézina, 2009; 2010) to the national secretariat of the CNFS; the major findings are shared here.

3. The **quality** of care is defined as "the degree to which health services for individuals and populations increase the likelihood of desired health outcomes and are consistent with current professional knowledge." As for **safety**, it is "the reduction of risk of unnecessary harm associated with healthcare to an acceptable minimum. An acceptable minimum refers to the collective notions of given current knowledge, resources available, and the context in which care was delivered weighed against the risk of non-treatment or other treatment." (Canadian Patient Safety Institute, n.d., n.p.)

4. Action research, or participatory action research (PAR) is a method intended to explore the perspectives of actors in different spheres of public life, with the understanding that these diverse realities are rich with meaning and the potential for action. Thus, action research integrates the knowledge and experience of different actor-participants, enabling them to better deal with complex issues and challenges. We invite readers interested in the subject to look at the studies in the following volume: Chevalier, J. M., Buckles, D. J., and Bourassa, M. (2013). *Guide de la recherche-action, la planification et l'évaluation participatives.* SAS2 Dialogue, Ottawa, Canada.

5. The questionnaire and the procedures used for data collection, analysis, and storage were approved by the committee responsible for evaluating the ethics of research on human beings in the faculty of graduate studies and research of the Université de Moncton, as well as the ethics committees of the universities involved in our study: Université Sainte-Anne, Collège universitaire de Saint-Boniface, Laurentian University, and University of Ottawa.

6. For reasons of confidentiality, data bases including the electronic addresses of students and new professionals were prepared by CNFS coordinators, in some cases, in cooperation with the registrar's offices of the institution. One of the effects of this procedure was to limit the control of the research team over the requests and, at times, to make it impossible to send reminders to people who had not yet responded.

7. A dialogic approach tries to integrate the knowledge of various actors (experts, citizens, professionals) in order to identity the priorities and to make decisions based on reason. "Dialogic democracy" is intended

to have logic emerge organically from dialogue and to reduce the "subjective" factors in decision-making. See: Callon, M., Lascoumes, P., and Barthe, Y. (2001). *Agir dans un monde incertain. Essai sur la démocratie technique.* Paris: Le Seuil; Lombard, E. (February 7, 2009). Démocratie dialogique: la logique du dialogue. *Observatoire des débats publics.* http://www.debatpublic.net/2009/02/07/democratie-dialogique-la-logique-du-dialogue/; Yankelovich, D. (2001). *The Magic of Dialogue: Transforming Conflict into Cooperation.* New York: Simon & Shuster; Stoyko, P., Henning, G.K., and McCaughey, D. (2006). *Creativity at Work: A Leadership Guide: Success belongs to me! CSPS Action-Research Roundtable on Creativity.* Canada School of Public Service.

8. Active offer refers to the notion of service equal in quality to that of the majority, which means, for example, that the wait time should be reasonable and similar to that of the majority, the use of bilingual forms, the availability of services in areas where official language minority communities (OLMCs) are located, the promotion of French language or bilingual organizations in the local media, etc. As specified in a document prepared for Service Canada, users are simply seeking services that those who speak the majority language receive. They want to have care in their own language, without delay, and adapted to their needs (Bouchard, Vézina, *et al.*, 2009, p. 62).

9. Office of the Commissioner of Official Languages (2016). *Annual Report 2015–2016.* Ottawa: Minister of Public Works and Government Services Canada.

10. Ethical and engaged leadership is associated with the knowledge to act and knowledge to live together. New professionals are called on to develop and practise leadership based on justice, compassion, and critical awareness. They become change agents and catalysts for innovation in their workplaces and their communities. Such leaders are committed and inspire other people in their organization to come together around a common vision, and thus contribute to an emerging culture of active offer (Lortie, Lalonde, & Bouchard, 2012, p. 12).

References

Betancourt, J. R., Green, A. R., Carrillo, J., E., & Ananeh-Firempong, O. (2003). Defining Cultural Competence: A Practical Framework for Addressing Racial/Ethnic Disparities in Health and Health Care. *Public Health Reports, 118*(4), 293–302.

Boelen, C. (2000). *Towards Unity for Health. Challenges and Opportunities for Partnership in Health Development. A working paper.* Geneva: World Health Organization.

Bouchard, P., & Vézina, S. (2010). *Rapport du Dialogue sur l'engagement des étudiants et des futurs professionnels pour de meilleurs services de santé en français dans un contexte minoritaire.* Consortium national de formation en santé. Retrieved from http://cnfs.net/upfiles/Rapport_projet_de_loutillage.Nov2010.pdf

Bouchard, P., & Vézina, S. (in collaboration with Paulin, C., & Provencher, M.). (2009). *L'outillage des étudiants et des nouveaux professionnels: un levier essentiel pour l'amélioration des services de santé en français.* Retrieved from http://www.offreactive.com/wp-content/uploads/2013/03/4outillage-des-etudiants-et-nouveaux-prof-levier-essentiel-web.pdf

Bowen, S. (2000). Access to Health Services for Underserved Populations in Canada. In *"Certain Circumstances:" Issues in Equity and Responsiveness in Access to Health Care in Canada* (A collection of papers and reports, pp. 1–60). Ottawa: Health Canada.

Bowen, S. (2001). *Language Barriers in Access to Health Care.* Ottawa: Health Canada. Retrieved from https://www.canada.ca/en/health-canada/services/health-care-system/reports-publications/health-care-accessibility/language-barriers.html

Bowen, S. (2015). *Impact des barrières linguistiques sur la sécurité des patients et la qualité des soins.* Final report prepared for the Société Santé en français.

Callon, M., Lascoumes, P., & Barthe, Y. (2001). *Agir dans un monde incertain. Essai sur la démocratie technique.* Paris: Le Seuil.

The Canadian Patient Safety Institute. (n.d.) *Effective Governance for Quality and Patient Safety.* Glossary of Terms. Retrieved from http://www.patientsafetyinstitute.ca/en/tools Resources/Governance PatientSafety/Pages/GlossaryofTerms.aspx

Chevalier, J. M., Buckles, D. J. & Bourassa, M. (2013). *Guide de la recherche-action, la planification et l'évaluation participatives.* Ottawa, ON: SAS2 Dialogue.

Consortium national de formation en santé. (n.d.). *Mission, valeurs et mandat.* Retrieved from http://cnfs.net/a-propos/mission-valeurs-mandat/

The Consultative Committee for French-Speaking Minority Communities. (2001). Report to the Federal Minister of Health. Retrieved from http://santeenfrancais.com/sites/ccsmanitoba.ca/files/cccfsm__report_to_the_federal_minister_of_health.pdf

The Consultative Committee for French-Speaking Minority Communities. (2007). *Towards a New Leadership for the Improvement of Health Services in French.* Report to the Federal Minister of Health. Retrieved from http://www.hc-sc.gc.ca/ahc-asc/alt_formats/hpb-dgps/pdf/olcdb-baclo/cccfsm/2007-cccfsm/2007-cccfsm-eng.pdf

Crozier, M. & Friedberg, E. (1977). *L'acteur et le système.* Paris: Seuil.

Fédération des communautés francophones et acadiennes du Canada. (2001). *Pour un meilleur accès à des services de santé en français.* Retrieved from http://www.fcfa.ca/user_files/users/40/Media/Pour%20un%20meilleur%20acc%C3%A8s%20%C3%A0%20des%20services%20de%20sant%C3%A9%20en%20fran%C3%A7ais.pdf

Friedberg, E. (1993). *Le pouvoir et la règle: dynamiques de l'action organisée*, Paris: Seuil.

Glouberman, S., & Mintzberg, H. (2002). *Gérer les soins de santé et le traitement de la maladie*. Revue Gestion, 27(3), 12–22.

Groupe de recherche et d'innovation sur l'organisation des services de santé. (2015, March). *Rapport du Forum de discussion intitulé Qualité, sécurité et langues officielles dans l'univers de la santé*. Département d'administration publique de l'Université de Moncton, Société Santé et Mieux-être en français du Nouveau-Brunswick, Consortium national de formation en santé—Secrétariat national et volet Université de Moncton.

Lalonde, G. (2004). Services en français: question de langue, d'équité et de santé, l'expérience de l'hôpital Montfort. *Le Bloc Notes*, 7(7). Retrieved from http://www.leblocnotes.ca/node/229

Landry, R., & Roussel, S. (2003). *Éducation et droits collectifs: au-delà de l'article 23 de la Charte*. Moncton, NB: Les Éditions de la Francophonie.

LeBlanc, P. (2008). *Rapport de l'évaluation sommative du projet de formation et de recherche du Consortium national de formation en santé*. Conseillers en gestion PRAXIS.

Lombard, E. (February 7, 2009). Démocratie dialogique : la logique du dialogue. *Observatoire des débats publics*. Retrieved from http://www.debatpublic .net/2009/02/07/democratie-dialogique-la-logique-du-dialogue/

Lortie, L., & Lalonde, A. J. avec la collaboration de Bouchard, P. à la recherche. (2012). *Cadre de référence pour la formation à l'offre active des services de santé en français*. CNFS. Retrieved from http://cnfs.net/upfiles/ Cadre_de_reference_CNFS_pour_formation_offre_active_ services_de sante_en_francais.pdf

Munoz, M., & Kapoor-Kohli, A. (2007). Les barrières de langue: Comment les surmonter en clinique? *Le Médecin du Québec*, 42(2), 45–52.

Office of the Commissioner of Official Languages. (2016). 2015–2016 Annual Report. Ottawa: Minister of Public Works and Government Services Canada.

Smith, P. C., Mossialos, E., & Papanicolas, I. (2008). Mesure des performances pour l'amélioration des systèmes de santé: expériences, défis et perspectives. Conférence ministérielle européenne de l'OMS sur les systèmes de santé : "Systèmes de santé, santé et prospérité", Tallinn, Estonia, June 25-27, 2008.

Stoyko, P., Henning, G.K., & McCaughey, D. (2006). *Creativity at Work: A Leadership Guide: Success belongs to me! CSPS Action-Research Roundtable on Creativity*. Canada School of Public Service.

Yankelovich, D. (2001). *The Magic of Dialogue: Transforming Conflict into Cooperation*. New York: Simon & Shuster, Touchstone Books.

PART II

POLICY LEVERS AND LEGAL MEASURES: THE INTERPLAY OF ACTORS

CHAPTER 3

French-Language Health Services in Canada: The State of the Law

Pierre Foucher, Faculty of Law, *University of Ottawa*

Abstract

This analysis of the legal framework of the active offer of French-language health care in Canada will examine its constitutional and legislative elements. The first part will explore the constitutional dimension, looking at aspects related to the *Canadian Constitution* and the *Canadian Charter of Rights and Freedoms* enshrined therein. In the second part, we will consider language laws at the federal level and in the provinces and territories. The study will show the asymmetrical nature of the legal model and the challenges it engenders.

Key Words: legal framework, law, health care, *Canadian Charter of Rights and Freedoms, Canadian Constitution.*

Introduction: Law, Language, and Health Care

In a study of the active offer of health care in the user's official language, a legal analysis allows us to establish the framework within which health care services themselves are provided. The law can create obligations for the state to fulfill, but it can also confer powers on service providers and define the limits of the exercise of these powers. A legal obligation to actively offer users health care in their official language is generally linked to the right to receive services in this language, enshrined in legislation. This chapter examines the legal framework within which institutions can provide an active offer of health services in the language of the minority.

Contrary to international law, Canadian law does not explicitly recognize the "right to health"[1] in official documents. The state is not legally obligated to give universal and free access to health care. Instead, for the state, it is a political choice expressed legally in laws and regulations that create or recognize health institutions, give them powers, provide the means to finance them, structure their actions, and establish their limits. Laws also establish language rights. The law can impose requirements to provide services in the minority language, and can also add the obligation to actively offer these services, so people in vulnerable situations who need care do not have to engage in a language battle to receive them.

This chapter presents the general constitutional framework in which the active offer of health care services is positioned, then reviews the laws that do or do not create obligations in this area. Because the linguistic, legal, and constitutional situation of Quebec is very different from that of the other provinces, we have chosen to not include it here.

Constitutional Framework of the Active Offer of Health Care in the Language of the Minority

Two aspects of the *Canadian Constitution* underpin the right to health care services in the official language of the minority community: federalism and fundamental language rights.

Federalism and Health

Canada is a federal state. However, health is one of the areas under the jurisdiction of both federal and provincial laws[2] and federal authority is secondary; provinces have the primary responsibility for regulating health care. Moreover, language is also an area of shared authority.[3] Every jurisdiction can thus adopt different language laws. This aspect of federalism will be addressed in the second part of the chapter. First, we will examine the scope of federal laws in this area.

Federal Funding

The most obvious way the central Government intervenes in health care is through the funds it spends under the Equalization program and the Canadian Health Transfer program. The Equalization program, the principle of which is protected under Section 36 of the

Constitution Act, 1982,[4] is based on the redistribution of the wealth generated by revenue from federal income taxes. The funds given to the provinces under this program are unconditional; provinces are free to spend the money on whatever programs and services they want, including health care.

The Government of Canada also makes abundant use of what is often called its "spending power" to increase access to health care services in French. This is a discretionary power of the federal government; it is not explicitly recognized in the *Constitution* but its legitimacy has been confirmed by the Supreme Court of Canada.[5] It allows the Canadian government to spend money in sectors the *Constitution* has already conferred to the legislative bodies of the provinces. The federal spending power for health is best illustrated by two major interventions: the Canada Health Transfer, and official language programs.

The *Canada Health Act* associates federal payments with five principles: public administration; comprehensiveness; universality, portability; accessibility.[6] Each of these conditions must be related to a financial matter; otherwise, it runs the risk of being considered by the Supreme Court as a means of regulating the sector, which the *Constitution* does not allow, rather than a condition for granting funds, which is permitted under the *Constitution*. The Commission on the Future of Health Care in Canada, in its final report, recommended that "governments, regional health authorities, health care providers, hospitals and community organizations should work together to identify and respond to the needs of official language minority communities." However, the Commission refused to recommend that access to health care in both official languages be made the sixth principle of the federal *Act.*[7]

The second component of federal funding is special official language funding programs; the Government's intervention is indirectly linked to Section 41 of Canada's *Official Languages Act.*[8] The Government's approach, geared to cooperation and coordination in federal/provincial/community initiatives, certainly respects shared jurisdiction, but does not provide any strong legal guarantees about the actual right to receive health care in one's own official language.

There are only a few legal measures to ensure provinces are accountable for the funds transferred to them to provide French-language health services, and little recourse for the Court to obligate provinces to respect their agreements, let alone sign them in the first place. It is not even certain that federal/provincial agreements are legal contracts; rather, they are political agreements.[9] In short, subject to the rights entrenched in the *Charter*, the *Constitution* does not seem to offer many binding legal solutions to the problem of whether there is a federal obligation to offer health care in French in Canada.

Direct Federal Jurisdiction

Aside from its spending power, certain matters under the jurisdiction of the federal government have an impact on health and it is these making it possible to regulate health and safety in a general sense.[10] Other areas under federal jurisdiction are secondary dimensions of access to health care. Because they are addressed to particular client groups who are under the responsibility of the Government of Canada—the military, veterans, detainees in federal penitentiaries, Aboriginals on and off reserves, marine hospitals, and young offenders in detention centres—health care may be offered through health facilities and medical centres established by the federal government of its own account. Services may also be provided to these "federal client groups" through agreements between the federal government and the provinces.

Language rights provided for by the *Charter* may also play a role in the area of health services.

Fundamental Language Rights and Language of Provision of Health Services

Since the *Lalonde* decision by the Ontario Court of Appeal, we would be justified in believing that Canadian constitutional law now recognizes the rights of linguistically homogenous health facilities.[11] In fact, nothing is less certain. First, the *Lalonde* decision deals with a government's decision to close an institution, not an obligation to create one. Next, *Lalonde* was based on Ontario's language law, supplemented by principles of interpretation, and not on a general constitutional right to linguistically homogenous health institutions. Finally, the Court was careful to mention that nothing in the text of the *Charter* stipulates that citizens have the right to health care in their own language, and that this omission was intended. However, certain language rights which are guaranteed under the *Charter* may apply indirectly to health care.

Language rights in the *Canadian Charter of Rights and Freedoms.*
Subsection 16(1) of the *Charter* states that English and French are
the official languages of Canada and have equality of status and
equal rights and privileges as to their use in all institutions of the
Parliament and the Government of Canada. Subsection 20(1) of the
Charter gives the public the right to receive services from and to communicate with federal institutions in English or French, either when
dealing with the head office or in other cases: when there is a significant demand for services or when, because of the nature of the office,
it is reasonable to expect them. Federal institutions delivering health
services must respect those language rights. English and French are
also the official languages of New Brunswick according to Subsection
16(2), and the public in New Brunswick has the right to receive services from the provincial government in English or French according
to Subsection 20(2). Furthermore, Section 16.1 states that the English
linguistic community and the French linguistic community in New
Brunswick have equality of status and equal rights and privileges,
including the right to distinct educational institutions and such
distinct cultural institutions as are necessary for the preservation
and promotion of those communities; this could include the institutions which provide health care, given the cultural dimension of
health facilities. So far, no other province has recognized the constitutional right to government services in English and French.

Subsection 16(3) of the *Charter* authorizes federal and provincial
laws to advance the equality of status or use of English and French.
This protects laws that might include, for example, distinctions related
to language (such as requiring the ability to speak one or both languages in public positions in the hospital, or guaranteeing the right to
care in English or in French only, which is considered discriminatory
when applied to other languages). Subsection 16(3) gives permission
but does not impose an obligation, either to create institutions or to
justify abolishing them.[12] Moreover, the *Charter* does not eliminate the
model of Canadian federalism: constitutional language rights correspond to the division of powers.[13] This creates an asymmetrical model
of rights, and asymmetry is a characteristic of modern federalism.

Unwritten constitutional principles. Certain constitutional principles are not written explicitly, yet they represent foundations of the
Constitution, the "vital unstated assumptions upon which the text is

based," "major elements of the architecture of the *Constitution* itself"; these underlying principles are not invented by the Courts, but can rather be deduced or derived from the text. They can generate specific legal obligations on the state, but they cannot create new rights.[14] The protection of minorities, and in particular linguistic minorities, is one of the unwritten principles.[15] It can be used to interpret language guarantees explicitly written in legislation, and to protect linguistically homogenous health institutions designated under a law. However, in our opinion, it cannot be used to force the government to create new institutions.

This, then, is the constitutional framework within which the federal Parliament and the provinces and territories adopt laws concerning health services and the language in which they are provided. The *Charter* creates linguistic obligations at the federal level and in New Brunswick; besides these obligations, federalism allows federal and provincial language laws to be adopted as ancillary to the primary jurisdiction. Thus, as we will see, laws on the language of health services are generally made under the jurisdiction of the provinces, which can decide whether to establish rights in this matter.

The Legislative Framework of the Active Offer of Health Services in the Language of the Minority

Since language is ancillary to the primary jurisdiction, and since health involves both federal and provincial powers, both federal and provincial laws come into play. However, some jurisdictions, as we will see, are more active than are others in dealing with the matter of language of health care.

The *Official Languages Act* and Health Care

Two components of Canada's *Official Languages Act* (*OLA*) are particularly relevant in the context of this research: the obligation of federal institutions to offer services in English and French, and the obligation of the government to take measures to preserve and promote official language minority communities.

Services Offered by Federal Institutions

Part IV of the *OLA* specifies federal constitutional obligations in the area of language. Section 22 in the *OLA* repeats almost word-for-word the text found in Section 20 of the *Charter*. It applies to offices of federal institutions, which may include those federal institutions delivering health care services (military hospitals, for example). It gives rights to the "public," which encompasses users of health care services. Finally, it sets out three different locations where services in the official language must be offered: in central or head offices, in areas where there is a significant demand for services, and where, because of the nature of the office, it is reasonable to expect services in both languages.[16]

Section 32 of the *OLA* delegates the responsibility for defining "significant demand" and "nature of the office" to the government, but provides for the definitions to be founded on certain criteria. The Regulation, which has been in effect since 1992,[17] sets out an essentially statistical method to assess the demand, calculated on the basis of a certain percentage or an absolute number of residents whose mother tongue is the minority official language in one of the census subdivisions served by that office.[18]

Subsection 24(1) of the *OLA* deals specifically with health services. A federal institution must ensure services are offered in both official languages in cases, specified in the Regulation, which are matters of health and safety. Section 8 of the Regulation contains detailed provisions on this subject. Paragraph (*a*) imposes bilingualism on services received in a clinic located in an airport, a train station, or a ferry terminal. As for services given by a federal institution outside these places, the general rule about significant demand applies. Meanwhile, Section 9 of the Regulation extends the linguistic obligation to services offered in national parks throughout Canada, subject to certain conditions: since the nature of the services is not specified in the regulation, the provision of emergency health care may or may not be included.

When a legal obligation to offer services in English and French exists, a federal institution must, according to Section 28 of the *OLA*, make an "active offer" of these services. This requires making it publicly known that services are available in the official language of the minority, by displaying signs, greeting people verbally in the language of their choice, or by introducing other relevant and appropriate measures. The institution must also ensure services are offered as promptly in the minority language as in the official language of the majority, and are of the same quality.[19]

In order to avoid a situation in which the federal government might indirectly evade its obligations by delegating a task to others, Section 25 of the *OLA* extends all federal linguistic obligations to anybody that acts "on its behalf." As a result, if a federal institution that must provide health services to a specific clientele (active military personnel, eligible veterans, First Nations, Métis, Inuit, inmates of federal penitentiaries, or others) chooses instead to make an agreement with a provincial institution to do so, Section 25 comes into play; the provincial institution has the same linguistic obligation as the federal institution itself. If the provincial language provisions are more favourable to the minority language, they will apply instead of the federal provisions.[20] And if a decision to delegate powers on a particular matter were to lead to a loss of language rights for its citizens, the federal institution would be in violation of the *OLA* and may be required to correct the situation.[21]

Positive Measures

The constitutional validity of federal spending powers was mentioned earlier: Section 41 of the *OLA*, which has been binding and actionable since 2005, entrenches this power in legislation. It specifies that the federal government is required to ensure that "positive measures" are undertaken to enhance the vitality of the English and French linguistic minority communities and assist their development, as well as to foster the full recognition of the equality of English and French, while respecting the jurisdiction and powers of the provinces. The Minister of Canadian Heritage can make agreements with the provinces to "encourage and assist provincial governments to support the development of English and French linguistic minority communities generally, and, in particular, to offer provincial and municipal services in both English and French," which includes health services; such agreements may also "encourage and cooperate with the business community, labour organizations, voluntary organizations and other organizations or institutions to provide services in both English and French and to foster the recognition and use of those languages."[22] Together, these provisions provide the legal foundation of the health component of the Action Plan for Official Languages.

The "positive measures" would probably include clauses on language in funding agreements the Government of Canada makes with provincial institutions or private entities requiring or urging them to find the means to make their services available in the official language of the province's minority. The legal source of the obligation originates, in this case, in the agreement with the federal government. This case should be distinguished from that of agreements whereby the provinces become agents of the federal government, and act "on their behalf" by providing health services to "federal clients"; in the latter case, the *OLA* applies directly to the federal institutions involved.

Language Laws and Policies in the Provinces and Territories and Health Care

The provinces are responsible for regulating health professions, for creating, maintaining, and managing hospitals, clinics, and other locations where health services are provided, and for regulating private organizations operating in the field of health care.[23] Therefore, it is the provinces that have the primary responsibility for organizing health care and determining the way health services are delivered. Because language is an ancillary power in relation to a primary jurisdiction, the level with constitutional jurisdiction over health can also regulate the language in which health services are offered. Our study is limited to the legal framework of the language of health care, and we will set aside the regulation of health professions and labour rights relating to language.

New Brunswick

New Brunswick has the most extensive legal provisions for French-language health care. Sections 33 and 34 of New Brunswick's *Official Languages Act*[24] specify the rights of members of the public in terms of health care. Section 33 stipulates that a health facility is subject to the general obligations, set out in Sections 27 and 28, to offer services and to communicate with members of the public in the official language of their choice. This means that each individual has the right to receive care in French or in English in every hospital, health centre, or other health facility belonging to one of the Regional Health Authorities in the province. Furthermore, because of the particular demography of the province, which comprises regions with a high Francophone majority, a high Anglophone majority, and bilingual regions, Subsection 33(2) stipulates that the Minister of Health, when establishing a provincial health plan, shall ensure that obligations to provide services in both official languages that arise from Sections 27 and 28 are met, as well as that the "language of daily operations" of the health facility are considered. Section 28.1 states that institutions subject to the obligation to serve the public in the official language of one's choice must make an "active offer" of these services, and take appropriate measures such as displaying signs or posters and communicating with the public in both languages. Section 34 indicates that, subject to the obligation to serve members of the public in the official language of their choice, Section 33 does not limit the use of one official language in "the daily operations" of a hospital or other facility. This concession to customs and language practices preserves the Francophone or Anglophone character of certain hospitals or medical centres, which must, nonetheless, serve the public in both languages. Indirectly, it recognizes linguistically homogenous health institutions.

The other piece of legislation affecting the language of health care in the province is the *Regional Health Authorities Act.*[25] Following a major restructuring exercise, New Brunswick established two Regional Health Authorities (RHAs). "Horizon" Network covers the south, west, and centre of the province, regions with strong Anglophone majorities, as well as a few facilities in southeastern New Brunswick which are primarily Anglophone. "Vitalité" Network covers the northwest, the north, and the northeast, where there are strong Francophone majorities, and the facilities in southeastern New Brunswick which are primarily Francophone. Thus, a form of linguistic duality has been preserved by the legislature. Subsection 19(1) recognizes that Horizon Network operates in English and Vitalité Network operates in French. Subsection 20(8) states that the board of the RHA should conduct their affairs in the language of operation of the RHA. Paragraph 19(2)(*a*) specifies that, despite this, RHAs must "respect the language of daily operations of the facilities under its responsibility." And Paragraph 19(2)(*b*) further specifies that the RHAs "provide health services to members of the public in the official language of their choice" throughout the network. Subsection 19(3), to our knowledge unique in legislation, charges the two RHAs with the responsibility to "improve the delivery of health services in the French language." Subsection 20(1) specifies the composition of the RHA boards (some of whose members are elected), and Subsection 20(1.1) instructs the Minister to "have regard to . . . the overriding interests of the official linguistic communities" when making appointments. Section 40 requires RHAs to provide simultaneous interpretation for any public meetings they hold. The regulation stipulates that meeting minutes be made available to the public in both official languages; as an exception, the minutes of meetings that are closed to the public are not published.[26]

Services referred to as "shared services" (supplies, clinical engineering, information technology, laundry) are provided by a Crown Corporation called "Service New Brunswick."[27] This agency provides Regional Health Authorities and hospitals with financial services, information technology, and supplies. It is subject to the *Official Languages Act*.

Ambulance services have also been a source of irritation for some. The *Ambulance Services Act*[28] gives the Minister of Health the responsibility to issue permits and make agreements for the delivery of ambulance services. Ambulance New Brunswick is a private corporation that offers front-line health services through a contract with the Department of Health; Ambulance New Brunswick acknowledges it is bound by the provisions of New Brunswick's *Official Languages Act*.[29]

In summary, the active offer of French-language health services in New Brunswick is subject to legal provisions that establish a model of judicial duality in health facilities and institutions. The facilities providing services are subject to the condition that the public has the right to receive care in the official language of one's choice anywhere in the province and at all times. There are still some grey areas, however: the true status of nursing homes, for example, which are private facilities regulated by the provincial government, remains undefined.

Ontario

Ontario represents the other provincial jurisdiction with a language framework for health care more favourable than most other provinces, although there is still work to be done. In the *French Language Services Act*,[30] Ontario opted for a system of designated services in designated regions, combined with the opportunity for facilities that are not government-based to apply to be self-designated if they offer services in a designated region. Section 5 of the *Act* states its principle that any member of public has the right receive services in French from any head or central office of "a government agency or institution" as defined under Section 1 of the *Act*; that section extends the definition of a "government agency" to include "a non-profit corporation or similar entity [or even an individual service provider] that provides a service to the public, is subsidized in whole or in part by public money, and is designated as a public service agency by the regulations." Finally, Subsection 8(a) allows the Lieutenant-Governor in Council to designate any "public service agency" through a regulation. This mechanism can apply to hospitals, clinics, nursing homes and special care homes, children's aid services, or any other organization that meets the criteria and asks to be designated. Regulation 398/93, as amended, includes a list of organizations designated according to these provisions, which are required to meet the obligations set out in Section 5. The designated organizations include several hospitals, community health clinics, seniors' centres operating programs on behalf of the Ministry of Health, and children's aid centres delivering services on behalf of the Ministry of Health.

The designation mechanism thus makes it possible to offer health care services to Francophones in their own language, through a wide range of semi-public, private, or community agencies. Many of these organizations are operated "by and for" Franco-Ontarians. The right to receive health services in French is not automatic, as it is in New Brunswick; instead it depends on a designation. A designation is made at the discretion of the Lieutenant-Governor in Council, but the Office of Francophone Affairs, which makes recommendations to the Government of Ontario, uses the following criteria. A designated agency must:

- offer French-language services on a permanent basis by employing people with requisite level of French-language skills
- guarantee French-language services can be provided for all or some services and during business hours
- ensure Francophones sit on boards of directors and committees in proportion to the Francophone population in the community
- have Francophones in senior management in proportion to the local Franco-Ontarian population
- make directors and senior managers accountable for the quality of French-language services
- demonstrate, every three years, how they have maintained this level of service. The board of each agency must submit a report detailing how this was accomplished to the ministry for which they are working.[31]

As for the management of health care services itself, besides the Ministry of Health, which falls directly under the definition of public services agency, health care is planned, organized, and funded by Local Health Integration Networks (LHINs) mandated to improve access to care. The *Local Health System Integration Act, 2006*[32] provides for the creation and operating structures of the LHINs. The *Act* stipulates LHINs respect the requirements of the *French Language Services Act* if they are in locations where they serve Francophone communities. It also provides for a French Language Health Services Advisory Council,[33] which was established by Regulation[34] and groups together organizations working in the area of, or with a special interest in, the delivery of French-language health services in the province. The council advises the Minister on matters related to "health and service delivery issues related to francophone communities" and on priorities to be integrated into the provincial plan. Furthermore, Article 16(1) states an LHIN "shall engage the community of diverse persons and entities involved with the local health system," while Subsection 16(4) stipulates that while doing so, it "shall engage the French language health planning entity" in its region. This was recommended by the French Language Services Commissioner in a special report published in May 2009.[35] Regulation 515/09 did, in fact, create "prescribe a French language health planning entity for the geographic area" of each LHIN.[36] It should be noted that these entities have a mandate to advise LHINs concerning, in particular, "the identification and designation of health service providers for the provision of French language health services in the area."[37]

Finally, Regulation 284/11 extends the obligations under Section 5 to any third-party entity that provides the public with a service "on behalf of" a government agency must do so according to the *Act*, subject to an agreement between the third party and the government.

Therefore, various acts prescribe mechanisms for formal consultations with Francophone communities regarding the active offer of French-language health services in the province,[38] but it is the designated health facilities themselves that ensure the direct delivery of health care and that must be designated in order for a true right to apply.

Manitoba

Section 23 of the *Manitoba Act, 1870*[39] created the obligation for the province to legislate in French and English, and the right to use either official language in the legislature and before the provincial courts. A language policy has been adopted; it applies to designated organizations "which provide health services, social services, or both," as well as designated regional health authorities. Regulation 131/2013[40] adopted under the *Regional Health Authorities Act*[41] lists the institutions and organizations designated for this purpose. A "Francophone" facility or program is defined as one in which "services are provided in both English and French, or in French only, and whose primary language of operation is French." Section 4 specifies that services in designated facilities "must comply with the government's French Language Services Policy." Moreover, a regulation obligates all Regional Health Authorities to submit to the Minister of Health "a proposed plan of French language services."[42] This plan lists the Francophone and bilingual facilities and programs offered in its region.[43] The Health Authorities must consult with the community and service providers before developing their plan.[44] The plans are approved by the Minister and the Health Authorities present that Minister with a report on the progress they have made.[45] Hence, there is a legal recognition of the provision of French-language services; in designated institutions, services must be offered actively, and in other Health Authorities and facilities, a plan must indicate what the organization intends to do. The Bill for the *Bilingual Service Centres Act*[46] foresees the creation of bilingual centres in each of the six regions designated under the policy; these centres will be able to offer a wide range of provincial services, including health services. Last, the *Francophone Community Enhancement and Support Act*[47] creates a more permanent legal framework for French-language services in the province. It establishes a Francophone Affairs Secretariat and a standing Francophone Affairs Advisory Council, and imposes the adoption of French-language services plans by government agencies, including those designated to offer health services in French.[48] It prescribes the active offer of French-language services whenever they are required.[49] In short, the legal situation in Manitoba is evolving and its policy on French-language services in the health system is gaining legal recognition.

Prince Edward Island and Nova Scotia

Prince Edward Island and Nova Scotia operate on the same legal model as Ontario, a *French Language Services Act.*[50] This type of law and the regulations accompanying it designate regions where designated services are offered in French.

On the Island, the designation would create a legal obligation to offer these services.[51] Although health services as such are not yet designated, the Department of Health already offers certain services in French, in accordance with Section 2 of the *Act*. All government institutions must respond in French to correspondence they receive in that language. They are obligated to hold at least one public consultation in French, or, if there is only one consultation, it must be bilingual. In addition, all government institutions have a French-language services coordinator.[52] Each institution must submit plans for the provision of French-language services, as well as an annual report on their progress. The Regulation identifies the "Department of Health and Wellness" as well as "Health PEI," the province's health authority, as government institutions subject to the *Act*, and therefore required to develop plans for French-language services. The *Act* also establishes a "French-language Services Co-ordinating Committee" that informs the institution of its priorities; health is one of them.

The legal structure is very similar in Nova Scotia. Institutions are designated pursuant to the *French-language Services Act* (*FLSA*) and the Regulation; this applies to the Department of Health and Wellness, as well as the nine former health authorities. The latter have been folded into a single entity, which is responsible for the provision of health care services throughout the province. Nevertheless, the *Act* that creates the new provincial health authority does not actually designate it under the legislation. On the other hand, the *FLSA*, which had previously designated the nine health authorities existing at the time, has not yet been modified and does not reflect the change.[53] Designated institutions submit plans to develop French-language services and the Minister responsible for overseeing them files an annual report on their progress. French-language service coordinators are appointed in each department and office of the government. It should be noted that these laws do not give people a right to receive services in French from the designated institutions; rather, it obliges the institutions to develop implementation plans and to report on them each year.

Newfoundland and Labrador, British Columbia, Saskatchewan, and Alberta

In Newfoundland and Labrador, a new French-language service policy was adopted in 2016.[54] A very brief document, it establishes the French Services Office, which coordinates French-language services within the government. It provides for training and translation services for provincial departments and institutions. Interpretation services are available in St. John's and in Labrador City; in other locations, the *Réseau Santé en français* (French health network) offers written material in French. In British Columbia, the *RésoSanté* health network publishes an online directory of health professionals who can provide services in French and who have self-identified by registering. Some institutions provide French-language services as well, including *La Boussole* community centre in Vancouver and the *Foyer Maillard* nursing home in Coquitlam. These resources have been supported financially by the federal government using its spending power. There are no laws or policies on French-language services in this province.

The policy framework for services in Saskatchewan is rather modest.[55] The province's *French-language Services Policy* applies to "the provincial government, its ministries, crown corporations, and other agencies." It specifies that correspondence with individuals or groups will be carried out in the official language preferred by the client, and signs and documents will be made available in both languages "when appropriate." As for services, it mentions that "the designation of bilingual positions [shall] be considered as a means to more effectively provide French-language services," and that "the inclusion of a French-language services component [shall] be considered when new Government of Saskatchewan programs and services are being developed." Nothing specific to health care is included. The Francophone Affairs Branch operates the French-language Service Centre, which serves as a single window for the public to access services and programs of the Government of Saskatchewan in French, particularly through Internet and telephone communication. Written materials on health issues have been published in French but there are no formally designated organizations. The application form for the provincial health insurance card is available in French. Any delivery or active offer of health care in Saskatchewan stems from administrative arrangements and partnerships between the French health network and provincial health authorities.

The same is true for Alberta. At the time of writing this chapter, a policy on French-language services was under way. A Francophone health centre, the *Centre de santé communautaire Saint-Thomas*, is located in the Francophone district of Edmonton, near the Campus Saint-Jean, the French-language faculty of the University of Alberta. The community health centre provides services from family physicians, nurses, dietitians, a social worker, a psychiatrist and an exercise specialist.

The Three Northern Territories

Canada's three territories, located in the North, are distinct in their structure from the provinces. However, the Government of Canada treats them as provinces in several respects, including matters related to health care delivery.

Yukon adopted a *Languages Act* in 1986.[56] Although it does not recognize official languages for Yukon itself—simply recognizing in Subsection 1(1) that French and English are the official languages "of Canada"—the *Act* sets out the language requirements of institutions of the Legislature and the Government of Yukon. Subsection 6(1) reproduces Subsection 20(1) of the *Charter*, simply adapting it to refer to Yukon: "Any member of the public in the Yukon has the right to communicate with, and to receive available services from, any head or central office of an institution of the Legislative Assembly or of the Government of the Yukon in English or French," and in other places when it is justified by a "significant demand" or "the nature of the office." Subsection 6(2) specifies that regulations can prescribe "circumstances in which . . . significant demand shall be deemed to exist or in which the nature of the office is such that it is reasonable that communications with and services from that office be in English and French." The *Prescribed Offices Regulation*, YOIC 2003/79, established the list of offices included in this category; no health institution is on the list. The *Hospital Act*[57] creates a "Yukon Hospital Corporation" and gives it a bilingual name ("*Régie des hôpitaux du Yukon*"), charged with operating the three hospitals in the territory "by a board independent of the Government." Section 10 of that legislation specifies that the *Languages Act* applies to the Corporation. The Yukon Hospital Corporation is responsible for providing medical and hospital care, pursuant to Section 2. Consequently, and at least in theory, Franco-Yukoners have the right to receive services in their own language in the health facilities in Whitehorse managed by the Yukon Hospital Corporation; to this point, only the Whitehorse General Hospital is included. Elsewhere, the institution would have to be designated by a regulation, and that has not yet been the case for other facilities.

In the Northwest Territories (NWT), the *Official Languages Act*[58] provides for nine Aboriginal languages as official languages, as well as English and French. Only measures related to French and English will be analyzed here. As in the Yukon legislation, Subsection 11(1) reproduces Subsection 20(1) of the *Charter*: The head office of government departments or agencies, as well as any other office where it is justified by "significant demand" or "the nature of the office" are required to offer services in French. A Regulation identifies four regions with a significant demand for French-language services: Yellowknife, Hay River, Fort Smith, and Inuvik.[59] The Health and Social Services Authorities of Fort Smith, Hay River, and Yellowknife are among the institutions designated in the Regulation. Eight Health Authorities, created by the Minister, offer health care to the population in facilities under their jurisdiction in accordance with Section 10 of the *Hospital Insurance and Health and Social Services Administration Act*. As a result, health facilities located in the four designated regions where there is "significant demand" for French-language health services are subject to the obligations set out in Section 11 of the *Act*. The *Fédération franco-ténoise* case[60] sheds light on some of the difficulties the Francophone community faced regarding the implementation of the *Official Languages Act* in the NWT at the time, and health care was one of the sectors subject to Judge Moreau's order in the first case. This aspect of the case was confirmed by the Court of Appeal, as health services are "confidential" services for which a direct, in-person, and immediate service is required.

Finally, Nunavut now has an *Official Languages Act*[61] that creates obligations on the part of the Government of Nunavut as well as the public organizations in the territory. The Department of Health is subject to the *Official Languages Act*. For the purposes of the *Act*, a "public agency" is an institution that meets the following three criteria: it is established by the laws of Nunavut, is subject to the direction of a Minister or the Executive Council, and is identified as a public agency under the *Financial Administration Act*. Because the *Financial Administration Act* does not designate health institutions, one of the three conditions is missing, so hospitals and clinics are not public agencies as defined by the *Act*. Nevertheless, the Government of Nunavut, through the Department of Health, can make agreements with hospitals for the provision of health services covered by insurance, certify health facilities, and authorize the creation of health facilities. Through these provisions, health centres and hospitals can be subject to the Nunavut's *Official Languages Act*.

Conclusion

The Canadian government has constitutional responsibility only for "federal client groups" and for federal institutions, which must offer services in the official language of the client's choice in accordance with the *Charter*. Institutions often delegate this responsibility to provincial institutions, and, in this case, the provincial institution must also offer services in the minority language, under the same conditions as in the federal institution. Furthermore, the Government of Canada uses its spending power to fund health care services in the language of the minority.

The provinces and territories are primarily responsible for the provision of health services, and for the linguistic dimension of these services. There are three basic models, characterized by different geometric structures. First, New Brunswick offers a general right to health care services in the language of the user's choice, in every region, in linguistically homogenous institutions. Next, some provinces have adopted laws making it possible to designate regions, services, and institutions. Finally, provinces that are less advanced in their progress towards language equality appear to be satisfied with an administrative policy creating an Office of Francophone Affairs that basically offers advice, information, and translation or interpretation services.

An active offer of health services in the language of the minority calls for an encompassing legislative framework. Besides health authorities, hospitals and clinics, we need to consider health professionals, their education and training, the designation of positions as bilingual or French, and staffing. Thus, a strategy for legislative progression can be imagined. It would start with mechanisms for designation (making it easier to identify points of service), continue through the right to work in health institutions that integrate a linguistic dimension, and finally reach the full right to health services in the language of one's choice, entrenched in an *Act* and, ultimately, in the *Canadian Constitution*.

While we are waiting for this to happen, official language minority communities are doing the best they can with the existing constitutional structure.

Notes

1. Art. 12 of the *International Covenant on Economic, Social and Cultural Rights*, GA XXI, /2200A, December 16, 1966, in effect since January 3,

1976, recognizes "the right of everyone to the enjoyment of the highest attainable standard of physical and mental health."

2. *Reference re Assisted Human Reproduction Act,* [2010] 3 SCR 457.

3. *Jones v. A.G. of New Brunswick,* [1975] 2 SCR 182.

4. Section 36 guarantees the principle of providing public services at reasonably comparable levels of taxation.

5. *Reference re Canada Assistance Plan,* [1991] 2 SCR 525.

6. *Canada Health Act,* R.S.C., 1985, c. C-6 art. 7.

7. Commission on the Future of Health Care in Canada, "Building on Values: The Future of Health Care in Canada," Saskatoon, Commission on the Future of Health Care in Canada, November 2002. Retrieved from http://publications.gc.ca/collections/Collection/CP32-85-2002E.pdf. Accessed February 18, 2017, pp. 171–172, Recommendation 28.

8. *Official Languages Act,* R.S.C., 1985, c. O-1, art. 41(1) and (2).

9. See Foucher, P., "Les droits linguistiques dans le secteur privé," in Michel Bastarache and Michel Doucet, ed., *Les droits linguistiques au Canada,* 3rd edition, Montréal: Yvon Blais Inc., pp. 840–842.

10. A rapid search reveals there are more than 300 different legislative or regulatory provisions at the federal level that impose obligations or offer choices regarding language in these matters.

11. *Lalonde v. Restructuring Commission* (2001), 56 OR 3d 577. The Court agreed that institutional completeness is a principle applying to the provision of services in the language of the minority. It overturned the decision to close Ottawa's Hôpital Montfort, the only French-language hospital in Ontario, because the decision violated provincial language laws.

12. *Lalonde, supra,* note 16, paragraphs 90–95.

13. *Conseil scolaire francophone de la Colombie-Britannique v. British Columbia,* [2013] 2 SCR 774; *Caron v. Alberta,* [2015] 3 SCR 511.

14. *Reference re Secession of Quebec,* [1998] 2 SCR 217, par. 54

15. *Id.* par. 79–82

16. See Klink, J., Ravon, P., Dubois, J., & Hachey, J.-P., *Le droit à la prestation des services publics dans les deux langues officielles,* in Bastarache and Doucet, *supra* note, pp. 451–471.

17. *Official Languages (Communications with and Services to the Public) Regulations* (SOR/92–48).

18. At the time of writing, the criteria identifying significant demand were being contested before the Federal Court.

19. Section 26 of the *OLA* deals with federal regulations in the area of health and safety. This provision does not seem to apply directly to the provision of health care as such, but rather to the regulation of health and safety. A quick search in the electronic data base of federal regulations, with the string "français anglais," generated 334 entries: http://laws-lois.justice.gc.ca/Recherche/Avancee.aspx. Accessed April 14, 2015.

20. *Société des Acadiens et Acadiennes du Nouveau-Brunswick and Paulin v. Canada (RCMP)*, [2008] 1 SCR 383.

21. *Canada (Commissioner of Official Languages) v. Canada (Department of Justice)*, [2001] FCT 239 *[Contraventions case]*.

22. *Official Languages Act*, para. 43(1) (*d*) and (*f*).

23. *R. v. Morgentaler*, [1993] 3 SCR 463; *Reference re Assisted Human Reproduction Act*, *supra* note 2.

24. *Official Languages Act*, SNB 2002, c O-0.5

25. *Regional Health Authorities Act*, RSNB 2011, c 217.

26. *Board Regulation, Regional Health Authorities Act*, NB Reg 2012-7, s. 5.

27. *Service New Brunswick Act*, SNB 2015, c 44.

28. *Ambulance Services Act*, SNB 1990, c A-7.3.

29. Office of the Commissioner of Official Languages for New Brunswick, Investigation Report, File Number: 2013–1992, Ambulance New Brunswick (ANB), March 2014.

30. *French Language Services Act*, R.S.O. 1990, c. F.32. The *Act* is scheduled to be revised in 2017, and it is possible that the entire province becomes a designated region (editor's note: information on revision not available at time of writing).

31. Office of Francophone Affairs, designation criteria. https://www.ontario.ca/page/government-services-french#section-2. Retrieved February 21, 2017. Note: the English version of the reference page does not mention "active offer" explicitly, as the French does.

32. *Local Health System Integration Act*, 2006, S.O. 2006, c. 4.

33. *Id.* para. 14(2)(2).

34. O. Reg. 162/07: French Language Health Services Advisory Council.

35. Office of the Commissioner of French Language Services, Ontario, *Special Report on French Language Health Services Planning in Ontario*, May 7, 2009.

36. Ontario Regulation 515/09.

37. *Id.*, para. 3(1)(d).

38. In March 2015, the *Regroupement des entités de planification* and the *Alliance des réseaux ontariens de santé en français* published a position statement on the active offer of French-language health services in Ontario. This *"Énoncé de position commune sur l'offre active des services de santé en français en Ontario"* can be found at: http://rssfe.on.ca/upload-ck/Enonce_OffreActive_10mars15_FR.pdf. Accessed February 21, 2017.

39. *An Act to amend and continue the Act 32–33 Victoria chapter 3; and to establish and provide for the Government of the Province of Manitoba*, 1870, 33 Vict., c. 3 (Can.).

40. *Bilingual and Francophone Facilities and Programs Designation Regulation*, Manitoba Regulation 131/2013.

41. *The Regional Health Authorities Act*, C.C.S.M. c. R34.

42. *French Language Services Regulation*, Manitoba Regulation 46/98 amended by Regulation 2013/138, s. 2.

43. *Id.*, para. 2(2)*a.1*).

44. ss. 2(3).

45. S. 6.

46. Bill 31, *Bilingual Service Centres Act*.

47. *The Francophone Community Enhancement and Support Act*, Manitoba, S.M. 2016, c. 9, adopted June 30, 2016.

48. *Id.*, Subsection 11(3).

49. *Id. ss.* 3(3).

50. *French Language Services Act*, PEI, SPEI 2013, c. 32; *General Regulations*, PEI Reg. EC845/13; *French-language Services Act*, SNS 2004 c. 26; Amended *An Act Respecting the Delivery of French-language Services by the Public Service*, SNS 2011 c. 9; *French-Language Services Regulations*, NS Reg 233/2006.

51. *French Language Services Act*, PEI, s. 3.

52. *Id.*, art. 9.

53. *Health Authorities act*, S.N.-S. 2014, c. 32.

54. *French Language Services Policy, Newfoundland and Labrador.* http://www. exec.gov.nl.ca/frenchservices/english/french_languages_services_policy .PDF. Accessed February 21, 2017.

55. *French-language Services Policy, Government of Saskatchewan*: https://www. saskatchewan.ca/government/government-structure/executive-council- and-office-of-the-premier/francophone-affairs-branch. Accessed February 21, 2017.

56. *Languages Act*, LRY 2002, c. 133.

57. *Hospital Act*, LRY 2002, c. 111.

58. *Official Languages Act*, RSNWT 1988, c. 56.

59. Regulation R-082-2006, as amended by R-079-2013.

60. *Fédération franco-ténoise v. Northwest Territories*, 2006 NWTSC 20 (Supreme Court), 2008 NWTCA 5 (Court of Appeal), application for leave to appeal dismissed on March 5, 2009 [2008] C.S.S.A. no. 432.

61. *Official Languages Act, Nunavut*, L.Nun. 2008, c. 10.

CHAPTER 4

The Co-Construction of the Active Offer of French-Language Services in Ontario's Justice Sector

Linda Cardinal, Martin Normand, and Nathalie Plante, *University of Ottawa*

Abstract

Since 2006, the justice sector in Ontario has benefited from its first strategic plan for developing the active offer of French-language services (FLS). This chapter deals with the representation of active offer that guides the strategic plan. It presents data from a review of the literature and from 12 interviews, conducted in 2012, with community and government actors participating in the management of the plan. The chapter shows that the principle of the active offer of FLS in the justice sector is not a neutral principle. Active offer is co-constructed by community and government actors; that is, it is subject to constant dialogue on its issues, which can arise from a managerial, judicial, and developmental perspective. Lastly, the chapter attempts to extrapolate lessons learned from the active offer of FLS in the justice sector to other areas of public policy, such as health and social services.

Key Words: active offer, justice sector, French-language services, strategic plan, Ontario, co-construction.

Introduction

In 2003, in Ontario, the active offer of French-language services (FLS) was a matter attracting particular attention in the justice sector. Not only had the Government of Ontario developed a strategic plan for the active offer of FLS, it also adopted a model of governance integrating key spokespeople of the Francophone community into the planning, implementation, and follow-up of the new plan. The objective of this chapter is to examine the representation of active offer guiding this new strategic plan in the area of justice in Ontario. Based on a review of the literature, as well as on 12 interviews with community and government actors participating in the management of the plan, the chapter shows that the principle of active offer is not neutral; in other words, it cannot be reduced to a management technique stripped of any deeper or symbolic meaning.[1] We will argue that active offer cannot be properly measured simply by calculating the number of services offered by the government to its Francophone population. Instead, active offer is first and foremost a policy instrument co-constructed by community and government actors, which is to say that it is the result of constant dialogue or debate among various actors. This chapter will show how this dialogue evolves and contributes to the co-construction of the active offer of FLS in the justice sector. We also intend to outline the lessons learned from this way of conceptualizing active offer, and see if they can be useful for other areas of public policy, such as health and social services. The chapter will also explore persistent challenges in the interactions between government and the community sector where the active offer of FLS is concerned.

The approach taken in this chapter is based on the instruments approach proposed by Lascoumes and Le Galès (2004; 2007), which refers to the choices and means through which governments govern their populations. To simplify the idea, the instruments approach (also called policy instruments approach or instrument-centred research) is used to study the policy choices made by governments, including those made in the area of language. All states have to ask themselves which language(s) will be privileged or given higher status within their borders, and which they will use to interact with their citizens. Even when a government decides to not formulate language policies, as is the case in the United States and Australia, it still has to act and communicate in a particular language or in particular languages. The states that do adopt language policies can favour or disfavour certain groups or minorities, as they can confer a status of official language on one or more languages spoken on their territory. When we apply the instruments approach to the area of language, we examine the tools developed by states, institutions, and organizations for the purpose of enacting language policies or directives. To give one example, census results are an important tool for generating data on a country's language composition. In Canada, the census includes several questions on language. The questions are designed to document the mother tongue of Canadians, the first official language they learned to speak and still understand, the language they speak at home, their understanding of French and English, and their ability to carry on a conversation in the other official language. The Government of Canada uses these data to organize service delivery in the two official languages of the country.

The numbers criterion is another tool used by governments in their management of services to the public in the area of language. To once again give an example from Canada: while Francophone minorities have the constitutional right to education in their own language, this right can only be exercised "where numbers warrant." This type of principle applies at the federal level as well as in the provinces. The latter have, in turn, developed specific tools to govern language use on their respective territories. Although these tools can regulate the delivery of services in French, policies also address Aboriginal languages in several provinces and territories, as well as certain non-official languages such as Gaelic in Nova Scotia or New Brunswick (Cardinal & Léger, forthcoming).

In 1986, when the *French Language Services Act* was enacted, the Government of Ontario chose to approach the delivery of FLS based on the principle of designated regions. Because of this decision, only the people living in these regions obtained the right to FLS in the various sectors under the jurisdiction of the provincial government. On the other hand, the government also opted to adopt the principle of active offer to guide delivery of FLS in these designated regions, notably in the justice sector.

Lascoumes and Le Galès (2004) agree that the choices and means chosen by states to govern their populations are not neutral. Indeed, the instruments approach is not intended to simply describe situations: it alludes to facets of public life guided by political debate, as well as power relations among actors. These representations also originate in the historical schemes of state action at the institutional and administrative levels (Cardinal & Sonntag, 2016). For example, the Province of Ontario has a long history of discriminating against its Francophone population, especially in the area of education. Historically, the discrimination has been rooted in Anglophone fears that Ontario would be overrun by French-Canadians moving into the province (Cardinal

& Normand, 2013). In the 1960s, when the Government of Ontario began to open more facilities and services to the Francophone population, its step-by-step or incremental approach to change was based on the fact that it was only reasonable and practical to offer services in French where numbers warranted. This approach to Francophones in Ontario continues to guide the development of FLS tools; we see it illustrated in the principle of designated regions where the application of active offer is limited to these specific regions.

In the first part of this chapter, we will present an overview of the situation of FLS in the justice sector in Ontario. The second part will show how the active offer of FLS was gradually established in the justice system. In the third part, we will specify key learning drawn from our study of the justice sector and how they apply to other sectors, such as health care and social services.

The Current State of FLS in the Justice Sector in Ontario[2]

Since the 1980s, the delivery of FLS in the justice sector has progressed considerably in Ontario. Before that, responsibility for FLS in judicial matters belonged to various advisory committees and an FLS Coordinator located in the Ministry of the Attorney General (Cardinal, Lang, Plante, Sauvé, & Terrien, 2005; Cardinal & Normand, 2013). In 1984, the Government of Ontario made a leap forward when it passed the *Courts of Justice Act*, which confirmed French and English would henceforth be official languages in provincial courts. In 1986, the *French Language Services Act*, previously mentioned, was enacted. These laws gave rise to, among other things, the formalization of the FLS Coordinator's status and the enactment of similar laws in other ministries, including those that governed judicial matters such as the Ministry of the Attorney General.

In 1995, the victory of the Conservative Party under Mike Harris—his platform had promised privatizing certain government services—led to considerable debate about the future of Ontario's public services. He merged the offices of two FLS Coordinators working in the Ministry of the Attorney General[3] and the Ministry of Community Safety and Correctional Services.[4] These two ministries encompassed numerous divisions, of which 11 would be part of the 2006 strategic plan. Moreover, in 2001, the justice sector was entrusted with both the Ontario Victim Services Secretariat (now Ontario Victim Services), in which the designated bilingual positions increased from one to 50, and the Ontario Native Affairs Secretariat. In 2003, Ontario Legal Aid was added to this list, then in 2004, the Ontario Human Rights Commission (Cardinal, Lang, Plante, Sauvé, & Terrien, 2005, p. 52).

These transformations broadened the mandate of the FLS Coordinator in the justice sector. Although the Coordinator's office was housed in the Ministry of the Attorney General, it also had responsibility for FLS offered throughout the newly expanded sector formed by the Conservative government, and for designing new programs and new ways of contributing to the sector and performing the tasks involved. At the same time, the Liberal government in Ottawa announced the forthcoming publication of an action plan for official languages. It also published the study *Environmental Scan: Access to Justice in Both Official Languages*, which described progress made in delivery of FLS in the judicial system throughout Canada (GTA Research, 2002). These important initiatives contributed to a renewed enthusiasm for official languages in the area of justice, in Ontario as well as across Canada. Thus, when the Ontario Liberal party returned to power in 2003, the time was ripe for real progress in the justice sector. Not only did the FLS Coordinator want the range of FLS to correspond more closely to the expectations of Francophones in the province, he also wanted to explore ways to integrate community actors in planning and service delivery into future initiatives to put an end to nearly 10 years of tense relations between the Francophone community and the former government. The FLS Coordinator took it upon himself to invite the *Association des juristes d'expression française* (AJEFO), the *Association française des municipalités de l'Ontario* (AFMO), *Action ontarienne contre la violence faite aux femmes* (AOcVF), the *Fédération de la jeunesse franco-ontarienne* (FESFO) and the *Fédération des aînés et des retraités francophones de l'Ontario* (FARFO)—organizations representing Francophone legal professionals, municipalities, activists working in the area of violence against women, youth, and seniors—to begin a consultation process with his Office for the purpose of developing a strategic and operational planning process for the active offer of FLS in all divisions of the justice sector. Without delay, these groups formed a Coalition that was quickly recognized by the Government of Ontario as the primary voice of the Francophone community on matters related to justice.

In 2005, the Office of the FLS Coordinator invited the University of Ottawa's *Chaire de recherche sur la francophonie et les politiques publiques* to prepare a status report on FLS in the justice sector in Ontario, accompanied by a statistical portrait of the Francophone community in the province, a series of recommendations, and a draft of a strategic plan (Cardinal, Lang, Plante, Sauvé, & Terrien, 2005). The results of this study were presented at the 2006 Francophone Stakeholders' Meeting attended by members of the Coalition and public servants. Other goals of this forum were to confirm the needs of the community, formulate guiding principles for the future development of FLS, and set out the first steps in a strategic planning exercise for the justice sector (Cardinal, Lang, & Sauvé, 2006). Active offer was among the forum's guiding principles.

At the end of 2006, the Government of Ontario published its *Strategic Plan for the Development of French Language Services in Ontario's Justice Sector*. Its objectives were to raise the awareness among Ontario Francophones about their FLS rights, improve and extend access to services, respond to the needs of various target groups, raise awareness of FLS among managers, develop new programs, and establish a governance structure integrating community participation in inter-ministerial cooperation. The plan was developed through a process characterized by community governance and continuous consultation with government officials and leading community organizations in the justice sector (Ontario, Office of the Coordinator of French Language Services for the Justice Sector, 2006). Because they had seats on the Steering Committee, the members of the Coalition would participate actively in the follow-up to the strategic plan, thereby guaranteeing that the needs of Francophones in the FLS planning process would be taken into account. Finally, follow-up would take place during an annual forum organized by the Office of the FLS Coordinator and attended by members of the Coalition and the government officials responsible for the different divisions of the justice sector.

First published in 2006, the plan has been reviewed and new plans have been published twice; the most recent plan covers the period up to 2016. At the time of writing, we are unable to say with certainty whether it will be renewed. At the time, the plan appeared to be the ideal structure to encourage new ways of conceptualizing and managing FLS delivery and ensuring its long-time sustainability. One of the new ways of doing things, through dialogue among community and government actors on the active offer of FLS, plays an important role in improving the planning process for FLS in the justice sector.

Co-constructing the Idea of the Active Offer of FLS

The idea of active offer in the justice system has a history that is part of a larger context of the application of the federal *Official Languages Act* (1969) and of the development of FLS in Ontario. According to François Charbonneau (2011, p. 43), in Canada, the legislator wanted citizens to have access to public services in the official language of their choice; before the law entered into effect, they did not have this choice. Without a law, Francophones could be restricted to English-language services because French-language services would simply not be available in their region.

On the other hand, as Charbonneau explains, language choices are often conditioned by external factors, which go far beyond the simple will to express a preference. Among these factors is the history of Francophone-Anglophone relations—the power relations between the two groups, or even assimilation. These factors also condition Francophones to not identify themselves as such, and to speak French in public only when they feel they have permission to do so. Cardinal, Plante, and Sauvé (2010) also noted this situation in their research on the justice sector in Ontario. Charbonneau explains this situation by referring to the concept of linguistic insecurity, meaning that the linguistic behaviour of Francophones is influenced by the phenomenon of linguistic minoritization (Charbonneau, 2011, p. 47). As well, Lafrenière, Grenier, and Corbeil (2006, quoted in Charbonneau, 2011, p. 47) consider that the more Francophones are spread out over a given territory, the more they tend to speak the language of the majority. According to these authors, the smaller the Francophone minority is, the less important Francophones might consider it is to have government services offered in their language (ibid., p. 48). In a minority context, according to Charbonneau (2011, p. 50), "the reflex to ask for FLS is practically non-existent, unless the conditions for it are created." Francophones will avoid asking for services in their own language because it might appear "as a whim, that is, a request for an unjustified privilege" (Charbonneau, 2011, p. 53). In such conditions, it is not surprising that some Francophones may perceive their proficiency in English as a form of prestige, while French unilingualism may be associated with ignorance (Tardif & Dallaire, 2010). Along the same lines, Deveau, Landry, and Allard (2009) emphasize that "asking to be served in French is a behaviour associated with a commitment to one's Francophone identity, and is relatively difficult for a person who has been socialized to believe that English is the main language, if not the only one, used in public institutions" (p. 88). Thus, Francophones are conditioned to choose to be served in English, even when they could be in a situation in which they could ask for services in French. As Charbonneau points out (2011), "evidently, offering French-language services only to citizens who ask for it directly is simply not enough to ensure that Francophones use French-language services" (p. 57).

At the beginning of the new millennium, this realization led several actors to put forward the idea of active offer, a dialogue then in its infancy. The Government of Canada defines the standards for active offer through the Treasury Board Secretariat, indicating that active offer must be founded on certain modalities such as to "provide clear visual and verbal indications that members of the public can communicate with and obtain services from a designated in either English or French" (Canada, Treasury Board Secretariat, n.d.). As for Ontario, the Office of the French Language Services Commissioner opted for innovation when, in 2010, it proposed a more subjective approach: active offer needed to make it possible for members of the Francophone minority to be "instantly recognized as full members of a strong and respected community that is taking its rightful place in Ontario society" (2010, p. 11). Added to this is the idea that "institutions provide reassurance to French-speaking members of the public not only as individuals but as members of a vibrant, dynamic Francophone community that has a future" (2010, p. 11). In their study on FLS in Nova Scotia, Deveau, Landry, and Allard (2009) concur with the Ontario Commissioner's view. These authors believe the more often Francophones in Nova Scotia receive services in French, the more they feel they contribute to the vitality of their community. The Office of Francophone Affairs (OFA) also makes a connection with the idea of vitality, explaining that cooperative action on active offer will contribute to enhancing well-being as well as the political, social, economic, and cultural vitality of the Francophone community in the province, which is the overarching goal of the *French Language Services Act* (Ontario, Office of Francophone Affairs, 2008, p. 4). Since this time, Ontario has established a close link between the behaviour and actions of Francophones, the vitality of their communities, and the FLS offered. Thus, active offer becomes an instrument to nurture a favourable representation of the French language and of Francophone minorities. As the Office of the French Language

Services Commissioner states: "Active offer makes it possible to reach those who hesitate to use French-language services in their daily lives and who are still walking the fine line between continuing to live as a Francophone and assimilation" (2010, p. 12). The concept of active offer encourages government institutions to leverage visibility, accessibility, and the availability of French-language services that meet the needs of the Francophone population. Understood this way, active offer is a tool that should enable action on several fronts: equity, justice, vitality, and self-representation.

Furthermore, contrary to the federal government, Ontario does not favour the concept of free choice. Its objective is to offer FLS, rather than to invite residents of Ontario to use the official language of their choice, since French is not an official language in the province. The provincial government subscribes to *de facto* bilingualism, that is, an idea of bilingualism that accepts the obligation to offer FLS where numbers warrant, in regions designated as bilingual. Nonetheless, at the beginning of the millennium, the resolution of the Hôpital Montfort court case, and the recognition of the courts that it is important for the Francophone community to manage its own institutions, pushed the province to take another look at the idea of active offer.[5]

In a document produced by the Council of Ministers in 2006, Tony Dean (the secretary at the time) affirmed that the Ontario Public Service was not fulfilling its obligations under the *French Language Services Act* (Ontario Public Service, *OPS Framework for Action: A Modern Ontario Public Service* 2006; in Ontario, Office of Francophone Affairs 2008, and in Ontario, Office of the Coordinator of French Language Services for the Justice Sector 2006). In 2008, the OFA published a manual for offering FLS, in which it is stipulated that active offer must be results-oriented, integrated into the service delivery model of the Ministry, and developed out of a dialogue with the population served, and must reflect the needs of this population. In addition, the OFA acknowledged that it should not have to be up to public to request FLS; members of the public service need to actively offer these services (Ontario, Office of Francophone Affairs, 2008).

Nevertheless, at the time, the French Language Services Commissioner felt that this definition did not go far enough and would not have a strong enough impact on Ontario's Public Service. He wanted the government to issue an actual directive about active offer, not merely issue guidelines. According to the French Language Services Commissioner:

> Obviously, this directive should provide for consultations with the Francophone community, planning from the moment that new programs and services are designed, and a results-based performance review. Such a directive should be accompanied by a strategy to promote French-language services. This strategy should be adapted and updated on a regular basis, as service offer changes and is updated. (Ontario, Office of the French Language Services Commissioner, 2010, p. 14)

The Office of the French Language Services Commissioner also provides its own definition of active offer, which it presents as a "clear signal" to citizens that wherever they live, they can receive services in French: "the agency's name and all of its posters, signage, brochures, literature, etc., are either bilingual or offered visually in English and in French." This also means "from the moment they begin interacting with the public, government employees staffing a service counter or answering the telephone proactively offer service in both languages." For the Commissioner, active offer means "creating an environment that is conducive to demand and that anticipates the specific needs of Francophones in their community" (Ontario, Office of the French Language Services Commissioner, 2010, p. 11).

In 2011, the Government of Ontario tried responding to this recommendation by adding a definition of active offer to a regulation adopted in 2011 governing FLS delivery by third parties. This regulation stipulates that:

> [E]very government agency shall ensure that a third party providing a service in French to the public on its behalf shall take appropriate measures, including providing signs, notices and other information on services and initiating communication with the public, to make it known to members of the public that the service is available in French at the choice of any member of the public. (Ontario, Ontario Regulation 284/11, n.d.)

For the OFA, this means that services in French are "clearly visible, readily available, easily accessible and publicized and that the quality of these services is equivalent to that of services offered in English"

(Ontario, Office of Francophone Affairs, n.d.). In 2013, the French Language Services Commissioner came to the fore, stressing that the measures adopted by the Government of Ontario were not sufficient. He reiterated his recommendation. In 2014, he also criticized the response of the government to his recommendation. In the Commissioner's opinion, the measures put in place by the Government of Ontario depended on the good will of each institution. He asserted "the current situation does not create an environment conducive to reaching those who are still hesitant to use services in French on a daily basis, nor to helping avert the constant threat of assimilation" (Ontario, Office of the French Language Services Commissioner, 2014, p. 8).

These debates are important to our understanding of the principle of actively offering FLS in the justice sector since 2003. Although the debates focus mainly on the practical aspects of active offer, the French Language Services Commissioner also contextualizes the government's actions in a broader framework, which uncovers the attitude and motivation of the government towards its responsibilities. Its focus on good will and voluntary action proves inadequate in ensuring a true active offer of FLS.

The issues raised by the French Language Services Commissioner can also be seen in the dialogue among various actors in the active offer of FLS within the justice sector. In 2006, during consultations in view of preparing the strategic plan, the actors listed a number of components to be included, stipulating that in active offer "Demand must be stimulated, using oral communication and written materials in designated places in order to promote FLS use. Active offer also includes integration of FLS into policy development from the outset" (Ontario, Office of the Coordinator of French Language Services 2006, p. 7). The different community and government actors involved were calling for actions that would not rely on good will, but instead on accountability. For community actors, the idea of introducing service models to guarantee FLS delivery is also at the centre of their representation of active offer. During consultations to prepare the plan, they included the principle of services offered by and for Francophones as an integral aspect of the active offer of FLS (Cardinal, Lang & Sauvé, 2006, p. 35), distinguishing this type of service from integrated services and services offered by Anglophone or bilingual groups. We should also mention that the *Réseau des Centres d'aide et de lutte contre les agressions à caractère sexuel* (CALACS, the network of rape and sexual assault centres for Francophones), administered by the *Action ontarienne contre la violence faite aux femmes* (AOcVF, an Ontario organization for action against violence towards women), is an example of a service in the justice sector by and for Francophones (Sirois & Garceau, 2007). AOcVF is one of the actors involved in managing the strategic plan. Its point of view is an integral part of the debates leading to the co-construction of active offer.

Once the plan was published, its principles continued to be a subject of dialogue among community and governmental actors. As part of the Steering Committee for the plan, these actors met annually and dealt with other issues as well, notably the matter of accountability. As part of the Advisory Committee's meetings, civil servants had to explain why they did not always take FLS into account when planning public services. They were also asked to say how they would ensure that FLS would be offered by a set date in the future. Thus, community actors considered civil servants accountable to the community. As one respondent interviewed for the study by Cardinal, Levert, Manton, and Ouellet (2013, p. 27) explained,

> [original: French] If they hadn't done what they said they would do, they would be shaking! I mean, they were really worried. The community had learned to be polite, but still to be firm, and I think they succeeded in having a good relationship, and I think it was a relationship that was something different, innovative, I think that led to faster changes and more French services. (Interview, University of Ottawa)

Because of the role of community actors, the principle of accountability was added to the details of active offer. Another respondent suggested:

> [original: French] Even the two colleges, now, the Ontario Police College and we also have the Ontario Fire College, both are part of the strategic plan, they have to be accountable to the team members. The members validate or don't validate, push for certain priorities, etc. (Interview, Public Servant 5, quoted in ibid, p. 27)

However, this accountability principle should not be taken for granted. For example, the findings from a survey of 1,000 employees working for the Ontario Ministry of the Attorney General by Cardinal, Plante, and Sauvé (2010) showed that even though the staff members know they are supposed to make an active offer of FLS, respondents do not actively offer them. They wait for Francophones to ask for services before offering them. The survey also revealed that respondents, including front-line staff, do not know if their office has active offer plans because these are not circulated. The data proved that the behaviour of managers could determine if FLS would be actively offered or not. The people who responded to the survey said, however, that they would like to have more tools available to develop their skills and enable them to actively offer services in French.

As part of our research, focus groups of service users were arranged, to determine if people knew they were entitled to receive FLS. The participants said they know they have a right to FLS. However, they admitted that they are often afraid to ask because they don't want to disturb the status quo. They further explained that their first contact with front-line staff is crucial. Often, they do not ask for the FLS that should be actively offered because they do not really feel that they are in an environment where the use of French is welcomed. On the other hand, non-verbal behaviour on the part of the employees could play a positive role in suggesting the opposite is true.

The responses about the active offer of FLS clearly show how this practice depends on representations linked to management principles such as accountability, and also show that they are more than a neutral management technique. Accountability relates to issues of legitimacy. Cardinal and Sauvé (2010) express the key role of accountability in the co-construction of the active offer of FLS this way:

> It's not that the work must be done over and over again, but that those responsible for service delivery must have a thorough understanding of the situation and needs of Francophones. Measures must be put in place to guarantee an active offer of FLS. As well as introducing these measures, it is important to integrate FLS into the structure of services, and to make them a basic component of the curricula. Francophones also must be informed and reminded of their right to FLS on a continuous basis. These services were put in place because it is important for Francophones to be able to be served in their own language. (2010, p. 8)

Since the responsibility for actively offering FLS belongs to the government, it follows that the government cannot limit itself to the existing demand. It must create a demand by fulfilling its obligations toward the Francophone community, and thereby mitigate the negative effects of managing strictly by numbers ("where numbers warrant . . .") and the discrimination that results. Thanks to the dialogue between community and government actors, and to the efforts of the Commissioner, the active offer of FLS in the justice sector has been co-constructed in a way that is far from technical. This co-construction builds active offer on the foundation of management principles, community aspirations, and a particular ideal of justice in the area of language.

Lessons and Applications of Experiences in the Justice Sector to Other Sectors

In a study of French-language health services in Ontario, researchers Bouchard, Beaulieu, and Desmeules (2012) describe the guideposts of active offer this way:

> At first sight, active offer may look like an invitation, verbal or written, to express oneself in the official language of one's choice. The offer to speak in the official language of one's choice must come before a request for services is made. For an offer to be active, it must be visible, audible, accessible (in speech), and obvious . . . and greetings and services for Francophones must be given automatically, like a reflex, and immediately. (2012, p. 46)

The authors suggest three aspects necessary for active offer: (i) visibility, (ii) accessibility, and (iii) availability of services. They specify that these three aspects neglect the aspect of service delivery.

> It seems opportune to emphasize the aspects of effective and quality delivery of health services in a minority language setting. Active offer also includes the ability to act upon this promise in French. . . . In fact, not only must services in French be actively offered, but staff must ensure that their accessibility and their delivery be of equivalent quality to those of services in English. (2012, p. 47)

Bouchard, Beaulieu, and Desmeules (2012) highlight the importance of an offer of "equivalent quality." The notion of equivalent quality can be considered an important condition of substantive equality. Understood as a principle of justice, active offer can contribute to countering inequalities between Francophones and Anglophones in Canada. As the same authors suggest, it is "a remedy or correct measure for inequalities made by proposing a concrete method to bring services closer . . . to the needs of the population." Active offer "represents a measure of equity designed to ensure compliance with the law, so that an equality of status corresponds to an equality of treatment" (2012, 44).

Research in the area of health care focuses more on the operationalization of active offer and less on the issues of co-constructing active offer. The definitions proposed are aimed at providing an accurate, detailed, and systematic method of providing active offer. However, one of the lessons we learned from our study of the justice sector and can extrapolate to other sectors, notably the health and social service sector, is that the active offer of FLS is a matter of representations. Active offer reflects different representations, depending on its context. Community actors may put the emphasis on how and on the type of services offered, while government actors must actively offer services within a set of integrated services. These different contexts influence the representation of active offer. They speak to the diversity of issues related to active offer that actors must take into account, and to the power relations among them. For this reason, the co-construction of active offer is always a work in progress. The research on the active offer of FLS in the justice sector illustrates the fact that there are important issues around accountability, and that they contribute to the minoritization of Francophones.

On the other hand, the experience of the justice sector also shows that the numerous legal victories of Francophones—we need only think of the Montfort case—have contributed to creating a context where these issues will be taken more seriously by the Government of Ontario. In addition, since the Liberal government, more receptive to the concerns of the Francophone population, came to power in 2003, the dialogue between the community and the different government actors opened up again. Finally, the involvement of intermediary actors highly committed to the development of FLS, such as the Office of the Coordinator of FLS for the Justice Sector, completes the list of elements fostering dialogue on active offer.

Meanwhile, the Coordinator of FLS believes civil servants should be more in tune with the community:

> [original: French] I have always told senior managers that it took the network [the Coalition] to put a face on, let's say, the Francophone community, because you know what I mean, it's like we, the senior managers, we are always sitting in our ivory towers, but we never get into the community. (Interview, Civil Servant 1, quoted in Cardinal, Levert, Manton, & Ouellet, 2013, p. 20)

For this public servant, the fact that government actors support and influence each other is important. The relationship of trust and respect that they develop among themselves should guide them in implementing the plan. This is how the dialogue enabling the co-construction of the active offer of FLS develops. However, many people must be convinced of its value before the various community and government actors will be able to sit at the same table and work together towards a common goal of actively offering FLS. Finally, given that there is an undeniable political dimension to co-construction, once the process is initiated, the dialogue must be nurtured by means of meetings between the actors. As we have seen, these meetings ensure accountability. They enable actors to work together to co-produce an opportunity for important debates, and for the kind of self-assessment and reflection that foster improvements in the way active offer is practised. These dimensions of co-construction of the active offer of FLS are important not only for the justice sector, but for all sectors targeted in the requirement to actively offer FLS. Having actors participate in the debate on active offer is an undeniable necessity. It is what makes it possible to co-construct the active offer of FLS. For example, the discussions are not exempt from verbal feuds and foul play. As one respondent explained, there are times when "you have to elbow your way into a discussion around the table":

> . . . sometimes [we] played a bit rough. Not with the other groups as much as with the funders. And it's always a fine line. I realized that if you don't throw a fit, or practically, at some point, not much is going to happen. At the same time, you have to be careful of your relationship with your inside allies. . . . As a Francophone, you don't necessarily have the same ability to

catch the attention of the media for a press conference, and then use that as a pressure tactic. . . . For me, anyway, I can't do that. That means, how can I get my way when I'm dealing with the government? So it's a fine line between blowing up and creating ties, and continuing to hammer out my message continually with the decision-makers and turning some of them into allies. (Interview, AOcVF, quoted in ibid., p. 27)

Community actors, then, can never assume they will be taken seriously. In addition, the turnover of staff in the government can also have a negative effect on the active offer of FLS: [original: French] "When senior managers change in the executive, all the work you've accomplished can be destroyed pretty quickly. This is what happened in the Ontario Victim Services Secretariat. After several years of working closely together, a change in senior staff made us take a huge step backwards" (Interview, AOcVF, quoted in ibid.).

In keeping with the French Language Services Commissioner, we recognize the dialogue between community and government actors relies too heavily on goodwill and that this is not sufficient. A "good discussion" between civil servants and community groups may have limited effect. The survey findings mentioned above are ample proof. Even though the active offer of FLS is governed by the principles of accountability and obligation, it lacks a more tightly structured approach that could include clearer policies, more explicit directives, and working tools to ensure that the methods government actors use to actively offer FLS have more lasting outcomes. These elements of analysis strike us as important, as they point to crucial issues that persist in the dialogue on the active offer of FLS.

Conclusion

Our intention in this chapter has been to examine the dialogue on the active offer of FLS in the justice sector. We were able to show that active offer is more than a management technique it is a principle conveying a certain understanding of FLS by community and government actors. Using the instruments approach, we can see FLS active offer is an object of reflection. Questions concerning its operationalization represent political issues, not simply matters of a technical nature. Active offer has an undeniably political dimension: the continuing debate on its meaning is connected with representations and with dialogue among different actors for the purpose of its co-construction.

The experiences of various actors in the context of the follow-up of the strategic plan for developing the active offer of FLS in the area of justice also includes learning that is relevant for other sectors, such as health and social services. First, the active offer of FLS must be developed through a process that brings the different actors involved together, and gives them an opportunity to take part in the co-construction of the active offer of FLS. Second, active offer must not rely only on the good will and voluntary action; it must be founded on policies, directives, planning, and accountability. Thus, there is ample material to continue a debate that is at once normative and pragmatic, and thereby to identify means of fostering active offer that do not depend solely on the good will of the actors present.

Notes

1. The data used here were collected in 2012 by Cardinal and her colleagues. They have previously been published in a research report by the Alliance de recherche, *Les savoirs de la gouvernance communautaire* (Cardinal, Levert, Manton, & Ouellet, 2013). This chapter makes use of the data already published in the report for this analysis of active offer.
2. The sections in this chapter quote extensively from Cardinal, Levert, Manton, and Ouellet, 2013, and are included with the authors' permission. This first section draws on pages 3 to 5.
3. In 2006, the centralization of the FLS portfolio in the justice sector combined FLS activities in five divisions of the Ministry of the Attorney General in the strategic plan: the Court Services Division, including the Support Unit to the implementation of the Law on Provincial Offences; the Criminal Law Division; the Ontario Victim Services Secretariat; the Office of the Public Guardian and Trustee; and the Office of the Children's Lawyer.
4. The divisions of the Ministry which participated later in the strategic plan were: the Ontario Provincial Police, Emergency Management Ontario, Adult Community Corrections Services, Adult Institutional Services, and the Public Safety Division.
5. In 1999, the Health Services Restructuring Commission established by the Government of Ontario recommended closing Hôpital Montfort, a hospital that served Francophones in Ottawa and eastern Ontario. The announcement of the closure gave rise to the SOS Montfort movement; leaders decided to appeal to the courts to prevent the government from closing the hospital.

References

Bouchard, L., Beaulieu, M., & Desmeules, M. (2012). L'offre active de services de santé en français en Ontario: une mesure d'équité. *Reflets: Revue d'intervention sociale et communautaire*, 18(2), 38–65.

Canada. Treasury Board Secretariat (n.d.) *Policy on Official Languages*. Retrieved from https://www.tbs-sct.gc.ca/pol/doc-eng.aspx?id=26160

Cardinal, L., Lang, S., Plante, N., Sauvé, A., & Terrien, C. (2005). *Un état des lieux. Les services en français dans le domaine de la justice en Ontario*. Ottawa: Chaire de recherche sur la francophonie et les politiques publiques.

Cardinal, L., Lang, S., & Sauvé, A. (2006). *Les services en français dans le domaine de la justice en Ontario: Rapport de la consultation des intervenantes et intervenants francophones, Toronto, 1, 2 et 3 mars 2006*. Ottawa: Chaire de recherche sur la francophonie et les politiques publiques.

Cardinal, L., & Léger, R. (accepted for publication). The Politics of Multilingualism in Canada. In F. Grin and P. Kraus (Eds.), *The Politics of Multilingualism: Linguistic Governance, Globalisation and Europeanisation*. Amsterdam: John Benjamins.

Cardinal, L., Levert, M.-È., Manton, D., & Ouellet, S. (2013). *La Coalition des intervenantes et intervenants francophones en justice: une innovation dans le domaine des services en français*. Ottawa: Alliance de recherche Les savoirs de la gouvernance communautaire.

Cardinal, L., & Normand, M. (2013). Distinct Accents: The Language Regimes of Ontario and Quebec. In J.-F. Savard, A. Brassard, and L. Côté, *Quebec-Ontario Relations: A Shared Destiny?* (pp. 119–144). Québec: Presses de l'Université du Québec.

Cardinal, L., Plante, N., & Sauvé, A. (2010). *De la théorie à la pratique: Les mécanismes d'offre de services en français dans le domaine de la justice en Ontario. Volume 2: Les perceptions des fonctionnaires et des usagères et usagers*. Ottawa: Chaire de recherche sur la francophonie et les politiques publiques.

Cardinal, L., & Sauvé, A. (2010). *De la théorie à la pratique: Les mécanismes d'offre de services en français dans le domaine de la justice en Ontario. Volume 1*. Ottawa: Chaire de recherche sur la francophonie et les politiques publiques.

Charbonneau, F. (2011). Dans la langue officielle de son choix: la loi canadienne sur les langues officielles et la notion de "choix" en matière de services publics. *Lien social et Politiques*, 66, 39–63.

Corbeil, J.-P., Grenier, C., & Lafrenière, S. (2006). *Les minorités prennent la parole: Résultats de l'Enquête sur la vitalité des minorités de langue officielle*. Ottawa: Ministère de l'Industrie.

Deveau, K., Landry, R., & Allard, R. (2009). *Utilisation des services gouvernementaux de langue française. Une étude auprès des Acadiens et francophones de la Nouvelle-Écosse sur les facteurs associés à l'utilisation des services gouvernementaux en français.* Moncton, NB: Institut canadien de recherche sur les minorités linguistiques.

GTA Research (2002). *Environmental Scan: Access to Justice in Both Official Languages.* Ottawa: Department of Justice. Retrieved from http://www.justice.gc.ca/eng/rp-pr/csj-sjc/franc/enviro/summ-somm.html

Lascoumes, P., & Le Galès, P. (2004). *Gouverner par les instruments.* Paris: Presses de Science pPo.

Lascoumes, P., et Le Galès, P. (2007). *La sociologie de l'action publique.* Paris: Armand Colin.

Ontario. Office of the Coordinator of French Language Services for the Justice Sector. (2006). *Strategic Plan for the Development of French Language Services in Ontario's Justice Sector.* Toronto: Ministry of the Attorney General, 26.

Ontario. Office of the French Language Services Commissioner (2010). *Annual Report 2009–2010: Open for Solutions.* Toronto: Queen's Printer for Ontario.

Ontario. Office of Francophone Affairs (2008). *Practical Guide for the Active Offer of French-language Services in the Ontario Government.*

Ontario. Office of the French Language Services Commissioner (2012). *Annual Report 2011–2012: Straight Forward.* Toronto: Queen's Printer for Ontario.

Ontario. Office of the French Language Services Commissioner (2014). *Annual Report 2013–2014: Rooting for Francophones.* Toronto: Queen's Printer for Ontario.

Ontario. Office des affaires francophones. Règlement 284/11 et l'offre de services en français. Retrieved from http://www.ofa.gov.on.ca/fr/loi-reglement284-11.html

Ontario. *Regulation 284/11 under French Language Services Act, R.S.O. 1990, c. F.32—Provision of French Language Services on Behalf of Government Agencies.* Retrieved from https://www.ontario.ca/laws/regulation/r11284

Sirois, G., & Garceau, M.-L. (2007). Le développement des services en français en matière de violence faite aux femmes: des pratiques à notre image. *Reflets: Revue d'intervention sociale et communautaire, 13*(1), 98–111.

Tardif, C., & Dallaire, C. (2010). La satisfaction des patients francophones de l'est de l'Ontario traités en réadaptation à domicile. *Francophonies d'Amérique, 30,* 61–88.

PART III

ACCESSIBILITY AND THE ACTIVE OFFER OF FRENCH-LANGUAGE SERVICES

The Health of Francophone Seniors Living in Minority Communities in Canada: Issues and Needs[1]

Louise Bouchard and Martin Desmeules,
University of Ottawa

Abstract

This chapter presents a profile of the socio-demographic characteristics and the health of Francophone seniors (aged 65 and above) living in minority language communities, and identifies the issues and the needs of this population. In the first section of the chapter, we discuss the minority context and its potential impact on the aging of the population, the social position of seniors, their health, and their access to services. The second section establishes the socio-sanitary profile of Francophone seniors in three large Canadian regions (Atlantic Canada, Ontario, and the West), based on data from the Canadian Community Health Survey—Annual Component (CCHS, combined cycles, 2003–2012). Finally, we discuss two issues that are, we believe, fundamental for this minority population: health literacy—the ability to adequately communicate in and navigate through the health system—and the active offer of services, which is a measure of equity and quality of care for people living in an official language minority community.

Key Words: Francophone seniors, linguistic minorities, socio-sanitary portrait, Canada, Canadian Community Health Survey (CCHS).

The Minority Language Context as a Determinant of Health

In the last few decades, a number of studies have demonstrated the importance of language and, more broadly, a minority language context as a determinant of health. To summarize, social determinants of health are the conditions in which people are born, live, and die, and the systems put in place to promote a better state of health. Looking more specifically at the impact of language on health, research on the linguistic and cultural barriers to health, especially in official language minority communities across the country (Bouchard & Desmeules, 2011; Bélanger, 2003; Bowen, 2001), testifies to the interest social scientists have in the issues faced by Francophones in these communities. In particular, this research shows that language barriers have a proven impact on access to and use of services (Flores, 2006; Yeo, 2004; Sarver & Baker, 2000; Hu & Covell, 1998; Solis *et al.*, 1990) and more broadly on the health of these populations (Leis & Bouchard, 2013; Bouchard *et al.*, 2009), as well as on the quality of care and services (Ava *et al.*, 2004; Woloshin *et al.*, 1997). In general, researchers recognize that "language barriers contribute to the risk of error in diagnosis (and/ or delays in diagnosis) and decrease the probability of adherence to treatment" (Beaulieu, 2010; CNFS, 2010; Tremblay, 2012).

Obstacles such as these can be even more overwhelming for an aging population facing increasing health problems, as is the case in official language minority communities in Canada. In all these communities, regardless of certain socio-demographic variations among provinces, the aging of the population is even more pronounced than in the majority language population. Studies (Bouchard *et al.*, 2011, 2012, 2013, 2015; Forgues *et al.*, 2011) have also found that the Francophone population in minority contexts is not only aging more rapidly, but is less wealthy and is culturally marginalized. Thus, they are more vulnerable when health problems occur. The effects of poor communication about health, combined with the effects of being a cultural minority—or even the very real threat of assimilation—have led us to examine possible solutions.

First, we know that efforts to close the literacy gap among Francophone seniors are necessary, as are efforts to enhance the active offer of French-language preventive, educational, and treatment services for these seniors living in official language minority communities.

Notes on Methodology

The descriptive data presented in this chapter are from the Canadian Community Health Survey (CCHS), a cross-sectional survey conducted by Statistics Canada that collects information related to health status, health care utilization, and health determinants for the Canadian population. The population surveyed in the CCHS includes individuals 12 years of age and over living in private households in the provinces and territories, excluding residents of Aboriginal reserves, certain remote regions, and military bases. In order to bridge the gaps associated with the low number of Francophone minority persons represented in the CCHS, several cycles were combined; this method has been validated by Statistics Canada as a way of increasing the accuracy of estimates (Makvandi et al., 2013). Despite the results of combined cycles, the number of Francophone seniors remains too low to present accurate findings for each of the provinces. Therefore, to show the regional variations in the data, findings are presented for Atlantic Canada as a whole, for Ontario and for the West as a whole, as well as for the overall population of Canadian seniors. To define the Francophone population, we created an algorithm allowing us to filter results based on four language variables shown in the CCHS: the language used for conversation, mother tongue, the language in which the interview was conducted, and the preferred contact language chosen for the survey. This method made it possible to identify and filter groups as clearly as possible, depending on their spoken and preferred language, and to select only those persons who identified themselves as French-speaking—both Francophones born in Canada and newcomers from other countries (Bouchard et al., 2009).

Socio-Demographic Portrait of Francophone Seniors

There are nearly a million Canadians identifying French as their mother tongue who live outside Quebec (Statistics Canada, 2011). Among them are 493,300 Francophones in Ontario (5.2% of the province's population); 233,530 in New Brunswick (34.7%); 68,545 in Alberta (3.1%); 57,280 in British Columbia (2%); 42,090 in Manitoba (6.3%); 31,110 in Nova Scotia (5.2%); 16,280 in Saskatchewan (3.7%); and 5,195 on Prince Edward Island (6.3%). In the Province of Newfoundland & Labrador (0.7%) and in the territories—Yukon (4.2%), Northwest Territories (2.7%), and Nunavut (1.4%)—there are 5,450 Francophones (Statistics Canada, 2011).

As in other countries in the Western world, Francophones living in Canada's official language minority communities are part of an aging population. The increasingly rapid rise in the numbers of aging persons is even more pronounced in minority communities: in 2006, the aging of the Francophone population was higher in every Canadian province (Forgues, Doucet, & Landry, 2011). In 2011, there were more than five million persons over 65 years of age, amounting to 14.1% of the total population (Statistics Canada, 2012); among Francophones living in minority communities, the proportion rose to 18% of the national population (CCHS, combined cycles, 2003–2012).

As well as this accelerated rate of population aging, Francophone seniors in official language minority communities also experience more pronounced economic instability than seniors in the Anglophone majority. In recent analyses, we found, for example, that Francophones aged 65 years and over are more likely than Anglophones to belong to the lowest-income quintile. Both language and belonging to the Francophone minority have been shown to be determinants of poverty (Bouchard *et al.*, 2013; Bouchard *et al.*, 2015). Furthermore, Francophone populations have fewer years of education and more often live in regions where the economic is less stable, which makes it more difficult to develop and access social and community resources (Bouchard & Leis, 2008; Bouchard & Desmeules, 2013).

The situation of seniors varies according to the region or province of residence. Data from the CHSS show that the proportion of Francophone seniors is 17% in Atlantic Canada, 18% in Ontario, and 20% in the West. Aging is also associated with the feminization of the population, as women seniors are proportionally more highly represented in the population than men. The population of Francophone seniors is over-represented in lower levels of education: 44% in Atlantic Canada, 31% in Ontario, and 29% in the West do not have a high school diploma, as opposed to 22% for the overall population. This population is also more likely to occupy lower income categories; more Francophone seniors are in the lowest-income quintile: (34% in Atlantic Canada, 28% in Ontario, and 31% in the West versus 28% for the overall population of Canada). In terms of their location, 53% of Francophone seniors in Atlantic Canada, 20% in Ontario, and 23% in the West live in rural settings. Nearly one senior in three lives alone, and the proportion is higher in the West (36%). Finally, the population of Francophone seniors includes a small proportion of immigrants (2% in Atlantic Canada, 11% in Ontario, and 9% in the West, compared to 33% in the overall population).

Table 1. Socio-demographic Profile of the Population

| | 65 yrs+ | Francophones 65 years and over | | |
	Canada (%)	Atlantic (%)	Ontario (%)	West (%)
65 years and over	15	17	18	20
Women	55	56	58	55
Men	45	44	42	45
No high school diploma	23	44	31	29
Low income (1st quintile)	28	34	28	31
Lives alone	28	26	29	36
Rural setting	20	53	20	23
Immigrant status	32	2	11	9

Source of data: CCHS: 2.1 (2003), 3.1 (2005), 4.1 (2007), 2008, 2009, 2010, 2011, 2012. Canada excluding Quebec and the Territories. Weighted data based on a sample of 7,640 Francophones and 157,312 Canadians aged 65 years and over.

Health Portrait of Francophone Seniors

The indicator of perceived health is often used by researchers as a means of describing the social aspects of the state of health in a population; it can, for example, provide information about such aspects as social isolation, a sense of inferiority, self-esteem, communication, and, of particular interest to us, manifestations of cultural and linguistic minoritization. Perception of health (Baillis *et al.*, 2003), combined with other indicators such as the need for help to perform everyday tasks and reports about activity limitations due to a chronic condition, contribute to a more accurate and objective reflection of the state of health and the need for services and care in a given population. More than one quarter of Francophone seniors perceive their health to be poor or very poor (31% in Atlantic Canada, 24% in Ontario, 27% in the West); a similar proportion of them state they need help with everyday tasks (29% in Atlantic Canada, 27% in Ontario and in the West); one out of every three reports his or her activities at home are reduced by a chronic condition (32% in Atlantic Canada, 34% in Ontario, 36% in the West). Excess weight and a sedentary lifestyle, factors that contribute to chronic diseases, affect more than half of them: 57% of Francophones in Atlantic Canada, 60% in Ontario, and 54% in the West state they are overweight or obese, and 60% in Atlantic Canada, 56% in Ontario, and 52% in the West state they are inactive. In terms of diet and nutrition, greater than half report they do not consume the recommended five daily portions of fruits and vegetables (53% in Atlantic Canada, 56% in

Ontario, 51% in the West). Finally, approximately 10% of Francophone seniors smoke every day or occasionally (8% in Atlantic Canada, 12% in Ontario, 11% in the West), and almost one senior in four reports drinking alcohol daily (10% in Atlantic Canada, 22% in Ontario, 21% in the West). In terms of mental health, 6% claim to have poor mental health (8% in Atlantic Canada, 6% in Ontario, 5% in the West).

Table 2. Perceived Health, Reduced Activities, and Lifestyle

	65 yrs+ Canada (%)	Francophones 65 years and over		
		Atlantic (%)	Ontario (%)	West (%)
Perceived poor health	25	31	24	27
Perceived poor mental health	6	8	6	5
Needs help with everyday tasks	27	29	27	27
Restricted activities	37	32	34	36
Overweight-obese	57	57	60	54
Inactive	57	60	56	52
Eats fewer than 5 servings of fruit and vegetables	55	53	56	51
Smokes regularly or occasionally	10	8	12	11
Drinks on daily basis	22	10	22	21

Source of data: CCHS: 2.1 (2003), 3.1 (2005), 4.1 (2007), 2008, 2009, 2010, 2011, 2012. Canada excluding Quebec and the Territories. Weighted data based on a sample of 7,640 Francophones and 157,312 Canadians aged 65 years and over.

Chronic Disease among Francophone Seniors

In response to questions about chronic disease, one of every two Francophone seniors claims to suffer from asthma (41% in Atlantic Canada, 50% in Ontario, 44% in the West), the most prevalent condition, followed by high blood pressure (49% in Atlantic Canada, 47% in Ontario, 43% in the West). Back problems affect more than one person in four (23% in Atlantic Canada, 29% in Ontario, 27% in the West). Diabetes affects 16% of Francophone seniors in Atlantic Canada, 19% in Ontario, and 16% in the West; heart disease afflicts a similar number (17% in Atlantic Canada, 21% in Ontario, and 18% in the West). Approximately one senior in twenty reports having cancer (7% in Atlantic Canada, 8% in Ontario and in the West); a stomach ulcer (7% in Atlantic Canada, 5% in Ontario, 4% in the West); a cardiovascular accident (CVA) (4% in Atlantic Canada, 5% in Ontario and the West); a mood disorder (6% in Atlantic Canada and the West, 5% in Ontario); or anxiety (6% in Atlantic Canada and Ontario, 4% in the West).

Table 3. Chronic Diseases

	65 yrs+ Canada (%)	Francophones 65 years and over		
		Atlantic (%)	Ontario (%)	West (%)
Asthma	45	41	50	44
High blood pressure	48	49	47	43
Bach aches (other than fibromyalgia and arthritis)	28	23	29	27
Diabetes	17	16	19	16
Heart disease	18	17	21	18
Cancer	7	7	8	8
Stomach ulcer	4	7	5	4
Cardiovascular accident (CVA)	5	4	5	5
Mood disorders	6	6	5	6
Anxiety	4	6	6	4

Source of data: CCHS: 2.1 (2003), 3.1 (2005), 4.1 (2007), 2008, 2009, 2010, 2011, 2012. Canada excluding Quebec and the Territories. Weighted data based on a sample of 7,640 Francophones and 157,312 Canadians aged 65 years and over.

Health Needs, Use of Health Services, and Difficulties Accessing Services

The vast majority of Francophone seniors have a family physician (97% in Atlantic Canada, 94% in Ontario and the West). Nevertheless, apart from those in New Brunswick (an officially bilingual province), most say they cannot speak French with him or her—the 69% in Atlantic Canada is offset by the lower figures of 33% in Ontario and 6% in the West. The most pressing need for health care is for routine care, according to statements by almost three-quarters of Francophone seniors (74% in Atlantic Canada, 67% in Ontario, 66% in the West). More than one third of Francophone seniors claim to need specialized care (33% in Atlantic Canada and the West, 35% in Ontario) and health information (32% in Atlantic Canada, 27% in Ontario, 33% in the West). One person in five expresses a need for urgent care (22% in the Atlantic and Western regions, 17% in Ontario) and one in ten needs non-urgent surgery (13% in the Atlantic and Western regions, 10% in Ontario). Difficulties in obtaining the necessary services are a reality for 10 to 20% of seniors, depending on the nature of the health care they need. The need for routine care is the most obvious, and about 7% of seniors (8% in Atlantic Canada, 7% in Ontario, 6% in the West) find it hard to obtain. Specialized care seems to be the most difficult type of service to receive (15% in Atlantic Canada, 16% in Ontario, and 19% in the West), followed by non-urgent surgery (10% in Atlantic Canada, 15% in Ontario, 12% in the West) and urgent care (16% in Atlantic Canada, 14% in Ontario, 9% in the West).

The proportion of Francophone seniors who state they received home care during the past year is 15% (20% in Atlantic Canada, 14% in Ontario, 13% in the West) and 34% indicate they were hospitalized (47% in Atlantic Canada, 29% in Ontario and in the West).

Table 4. Needs, Use, and Difficulty Accessing Health Services

	65 yrs+ Canada (%)	Francophones 65 years and over		
		Atlantic (%)	Ontario (%)	West (%)
Has a family physician	96	97	94	94
Usually speaks French with physician	2	69	33	6
Need for routine care	64	74	67	66
Need for specialized care	39	33	35	33
Need for health information	39	32	27	33
Need for urgent care	21	22	17	22
Need for non-urgent surgery	11	13	10	13
Difficulty obtaining routine care	9	8	7	6
Difficulty obtaining specialized care	18	15	16	19
Difficulty obtaining information	12	10	10	13
Difficulty obtaining urgent care	16	16	14	9
Difficulty obtaining non-urgent surgery	16	10	15	12
Home care	14	20	14	13
Hospitalization	35	47	29	29

Source of data: CCHS: 2.1, 3.1, 4.1, 2009 and 2011. Canada excluding Quebec and the Territories. Weighted data based on a sample of 3,630 Francophones and 36,380 Canadians aged 65 years and over.

To summarize, the situation of Francophone seniors is more affected by the rate of aging (18%); a larger proportion of them lack a high school diploma (34%); they live in the lowest-income quintile (30%); are alone (30%); and live in a rural setting (30%). These social determinants have an important influence on the state of health of Francophone seniors and their use of social services and health care. Significant numbers perceive themselves to be in poor health (27%) and need help with everyday tasks (28%); say their activities are restricted by a chronic condition (34%); are sedentary (56%); and report being overweight or obese (58%). These factors contribute to the burden of chronic disease. Although the majority have a family physician (95%), only 38% overall say they speak French with their doctor; however, there is a wide variation depending on the status of the official languages in the provinces. A substantial percentage (69%) of Francophone seniors say they need routine care; a large majority of them are quite fortunate in that these services are not difficult to obtain. All the same, between 10% and 20% of these seniors do experience problems with obtaining health care. Interestingly, one senior out of every three (34%) was hospitalized during the year preceding the survey. This portrait is coloured by regional variations. Francophone seniors in the Atlantic provinces are the most vulnerable socio-economically; more of them say they are in poor health and that they require routine care and home care. On the other hand, this is the region where the largest proportion of Francophone seniors can speak French with their family physicians, given New Brunswick's status as an officially bilingual province.

The Issue of Health Literacy: Incidence among Francophone Seniors

The level of health literacy refers to the capacity of a patient to understand the treatment and care she or he receives and it is recognized as a core determinant of health:

> Importantly, we now understand that poor health literacy adversely affects people's health. Literacy has been shown to be one of the strongest predictors of health status along with age, income, employment status, education level and race or ethnic group. (Jakab in Kickbusch *et al.*, 2013, p. iv)

The people who are the most at risk for having a lower level of literacy are, first and foremost, those with the least education. As we pointed out earlier, more than a third of Francophones 65 years and over have not graduated from high school. In previous empirical studies, we noted the importance of health literacy for seniors living in official language minority communities in different regions of Ontario (Bouchard *et al.*, 2012a). Difficulties having access to social services and health care to meet the user's linguistic and cultural needs, especially in rural areas or in settings where the minority community was extremely small, were clearly identified. These problems are closely intertwined with the literacy gaps among Francophone seniors and lead to increased difficulties in communicating with health professionals, thereby aggravating the harmful effects of language barriers on health.

Gaps in education among Francophone seniors suffering from one or more chronic disease(s) affect their comprehension and their communication with health professionals, which may compromise the quality of services received and thus their health. Although the specialized language of medicine may make the patient feel insecure, this problem is exacerbated if communication is, in addition, made more difficult by the lack of linguistic concordance between the professional and the senior (Bouchard *et al.*, 2010, p. 19).

In minority language contexts, the low level of literacy among seniors has a high impact on matters of health. In their 2012 analysis for the Public Health Agency of Canada, Mitic and Rootman revealed literacy deficits are even more pronounced in a second language. As defined above, literacy refers to general knowledge about health and being able to understand health issues, and thus is connected to the ability of individuals to obtain necessary health services and to apply medical advice and information correctly.

The conceptual model produced by the Regional Office for Europe of the World Health Organization (WHO) breaks health literacy into sub-categories: these include access and the ability to obtain information about medical care and services, prevention, illness, and health promotion, as well as being able to understand the information, evaluate it, and apply it to one's own situation (Kickbusch *et al.*, 2013; Sørensen *et al.*, 2012).

Table 5. The European Health Literacy Survey: The 12 Subdimensions as Defined by the Conceptual Model

Health literacy	Access or obtain information relevant to health	Understand information relevant to health	Appraise, judge, or evaluate information relevant to health	Apply or use information relevant to health
Health care	**1)** Ability to access information on medical or clinical issues	**2)** Ability to understand medical information and derive meaning	**3)** Ability to interpret and evaluate medical information	**4)** Ability to make informed decisions on medical issues
Disease prevention	**5)** Ability to access information on risk factors	**6)** Ability to understand information on risk factors and derive meaning	**7)** Ability to interpret and evaluate information on risk factors	**8)** Ability to judge the relevance of the information on risk factors
Health promotion	**9)** Ability to update oneself on health issues	**10)** Ability to understand health-related information and derive meaning	**11)** Ability to interpret and evaluate information on health-related issues	**12)** Ability to form a reflected opinion on health issues

Source: Adapted from "Health literacy and public health: a systematic review and integration of definitions and models," by K. Sørensen et al., 2012, *BMC Public Health*, 12, p. 80.

Furthermore, the effects of deficits in health literacy, or simply partial understanding, may be direct or indirect, as shown in research (Petch *et al.*, 2004) summarized in the DÉAAC report on aging, literacy, and health (Racine, 2008):

> Although the direct repercussions are more obvious [for example the inability to read or to understand a prescription] . . . the indirect consequences are no less significant. These are such problems as . . . stress, vulnerability, poor lifestyle, and longer and more frequent hospital stays. (Racine, 2008, p. 20)

Finally, we should point out that development of health literacy skills is a matter of concern to all those who work in the health system, as well as the users themselves, of course. We recognize that **citizens** need to be making decisions about their health for themselves, not merely responding to decisions made for them by others; **patients** should be truly engaged and empowered to engage in care decisions; **professionals** have a responsibility to tailor their communication to meet the needs of their patients and see it as their responsibility to foster their health literacy; and **politicians** need to incorporate the notion and paradigm of health literacy into their design of policy, their research agendas, and their objectives for population health (Mitic & Rootman, 2012; Kickbusch *et al.*, 2005).

It is undeniably important that if we are to improve health services for the entire population of seniors (and in particular for Francophone seniors in official language minority communities), we must encourage all actors to consider the importance of health literacy and to help all seniors develop health literacy skills. This communication issue has a tangible impact on health (health promotion, quality of care, prevention) and disproportionately affects Francophone seniors who live in minority communities. They face a triple challenge in literacy: they are very often socialized in their second language, English; they have less education; and they are insufficiently equipped to understand the specialized language of medicine. In this regard, we feel it pertinent to reiterate certain recommendations offered in our earlier research (Bouchard *et al.*, 2012a), namely: actively offer services in French; train and fund "facilitators"; create, evaluate, and adapt communication tools; establish more local services; train service providers on language rights; and, finally, create an online or print lexicon of medical terms in French and English.

The Issue of the Active Offer of French-Language Health Services: A Step toward Equity

Research conducted with Ontario health professionals in 2011–2012 on the concept of the active offer of French-language services allows us to identify several options designed to mitigate the disparity of health outcomes among Francophones in official language minority communities. From the outset, we thought it wise to adopt a working definition of the approach:

> Active offer can be defined as a verbal or written invitation to users to express themselves in the official language of their choice. The active offer to speak their language must precede the request for such services. For active offer to exist, the offer must be visible, audible, accessible (spoken), and clear, and greetings and services for Francophones must be automatic, like a reflex, and immediate. (Bouchard *et al.*, 2012b, p. 46)

This definition integrates several elements reflecting the characteristics of a person's experience as a member of a minority that are even more prevalent for members of an aging population. We have every reason to believe the active offer of services in French encourages Francophones to choose health services in their own language (Bouchard *et al.*, 2012a; Forgues & Landry, 2014; Deveau *et al.*, 2014), and that an approach focused on waiting for a person's request for services in French is a less effective option. In a situation where they are vulnerable, Francophone seniors are less likely to demand services in their mother tongue even if the services exist—unless they are offered explicitly. This stems from their experience of being culturally marginalized. "To dare to assert oneself or to advocate for one's rights in a minority context, one has to not only believe the situation is unjust, but also trust that it can change" (Forgues & Landry, 2014, p. 98).

The fact that it is necessary to not merely respond to a request for services in French but to instinctively offer them "up front" has been recognized by the Consultative Committee for French-Speaking Minority Communities (CCFSMSC), the Official Language Community Development Bureau, and the Ontario Office of the French Language Services Commissioner, among others.

Our own research led us to make five necessary recommendations (Bouchard *et al.*, 2012b) for promoting an active offer of French-language services: a working definition of active offer; a communication strategy for active offer; measures to ensure the system is accountable for providing French-language services (FLS); a commitment to FLS on the part of service providers; and finally, the development of tools and practices for active offer that are shared and readily available.

The necessity of offering actively—visibly, audibly, and in a way that is clearly understood—has also been emphasized by the Regional Office for Europe of the WHO:

> Providing signage in minority languages not only helps ethnic minority patients find their way around hospitals but also creates a sense of belonging and inclusiveness. Although plain language is important in conveying messages, other means of communication such as images, photographs, graphic illustrations, audio and videos should be considered in producing materials. (Kickbusch *et al.*, 2013, p.19)

In our opinion, this type of approach, while it may vary among different regions, is very promising. Developing active offer in this way would contribute to better and more effective services and, ultimately, to better health in official language minority communities across Canada.

Conclusion

In this short chapter, we reviewed the specific situation of Francophone seniors living in official language minority communities as it relates to their state of health and their access to services. This review was intended to remind us of the disadvantages experienced by these groups in terms of both the major social determinants of health and access to resources in their own language, despite the fact French is recognized by the federal government as an official language. With this situation in mind, we were interested in learning more about two issues: health literacy and the active offer of services, including information that is written in appropriate language and culturally sensitive. In our view, it is vital that these issues—though utterly distinct in each Canadian region, province and territory—be addressed if we are to plan for a future in which health services are fair, equitable, and offered in the minority official language.

Notes

1. Our research program was supported by the Ontario Ministry of Health and Long-Term Care and its Applied Health Research Network Initiative (AHRNI) and the *Réseau de recherche appliquée sur la santé des francophones de l'Ontario (RRASFO 2009–2014)*. The analyses were conducted by Data

Services at Carleton, Ottawa, Outaouais (CDR-COO), a member of the Canadian Research Data Centre Network (CRDCN). We would like to thank Ewa Sucha, who is responsible for data processing for the CCHS.

References

Ava, J.-B., *et al.* (2004). The effect of English language proficiency on length of stay and in-hospital mortality. *Journal of General Internal Medicine,* 19(3): 221–228.

Baillis, D. S., Segall, A., & Chipperfield, J. G. (2003). Two views of self-rated general health status, *Social Science & Medicine,* 56: 203–217.

Beaulieu, M. (2010). *Formation linguistique, adaptation culturelle et services de santé en français.* Ottawa, Société Santé en français et CNFS.

Bélanger, M. (2003). *Access to Health Care for the Official Language Minority Communities: Legal Bases, Current Initiatives and Future Prospects,* Standing Committee on Official Languages, Canada.

Bouchard, L., Batal, M., Imbeault, P., Sedigh, G., Silva, E.E., & Sucha, E. (2015). Précarité des populations francophones âgées vivant en situation linguistique minoritaire. *Minorités linguistiques et société / Linguistic Minorities and Society,* 6: 66–81.

Bouchard, L., Chomienne, M.-H., Benoit, M., Boudreau, F., & Lemonde, M. (2010). *Rapport de recherche du CNFS. Impact de la situation linguistique minoritaire sur les soins de santé pour des personnes âgées francophones de l'Ontario souffrant de maladies chroniques: une étude qualitative exploratoire.* Ontario.

Bouchard, L., Chomienne, M.-H., Benoit, M., Boudreau, F., Lemonde, M., & Dufour, S. (2012a). Do chronically ill, elderly Francophone patients believe they are adequately served by Ontario's health care system? Exploratory study of the effect of minority-language communities. *Canadian Family Physician,* 58, December: e686–e687. Retrieved from http://www.cfp.ca/content/58/12/e686.full. Accessed February 8, 2017.

Bouchard, L., & Desmeules, M. (2011). *Minorités de langue officielle du Canada: égales devant la santé?* Montréal: Presses de l'Université du Québec.

Bouchard, L., & Desmeules, M. (2013). Les minorités linguistiques du Canada et la santé, *Healthcare Policy / Politiques de santé,* 9 (special number): 38–47.

Bouchard, L., Desmeules, M., & Beaulieu, M. (2012b). L'offre active de services de santé en français in Ontario: une mesure d'équité. *Reflets: revue d'intervention sociale et communautaire,* 18(2), 36–65.

Bouchard, L., Gaboury, I., Chomienne, M.-H., Gilbert, A., & Dubois, L. (2009). La santé en situation linguistique minoritaire. *Healthcare Policy / Politiques de santé,* 4(4), 36–42.

Bouchard, L., & Leis, A. (2008). La santé en français. In J.-Y. Thériault *et al.* (Eds.) *L'espace francophone en milieu minoritaire au Canada: nouveaux enjeux, nouvelles mobilisations*. Montréal: Fides.

Bowen, S. (2001). *Language Barriers in Access to Health Care / Barrières linguistiques dans l'accès aux soins de santé*. Health Canada Minister of Public Works and Government Services, Canada.

Deveau, K., Landry, R., & Allard, R. (2009). *Utilisation des services de langue française. Une étude auprès des Acadiens et francophones de la Nouvelle-Écosse sur les facteurs associés à l'utilisation des services gouvernementaux en français*. Moncton, NB:, Institut canadien de recherche sur les minorités linguistiques.

Flores, G. (2006). Language barriers to health care in the United States. *New England Journal of Medicine*, 355(3), 229–231.

Forgues, É., & Landry, R. (2014). *L'accès aux services de santé en français et leur utilisation en contexte francophone minoritaire*. Moncton, NB:, Institut canadien de recherche sur les minorités linguistiques.

Forgues, É., Doucet, M., & Noel, J.G. (2011). L'accès des aînés francophones aux foyers de soins en milieu minoritaire, un enjeu linguistique en santé et mieux-être. *La Revue canadienne du vieillissement*, 30(4), 603–616.

Hu, D. J., & Covell, M. (1998). Health care usage by Hispanic outpatients as a function of primary language. *Western Journal of Medicine*, 144: 490–493.

Kickbusch, I., Pelikan, J.M., Apfel, F., & Tsouros, A.D. (Ed.) (2013). *Health Literacy: The Solid Facts*. Copenhagen: World Health Organization, Regional Office for Europe.

Kickbusch, I., Wait, S., & Maag, D. (2005). *Navigating Health: The Role of Health Literacy*. Retrieved from http://www.ilonakickbusch.com/kickbusch-wAssets/docs/NavigatingHealth.pdf, p.16. Retrieved Feb. 8, 2017.

Leis, A., & Bouchard, L. (2013). Éditorial: La santé des populations de langue officielle en situation minoritaire. *Revue canadienne de santé publique*, 104(6), supplement 1: S3—24.

Makvandi, E., Sedigh, G., Bouchard, L., & P.-J. Bergeron (2013). Methodological issues in analyzing small populations using CCHS cycles based on the official language minority studies. *Canadian Journal of Public Health*, 104(6), S55–S59.

Mitic, W., & I. Rootman, I. (Eds.). (2012). *An Inter-sectoral Approach for Improving Health Literacy for Canadians*. Victoria: Public Health Agency of Canada.

Petch, E., Ronson, B., & Rootman, I. (2004). *Literacy and Health in Canada: What We Have Learned and What Can Help in the Future? A Research Report*. Ottawa: CIHR. Retrieved from http://www.cpha.ca/uploads/portals/h-l/literacy_e.pdf. Retrieved February 9, 2017.

Racine, A. (Ed.) (2008). *Étude exploratoire sur l'analphabétisme en lien avec la santé et le vieillissement de la population*. Québec: Ministère de l'Éducation, du Loisir et du Sport, Direction de l'éducation des adultes et de l'action communautaire (DEAAC).

Sarver, J., & Baker, D.W. (2000). Effect of language barriers on follow-up appointments after an emergency department visit. *Journal of Internal Medicine*, 15(4), 256–264.

Solis, J., Marks, G., & Shelton, D. (1990). Acculturation, access to care, and use of preventive services by Hispanics: Findings from HHANES 1982–84. *American Journal of Public Health*, 80, supplement: 11–19.

Sørensen, K., Van den Broucke, S., Fullam, J., Doyle, G., Pelikan, J., Slonska, Z., Brand, H., & Consortium Health Literacy Project European (HLS-EU). (2012). Health literacy and public health: A systematic review and integration of definitions and models. *BMC Public Health*, 12:80. http://doi.org/10.1186/1471-2458-12-80. Retrieved April 17, 2015.

Statistics Canada (2012). The Canadian Population in 2011: Age and Sex. Analytical document. Retrieved from http://www12.statcan.gc.ca/census-recensement/ 2011/as-sa/98-311-x/98-311-x2011001-eng.pdf. Accessed June 9, 2015.

Statistics Canada (2012). Population according to mother tongue and age groups, (65 years and over), percentage breakdown (2011), for Canada, provinces and territories. Retrieved from http://www12.statcan.gc.ca/census-recensement/2011/. Accessed June 18, 2014.

Tremblay, S. (2012). *Étude sur les services de santé linguistiquement et culturellement adaptés: portrait pancanadien*. Ottawa: Société Santé en français.

Woloshin, S., Schwartz, L.M., Katz, S.J., & Welch, H.G. (1997). Is language a barrier to the use of preventive services? *Journal of General Internal Medicine*, 12(8), 472–477.

Yeo, S. (2004). Language barriers and access to care. *Annual Review of Nursing Research*, 22(1), 59–75.

The Experience of Francophones in Eastern Ontario: The Importance of Key Facilitators (Service Users and Providers) and the Influence of Structures Supporting the Health and Social Services System[1]

Marie Drolet, Jacinthe Savard, Sébastien Savard, Josée Lagacé,
Isabelle Arcand, Lucy-Ann Kubina, and Josée Benoît, *University of Ottawa*

Abstract

This chapter describes the experiences of Francophones in eastern Ontario in terms of access to social services and health care. The experiences and perspectives of 40 parents, seniors, and caregivers were collected through semi-structured interviews. Qualitative analysis of the transcripts, as well as visual analysis of the trajectories of a subgroup of nine participants, made it possible to identify facilitators and challenges these users experienced in accessing French-language services, either from their perspective or that of their caregivers. More specifically, this chapter emphasizes elements that facilitate access; these are discussed in order to share the lessons learned, which can contribute to improvements in social services and health care in official language minority communities.

Key Words: access to services in French, Ontario Francophones, qualitative analysis.

Introduction

This chapter describes the experience of Francophones in eastern Ontario who access social services and health care. Connecting this analysis to the sociology of organizations presented in Chapter 1, this chapter begins by outlining the context of the current state of French-language services in Ontario. This is followed by an analysis of the actors and systems of action that define the social space in which services are offered, and then by a review of theoretical reference points on the idea of minority identity. The contextualization will allow for a better understanding of the service trajectories reported by the participants in this study, which are discussed in the second part of the chapter.

The Context of French-Language Services in Ontario

According to the 2011 Census (Statistics Canada, 2015), Ontario's Francophone minority represents 4.3% of the population. In calculating the numbers, Statistics Canada includes 500,275 people who speak French as their first official language and half of the 84,225 people who learned French and English simultaneously.

The *French Language Services Act* of 1986 (Office of the French Language Services Commissioner, 2009) guarantees the public the right to receive services in French from the ministries and organizations of the Government of Ontario located in 26 designated regions. However, organizations that are partially funded by the province and provide services to the public (such as hospitals, children's aid societies, and long-term care facilities for seniors) are not automatically covered by the *French Language Services Act*; these facilities can, however, voluntarily ask for a designation. The designation may be complete ("designated") or partial ("partially designated," which means certain services or programs are offered by the organization but not by others). Under some circumstances, facilities may be strongly urged to ask to be designated by the Local Health Integration Network (LHIN) and the French Language Health Planning Entity in their region. The mandate of the French Language Health Planning Entities is to advise the LHINs on the organization of French-language services in their region (Ontario Ministry of Health and Long-Term Care, 2012), whereas the mandate of the LHINs is to improve coordination and cooperation within Ontario's health system.[2] To accomplish this, they have control over the distribution of the majority of resources within their boundaries, with the exception of physicians, who are covered by the Ontario Health Insurance Plan (OHIP).

Health services covered also include certain social service organizations, such as community support services. For example, Champlain LHIN (Eastern Ontario) is responsible for planning, coordinating, and financing services in the following sectors: hospitals; home care agencies and community care access centres; mental health and addiction agencies; community support services (e.g., Meals on Wheels); community health centres; and long-term care facilities or residences (Champlain LHIN, n.d.).

Actors in the System

According to Champagne, Contandriopoulos, Picot-Touché, Béland and Nguyen (2005), the health and social services system can be conceptualized as an organized system of actions, located in a concrete geographical and temporal context:

> Its structure is formed by the interaction of a particular physical structure (buildings, architecture, technical platforms, public and private financial resources), an organizational structure defined by provincial and federal laws, the regulations in effect, the operating rules adopted over time (governance), and a specific symbolic structure (representation of health, life, disease, collective values and norms). It delineates a structured social space in which four large groups of actors (professionals, managers, commercial representatives and political representatives) interact in order to accomplish one or several collective projects that contribute to achieving the objectives of the health service system. The primary goal of the health system is to reduce the duration and intensity of disease by enabling any person suffering from an illness to have free and equitable access to quality health care and social services. (p. 18)

This analytical framework proves to be very useful for understanding the various structures that influence the organization of services and access to them, as the way they are organized has an impact on the experience of service users navigating the health and social service system, including minority official language users. Nevertheless, some important actors are missing from this analytical framework: the persons using these services and their caregivers.

Improving the System: The Interaction Between
Two Actors—Provider and Service User

To improve the health system, as well as specific practices in health care and social services therewith in, the Ontario Ministry of Health and Long-Term Care (2007) decided to look for better ways to manage chronic health problems. This meant thinking differently about the way care and services were distributed. The design of the restructuring was founded on two evidence-based models in the area of chronic illness: (1) the Chronic Care Model (CCM) developed by Wagner and his colleagues in 1996 and used internationally (Wagner, Austin, & Korff, 1986); and (2) a variation of this model developed in Western Canada by Barr and her colleagues in 2003 and known as the Expanded Chronic Care Model (ECCM) (McCurdy, MacKay, Badley, Veinot, & Cott, 2008).

The basis for the realignment in the Chronic Care Model is to create a dynamic relationship between the care and service provider (physician/health and social service team) and the person who receives the care and services (as well as his or her caregivers). The goals of integrating the relationships into the model are to improve the quality of the services, to adopt an approach more focused on meeting the needs expressed by the user and the caregiver, and to obtain better outcomes (Bodenheimer, Wagner, & Grumbach, 2002). The productive interactions between these two partners (provider and user) change the paradigm of urgent and short-term health care (expert provider and passive user) and transform it into cooperation among the caregivers, the service user, and the providers of health care and social services (Bodenheimer et al., 2002). The provider becomes proactive, open to networking: an approach with multiple components. The service user and caregivers, better informed and equipped to manage the former's chronic health condition, are also invited to be proactive and to undertake behavioural and lifestyle changes (Wagner et al., 2001). From this starting point, a new arrangement of actors will take shape.

The Expanded Chronic Care Model promotes not only this interaction between a well-informed and well-equipped user and a well-prepared and proactive service team, but also the use of community resources, the creation of supportive environments, enhanced community participation, and the development of public policies that foster health and wellness (Barr et al., 2003). The Ontario framework, inspired by the model, strives to improve the health of the population—and especially of under-served groups, including Francophone minority language communities—by attaching value to and encouraging productive relationships among community members, service providers, health and social service organizations, community workers, and community organizations (Ontario Ministry of Health and Long-Term Care, 2007).

Social Identity and Minority Groups

Can people who live and work in minority language settings (users and service providers) become proactive while navigating the channels of the social services and health care system and thereby promote better access to safe, quality services provided in the minority language? Theories of social identity and minority groups help us to understand that becoming proactive while living in a minority community is, in itself, a complex phenomenon. Social identity is constructed through intergroup contacts in which individuals define their identity, to themselves and to others, in relation to the characteristics of their group of origin (Hogg & Abrams, 2003). People from the same group compare themselves favourably to other significant groups, characterizing themselves and their group in positive ways (Tajfel & Turner, 1986). Members of a given social group possessing particular assets are highly motivated to preserve them.

A dominant group in a given society will consider minority groups less important (Tajfel, 1978). To protect its positive identity, the minority community will be inclined to view itself as homogenous and consensual. Its members will tend to be more passive, to not stand out, to conform to norms including those of their own group, to turn inward toward their own community, ignoring certain individual differences in order to survive (Hogg & Abrams, 2003). When a person's social identity does not enable a positive self-image to develop, an individual may leave the minority group and join the majority group which is more highly valued and offers additional opportunities (Tajfel & Turner, 1986). People may go as far as allowing themselves to be assimilated to ensure they have access to a process of social integration into the new group and to achieve their personal aspirations. Between majority and minority language groups, the number, social status, and economic and political power are unequal; the majority group therefore appears attractive, as it has more resources and makes social insertion easier than the minority group.

Living in an English-dominant North American context, Francophones in official language minority communities face two challenges: the need to navigate daily between French and English, and the challenge to maintain the quality of their language of origin. Some people who are firmly rooted in a minority community speak a French coloured by English words and structures; that is, a non-standard language, which is used to communicate in familiar settings (Gérin-Lajoie & Labrie, 1999). This language not only marginalizes them, it arouses in them a sense of linguistic insecurity, which in turn leads to individuals (1) having negative reactions toward the way they learned to speak in their home environment; (2) alternating regularly between the minority and majority languages; and (3) making considerable efforts to correct their accents or vocabulary (Desabrais, 2010). Being confronted regularly with the limitations of their language makes them deeply conscious of their minoritization and the forms of language needed to advance to higher levels in the social hierarchy (i.e., standard majority and minority languages).

Objectives of the Study

As a result of these challenges, and in the wake of the question raised previously, the objective of this study was to learn how actors in a minority official language community (users and service providers) can become proactive within the various layers of social services and health care, act in a way that promotes better access to these services, and thus counteract the rather negative theoretical view of minority groups. While the study has attempted to understand the facilitators and the challenges associated with access to social services and health care in French experienced by Francophone service users, we deal with specific aspects in more depth in this chapter: the way key facilitators (caregivers or professional service providers) are able to overcome the obstacles to access they encounter, and the influence of structures that frame the delivery of these services on access to services in French. Emphasis will be placed on the elements that facilitate access in order to outline how to improve social services and health care in Ontario and, more broadly, services in official language minority communities in a wide range of contexts. This may be achieved through acquiring a better understanding of the social actors who, through their strong and dynamic presence, play key roles in improving the situation of the individual or the state of the system.

Methodology

Participants

Between summer 2012 and spring 2014, we met 40 caregivers in the Greater Ottawa Area: 24 parents of school-age children or youth (aged 6 to 18) experiencing difficulties with communication and social integration, as well as 16 caregiver-senior dyads (i.e., caregivers) of seniors 65 years of age and older who were having difficulties with communication resulting from a neurological injury. The parents were recruited with the help of resource people in a community social services centre, a community clinic, and a Francophone school board. The seniors and their caregivers were reached through a community clinic, a day centre, and a community services centre. Recruiting seniors and their caregivers proved to be more complicated. We learned that family members and friends who cared for seniors are overwhelmed by their daily responsibilities; this explains the smaller number of caregivers who participated. In the remainder of this chapter, the term caregiver will be defined in its broadest meaning, encompassing the reality of parents and people who are close to the senior and provide care and services. It is a well-known fact that parents are often the first in line to ask for services for their children. In the same vein, seeking out services that are needed and appropriate is one responsibility among many that caregivers perform for seniors.

We also interviewed a subgroup of nine caregivers or caregiver-senior dyads for a second time in order to better understand the pathways they followed through the health and social service sector.

Data Collection

Data were collected in semi-structured interviews coordinated by a research associate with a doctorate in education. The interviews were conducted by four research assistants, three of whom were graduate students in social work, and an occupational therapist with a master's in occupational therapy and more than 20 years of experience. They were assisted by a fifth team member who had completed a doctorate in education. Each of the interviews lasted between 60 and 90 minutes and took place either in the participant's home or in an office at the university, depending on the preference of the user or caregiver.

An interview grid designed by the research team investigated the following: the participant's background (family and community environment); the reasons that led the parent, senior, or caregiver to decide to obtain social services or health care for the child or senior; their use of different services and their service trajectories; the care they received; the successes and the difficulties they encountered; as well as their experience with the services they received in terms of the language in which they were provided. This protocol ensured that the interviews were sufficiently structured to suggest themes for discussion and, at the same time, were sufficiently flexible to let the participants speak freely during the interviews.

In a second interview involving a subgroup of participants, a diagram depicting each one's trajectory of service use (as the research team had interpreted it) was presented to them. The diagram was discussed to validate its accuracy and provide an opportunity to add clarifications or new information. Supplementary questions were added that addressed how important it was for participants to receive services in French, and the reasons for service interruptions or terminations.

Data Analysis

The interviews were recorded on audio tape, and transcribed in their entirety. The transcriptions were then imported into NVivo 10 (QSR International, 2012) data analysis software. Three research assistants coded interview data using a predetermined procedure: (1) a first reading of 20% of the transcriptions for the purpose of identifying categories (general annotation) and emerging themes (annotation specifying what is discussed) (Paillé & Mucchielli, 2008); (2) reaching an inter-rater consensus on the categories and themes among the research team members, who represented six different professions in the social services and health care sectors; (3) developing a list of codes (abbreviated forms of categories and themes); (4) validating the list of codes with the various members of the research team; and (5) coding the remainder of the data according to the list of codes identified, while leaving room for new codes to emerge. Thus, the data were analyzed deductively and inductively; each interview was examined thoroughly, then intergroup comparisons were made

(Huberman & Miles, 2002). The analyses showed that the data had reached saturation.

Complementary to the coding exercise was a visual analysis of the trajectories of the 12 participants who completed two interviews. To produce the diagram, the services requested and received by participants were placed in chronological order, indicating the language in which the services were received. The type of facility offering each service was noted, as was the status of that facility under the *French Language Services Act* (designated, partially designated, or non-designated). The means through which the participant accessed the service (referred by a professional, decided personally by the senior or the caregiver, etc.) were added, as well as the reasons for which the service was not received, or at least was not received in French.

In this chapter, we present an analysis of the transcriptions of participants noting critical incidents—that is, unexpected and sudden events that required the ability to adapt (DeBoer, 2011; Sharoff, 2008). When these incidents occurred, their problem-solving skills proved to be effective for obtaining services in French. We also highlight the structural elements associated with points of interruption/discontinuation and continuity in the access to services in French, which appeared in the visual analysis of the trajectories.

Results: Acting in a Way That Promotes French-Language Services

The experience of people living in an official language minority community (parents, seniors, and caregivers of seniors) in the context of each one's trajectory through health care and social services is punctuated with both obstacles and successes. Based on critical incidents and service trajectories, the results demonstrate the conditions for successful access to safe, quality services in French. Overall, it appears these conditions exist when caregivers with several assets or qualities meet professionals who are committed to providing quality health care and services and, in addition, are aware of the importance of language to the actual quality. This observation is in line with the Extended Chronic Care Model and the adaptation of this model in Ontario, both described above. While the analysis of trajectories identifies certain structural elements that influence the access to services in French, the analysis of critical incidents shows that when obstacles occur, service trajectories develop through turning points related to the actions of key facilitators. These include the caregivers themselves, as well as health professionals and social workers.

The Analysis of Critical Incidents: Turning Points

Interviews that addressed the turning points in social service and health care trajectories referred to triggers that signal a need for services, and opportunities to make links between services in order to benefit from networks of professionals, organizations and services.

Triggers

Triggers in the channels through social services and health care take diverse forms and can be different for children and for seniors who use services. Even though the people involved in the lives of service users may suspect that something is less than optimal, participants in this study usually identified an event or a critical incident that alerts them to needs and starts them on a search for services. Parents of children reported that the initial trigger occurred when a teacher or daycare staff member noticed an anomaly or difficulty—often behavioural in nature—and commented on it to parents/caregivers, thereby making them aware of a need and setting them off to seek services. The interviews showed that in seniors' experiences, the initial trigger is often a particular incident that results in a crisis, leading to the realization that their faculties have declined and services are needed.

Respondents shared many examples of times they received important information from a professional, which triggered their awareness of a need or of the severity of a problem, as this passage illustrates:

> [original: French] I told [the geriatrician] "We're going to Boston for a week." And he looked at me and said: "No way . . . It's too dangerous, you're going to change her surroundings and when you get back, she'll lose even more." I didn't know that. . . . He was right. (B012-E1)

This kind of trigger has an influence on what happens next and on the direction the trajectory takes afterwards, as the awareness shapes subsequent decisions made by the person's caregiver.

Links and Networking

Besides the events that activated the search for services, the triggers in the course of services often take the form of links between points of service and organizations. The linkages depend on several conditions that promote networking among people in the minority language community. The elements are sometimes associated with caregivers, or with health professionals or social workers, and at other times with organizations or facilities that provide services.

Caregivers and Seniors

The capacity to link to care and services, especially in French, stems partly from qualities that some caregivers possess. Of particular importance is their open-mindedness, which encourages them to explore every avenue of services offered by support groups, community organizations, and other service providers. These avenues may be useful because they offer services that meet an identified need, or because they lead to other options. Caregivers who find effective paths through the system, especially those who locate French-language services, are proactive: they take charge of the situation by using every opportunity to ask questions of the professionals they meet, and by creating close connections to professionals who seem to be proactive themselves. As one respondent explained, [original: French] "The case manager who was supposed to be looking after our file didn't call us back. When people don't move fast or when I don't get my calls returned, I call my contact person again. Then things get moving!" (B003-E2)

Health and Social Service Providers

Clearly, the ability of health professionals and social workers to network may also create important turning points in effective service trajectories. The service users we met mentioned the communication skills of key professionals. They found that these service providers, who engage in sustained and effective communication with them, as well as with their colleagues and other organizations, help them to find better supports. Respondents illustrated this idea by sharing examples of professionals who know the health care and social services system thoroughly and, in particular, *where* to find French-language services. They are able to offer good advice on options to explore and are especially helpful when users or caregivers feel they are at a dead end. While respondents navigate their way through health and social services by trial and error, they place inestimable value on advice from someone who knows the pathway and can show them a short cut. One caregiver exclaimed: [original: French] "I would have never found that by myself!" (B007-E1)

Inter-Organizational Collaboration

Finally, networking among organizations that offer health care and social services makes it possible to locate services in French more readily. [original: French] "When I said I was Francophone . . . she told me: 'Listen, I'm going to give your name to a Francophone who works here right away.' The guy phoned me five minutes later!" (B001-E1). The participants stressed how helpful and cooperative the links between organizations offering French-language services are for them. They gave several examples of times when services are streamlined because there are agreements or understandings among organizations. This can be seen in the example of a service provider in a designated facility who directs the user toward other facilities that are designated or partially designated to offer services in French.

> [original: French] It was them [social worker at X Hospital, designated] who told us about Y Centre, which is designated. . . . They told us: "Go register there . . ." They're the ones who linked us up with Z agency for home care services, which is partially designated. (B011-E2)

Structural Elements of Trajectories

Through an in-depth analysis of the structural elements in the trajectories, it becomes obvious that when a need for services is identified in a child who attends a Francophone school, professionals in the school generally refer the child to services offered in French. The lack of resources available sometimes causes interruptions in the trajectories; accordingly, both caregivers and service providers make efforts to bypass or overcome them. In any case, since schools are organized along linguistic lines in Ontario, social workers, health professionals, and educational professionals who work in Francophone school districts are usually aware of the Francophone or bilingual resources that exist in the public and private sectors.

Services for seniors, on the other hand, are not organized according to language, hence much less consistency is observed in the referrals of Francophones to services in their language. This realization led our team to analyze the trajectories of nine seniors in more detail. The channels they pursue through the system reveal some important structural elements concerning access to social services and health care in French.

In terms of symbolic structure, some users attribute more importance than others to obtaining services in their language. A clear request generally ensures better continuity in access to services in French, although it does not actually guarantee it. Access to services in French is also modulated by the availability of the services, as will be seen later.

With respect to the organizational structure of social services and health care, we can see some of the effects of the legal framework that governs French-language services in Ontario. In the nine trajectories analyzed in detail, services received from designated facilities are always available in French. On the other hand, in partially designated facilities, participants almost always experience interruptions: either the services are not available in French at certain times of the day, or only some services are offered in French.

The choice to go to a designated facility for specific care or services is not always up to the individual or to the professional providing advice. Some services are not offered in designated facilities. For example, when she had a cerebral vascular accident (CVA), B008 went to a community hospital that was designated under the *French Language Services Act*. Because the treatments required for a hemorrhagic CVA were not available there, she was transferred to a partially designated university hospital where services in the neurology department were apparently not offered in French. The situation had an impact on the respondent: [original: French] "I didn't like that, that hospital (university hospital with neurology services). It was all in English." (B008-1)

Furthermore, the public health and social services system appears to lack resources to respond to the multiple needs of the population, regardless of the language of service. In a context such as this, many people are unable to receive the full range of services necessary for their health condition(s); instead, they receive the maximum available according to rules determined by budget restrictions. The people who are most proactive in demanding and justifying their need for services seem to succeed better in obtaining the services they need. The even more evident shortage of resources offering French-language services may result in a lack of continuity in services offered in French at certain times (e.g., on weekends or during vacation periods), less frequent access to specialists who speak French, or the need to ask a professional who does not speak the language for a second opinion if the user desires one.

When they reach the limit of public services, several people turn to private services or community organizations to meet their needs. Private services are not covered under the *French Language Service Act*. Finding service providers who speak French is often difficult, and some respondents decided to accept services in the language of the majority (for example, private overnight care [B001], private physiotherapy [B008], respite lodging [B011]). Community support groups can present good opportunities for networking; even when their activities take place in the majority language, participants from the minority language group may enjoy a chance to share services available in their language.

To summarize the situation, certain structural elements seem to facilitate access to services in French: the importance placed on language of service by participants or the professionals they meet; visiting a facility that is (fully) designated under the *French Language Services Act*; and networking among minority language speakers to share knowledge of existing resources in French.

Key Facilitators

Proactive Actors

In the service trajectories described to us, we saw that certain people are particularly effective in locating French-language services. These key figures can be seen as facilitators or facilitators in the respondent's route through the system. They include the caregivers and seniors themselves, as well as the health professionals and social workers whose efforts make it possible or easier to access services in French. The experiences shared by respondents reveal many characteristics and actions that define a key facilitator.

Caregivers

Interviews showed that certain qualities in caregivers are crucial in obtaining social services and health care in French. In several of the trajectories, we witness the tenacity of caregivers who take charge of the situation and insist on receiving services needed by the child or senior for whom they are caring. Participants told several stories about doing Internet searches and making numerous phone calls, contacting many different people, and asking questions repeatedly in order to take full advantage of the services available. Other qualities appear to be beneficial to the service trajectories, but they are not the norm for caregivers' behaviour. For example, some caregivers have experience in management or inside knowledge about the health and social service system, thereby allowing them to navigate more easily therein and obtain services needed by the child or senior they are supporting.

> [original: French] We're lucky my sister works in the system [as case manager], because if that wasn't the case, we would've had to start with the family doctor. And I don't know if our family doctor knows everything that's available. . . . I don't know what I would have done on my own. (B009-E2)

Health and Social Service Providers

Results show that the competency of health professionals and social workers is a decisive factor in the trajectories of people who use their services. Respondents told compelling stories about the explicit commitment of certain staff members they encountered when they tried to find services in French. The people distinguishing themselves most are those who make themselves available to listen to their clients' needs, advocate for them, maintain regular contact with their family members or support network, monitor closely and follow up on their situation, and ensure that they obtain the information and services they need. Besides this, key figures encourage the people they serve to find out about and take advantage of existing services and to be insistent in order to improve their chances of obtaining them.

> [original: French] The speech-language therapist and the prin-
> cipal encouraged me to ask for the speech-language therapist at
> the school board. Otherwise [child-user] would stay on the
> waiting list forever. The school really encouraged me a lot and
> supported me. . . . There was a need, and that principal saw it.
> (A014-E2)

The data emphasize the proactive capacity of service providers who play an important role in the service trajectories described. Their actions demonstrate a proactive approach centred on the person concerned, an ability to adapt strategies to target needs, and a high level of responsiveness and attention in order to tune into emerging needs. Several respondents also highlighted the humanity of the key person—that is, his or her ability to show empathy, openness and respect. They adapt to the needs and to the level of knowledge and language of the user and of the caregiver, making the care provided more accessible to them.

> [original: French] She [service provider] explained the test. She
> didn't talk to me like I was dumb, she wasn't condescending. . . .
> "Oh, wow! Yes, OK, I get what you're doing!" *Interviewer: Did
> you feel more involved that way?* Oh yes, oh yes, yes. And [child],
> he understood what was happening, too. He was less scared. He
> really liked going there. He wasn't afraid. (A012-E1)

Scope of Action

In the course of analyzing the data from interviews, we noticed with great interest that interactions with service providers who are engaged, proactive, sensitive, and encouraging have an extremely positive effect on the experience of the service users and caregivers. The importance of the role of these champions can be seen in the relief of respondents facing numerous difficulties in their attempt to get the social services and health care they need, especially in French. The users expressed their belief that they would have never reached such a positive conclusion without the support of these key profes-sionals. Moreover, several comments in the transcripts attest to the trust that users and caregivers have in the professionals who repre-sent key facilitators in their trajectories: [original: French]: "They didn't call me back. I went back to [the key professional], she told me, 'Don't worry, I'll look after it, things will get moving'. . . . Dear Lord, right then I knew it. 'Phew, she's going to call me back.'" (B003-E2). The interviews also illustrate the affective benefit these key figures have on the service users and caregivers interviewed. Several expressed a deep appreciation of these people, who have a major influence on their service trajectories. Their gratitude is, in part, linked to the connections that can generate new avenues to explore as they seek French-language services. It is also tied to the fact they are able to count on reliable and dedicated service providers.

In short, the experiences of the people who took part in this study reveal that the trajectories of social services and health care in French are complex and follow a meandering zigzag path. They are profoundly influenced by turning points that assume the form of triggers and links, which can be initiated by caregivers or service providers and may be supported by networks of organizations and programs that offer services in French. The experiences recounted by respondents also illustrate the central place occupied by key facilitators in the service trajectories that, in turn, are influenced by tenacious, proactive caregivers and engaged, empathetic service providers. The personal characteristics we identified in key individuals are clearly distinct from theories of minority identity. We would have expected that caregivers (and sometimes even professionals in minority language settings) would tend to be passive and conform to the behaviour and actions of the majority, and that they would not insist on receiving services in the minority language. Instead, proactive and cooperative interactions among users or caregivers and service providers truly seem to have made a difference to their experiences.

Discussion: Improving Social Services and Health Care in Official Language Minority Communities

This chapter draws from the experiences and perspectives of 40 parents, seniors, and caregivers who live in minority-language communities. The parents and caregivers are responsible for children and seniors who use French-language health and social services. Through an analysis of their service trajectories and critical incidents, we seek to identify the conditions that result in a successful active offer of services in French. A better understanding of these conditions will make it possible to provide safe, quality French-language services to people in official language minority communities, as part of the continuum of care and services in the health and social services sector.

The results clearly indicate both the advantages and the limitations of designating facilities under Ontario's *French Language Services Act* (1986) to offer services in French. It seems that in fully designated facilities the active offer of services in French is practised, while in partially designated facilities the active offer is not systematic. Although the list of partially designated facilities is public, it does not indicate which of the services or programs in each one are designated. Thus, it is not possible to know if any gaps in access to services in French in these facilities are due to the fact that the particular program is not designated, or to the poor implementation of the designation. It is possible that a partial designation is insufficient to create an organizational culture that promotes active offer, either in the designated programs or by bilingual service providers in other programs. In this context, the active offer of French-language services becomes dependent on the good will of the staff. In a situation where clients feel vulnerable and do not have all the information they need, they will be unable to figure out if they should expect to be served in their own language or not. They will be less likely to ask for services in French. Moreover, if they do ask for them but do not receive them, they will accept the answer without argument, as has been shown in the theoretical studies of social identity and minority groups (Hogg & Abrams, 2003; Tajfel, 1978; Tajfel & Turner, 1986).

In line with the Extended Chronic Care Model and the adaptation used in Ontario, numerous conditions for success are put in place when caregivers with specific personal qualities meet health and social service professionals who are committed to offering quality social services and health care and who recognize the importance of providing services to users in their own language. We have demonstrated the way the respondents' service trajectories changed course because of key facilitators (including the caregivers themselves) as well as health and social service professionals. These key figures may be Francophone, bilingual, or Francophile.

The respondents illustrated numerous turning points that underscore the action of key facilitators who are able to offer relevant and valuable information, thereby raising awareness of a need for appropriate services and launching the search. Once again, networking among people who speak the same language creates connections between caregivers and seniors, as well as connections with professionals and public or community organizations (Savard *et al.*, 2013). The networking and links often serve to initiate services or provide information on French-language services. The interviews also revealed the crucial role key facilitators play in paving the way towards services. Certain qualities in caregivers stand out, particularly their tenacity and their experience in management and knowledge of the health and social services system (Drolet *et al.*, 2015). Furthermore, the experiences they recounted emphasize the importance of the proven competency of professionals—especially their commitment and their proactive attitude. These qualities make service providers better able to support users and their families in their service trajectories, with the accent on ensuring as much of their experience as possible takes place in their own language.

The analysis presented here highlights the action of proactive parents and caregivers who take charge of their trajectories through the health and social services system in a minority language community. Our objective in doing so is to underline the conditions for success in the social service and health care trajectories of individuals who live in official language minority communities. The theoretical reference points of social identity and minority groups (Hogg & Abrams, 2003; Tajfel, 1978; Tajfel & Turner, 1986) suggest that people who speak a minority language tend to be passive and follow the lead of the majority, and do not insist on receiving services in their own language. On the other hand, a certain number of people who took part in this study do persevere in their efforts to obtain services in their own language and are often supported by proactive service providers. All the same, it should still be kept in mind that this proactive behaviour is not typical of the parents, seniors, and caregivers we met (nor of the population of minority official language speakers overall) in terms of asking for services in their language (Drolet *et al.*, 2015; Forgues & Landry, 2014). Instead, the strategies and attitudes they demonstrate emphasize the conditions we should encourage in order to support successful service trajectories. This is one way we can improve minority-language services.

Conclusion

This study demonstrates that access to social services and health care in official language minority communities is fostered both by structures that facilitate the organization of these services and by the perseverance of committed and proactive users and service providers. *Preventing and Managing Chronic Disease: Ontario's Framework* describes four important sub-dimensions that are prerequisite to successful implementation of the Framework's practice and system changes: strong leadership; aligned resources and incentives; commitment to quality improvement; and accountability for outcomes (Ontario Ministry of Health and Long-Term Care, 2007). The leadership of social and community actors is helpful in stimulating the request for services in the minority official language. Leadership in organizing services has also been shown to be crucial in stimulating the active offer of services in official language minority communities and the kind of organizational culture that supports it, thereby ensuring that services in the minority language are available as part of the continuum of care that an individual may need.

Leadership in the political arena and legal efforts in the area of language rights are undeniably vital. We must continue deepening our understanding of the benefits and limitations of the designation (full or partial) of facilities. Analyzing these influences in the future will help us find more and better ways to encourage professionals and managers in their efforts, as well as to give organizations the boost they need to foster the active offer of services to users in Francophone minority communities, especially in a province such as Ontario.

In summary, our study shows that political and legal structures facilitate access to official language services in minority settings, heighten awareness and autonomy among service users and caregivers, and also raise greater awareness and accountability among service providers. These positive outcomes make it possible to bridge existing gaps in the formal mechanisms where services in the language of the minority can be obtained.

Notes

1. This study was made possible through the financial support of the *CNFS—Secrétariat national*, which is funded by Health Canada under the *Roadmap for Canada's Official Languages 2013–2018* program.
2. This chapter deals with both health and social services: that is, practices in health care and in social services. However, we will use the term "health system" when discussing the specific elements under the jurisdiction of the Ministry of Health and Long-Term Care.

References

Barr, V. J., Robinson, S., Marin-Link, B., Underhill, L., Dotts, A., Ravensdale, D., & Salivaras, S. (2003). The expanded chronic care model: An integration of concepts and strategies from population health promotion and the chronic care model. *Healthcare Quarterly, 7*(1), 73–82. doi: 10.12927/hcq.2003.16763

Bodenheimer, T., Wagner, E. H., & Grumbach, K. (2002). Improving primary care for patients with chronic illness: The chronic care model, part 2. *JAMA, 288*(15), 1909–1914. doi: 10.1001/JAMA.288.15.1909

Boudreau, A., and Dubois, L. (2008). Représentations, sécurité/insécurité linguistique et éducation en milieu minoritaire. In P. Dalley, and S. Roy, (Eds.). *Francophonie, minorités et pédagogie* (pp. 145–176). Ottawa: Les Presses de l'Université d'Ottawa.

Boudreau, F. (1999). Langue minoritaire et services de santé mentale en l'an 2000: droits et besoins des Francophones de Toronto. *Reflets: Revue d'intervention sociale et communautaire, 5*(2), 123–154. doi: 10.7202/026273ar

Champagne, F., Contandriopoulos, A., Picot-Touché, J., Béland, F., & Nguyen, H. (2005). *Un cadre d'évaluation globale de la performance des systèmes de services de santé: Le modèle EGIPSS.* Montréal: Groupe de recherche interdisciplinaire en santé de l'Université de Montréal.

Champlain LHIN (n.d.). *About Us.* Retrieved February 2, 2017 from http://www.champlainlhin.on.ca /AboutUs/Intro.aspx. French version: RLISS de Champlain (n.d.). *À propos de nous.* Accessed July 15, 2015.

DeBoer, G. E. (2011). The globalization of science education. *Journal of Research in Science Teaching, 48*(6), 567–591. doi: 10.1002/tea.20421

Desabrais, T. (2010). L'influence de l'insécurité linguistique sur le parcours doctoral d'une jeune femme acadienne: une expérience teintée de la double minorisation. *Reflets: Revue d'intervention sociale et communautaire, 16*(2), 57–89. DOI:10.7202/1000314ar

Drolet, M., Arcand, I., Benoît, J., Savard, J., Savard, S., Lagacé, J., Lauzon, S., & Dubouloz, C-J. (2015). Agir pour avoir accès à des services sociaux et de santé en français: Des Francophones en situation minoritaire nous enseignent quoi faire! *Revue canadienne de service social, 32* (1 & 2), 5–26.

Forgues, É., & Landry, R. (2014). *L'accès aux services de santé en français et leur utilisation en contexte francophone minoritaire.* Moncton, NB: Institut canadien de recherche sur les minorités linguistiques (ICRML).

Gérin-Lajoie, D., & Labrie, N. (1999). Les résultats aux tests de lecture et d'écriture en 1993-1994: une interprétation sociolinguistique. In N. Labrie, & G. Forlot (Eds.). *L'enjeu de la langue en Ontario français* (pp. 79–108). Sudbury, ON: Prise de Parole.

Hogg, M. A., and Abrams, D. (2003). Intergroup behaviour and social identity. In M. A. Cooper, & J. Cooper, (Eds.). *The SAGE Handbook of Social Psychology* (pp. 407–431). London: SAGE Publications Ltd.

Huberman, A. M., and Miles, M. B. (2002). *The Qualitative Researcher's Companion: Classic and Contemporary Readings*. Thousand Oaks, CA: SAGE Publications.

Krippendorff, K. (2012). *Content Analysis: An Introduction to Its Methodology*. Thousand Oaks, CA: SAGE Publications.

McCurdy, B., MacKay, C., Badley, E., Veinot, P., & Cott, C. (2008). *A Proposed Evaluation Framework for Chronic Disease Prevention and Management Initiatives in Ontario*. Toronto: Arthritis Community Research & Evaluation (ACREU).

Office of the French Language Services Commissioner. (2009). *2008–2009 Annual Report: One Voice, Many Changes*. Toronto: Queen's Printer for Ontario.

Ontario Ministry of Health and Long-Term Care (2007). *Preventing and Managing Chronic Disease: Ontario's Framework*. Retrieved from http://www.health.gov.on.ca/en/programs/cdpm/pdf/framework_full.pdf. Accessed February 5, 2017.

Ontario Ministry of Health and Long-Term Care. (2012). *French Language Health Services. French Language Health Planning Entities under the Local Health System Integration Act, 2006 and Regulation 515/09*. Retrieved from http://health.gov.on.ca/en/public/programs/flhs/planning.aspx

Paillé, P., & Mucchielli, A. (2008). *L'analyse qualitative en sciences humaines et sociales*. Paris: Éditions Armand Colin.

QSR International. (2012) NVivo qualitative data analysis software. Version 10, 2012.

Savard, S., Arcand, I., Drolet, M., Benoît, J., Savard, J., & Lagacé, J. (2013). Les professionnels de la santé et des services sociaux intervenant auprès des francophones minoritaires: l'enjeu du capital social. *Francophonies d'Amérique*, (36), 113–133. doi:10.7202/1029379ar

Savoie-Zajc, L. (2009). L'entrevue semi-dirigée. In B. Gauthier (Ed.), *Recherche sociale: De la problématique à la collecte de données* (5th ed., pp. 337–360). Québec, QC: Presses de l'Université du Québec.

Société Santé en français. (2012). *Destination santé 2018: qualité, sécurité et mieux-être en français*. Ottawa: Société Santé en français.

Sharoff, L. (2008). Exploring nurses' perceived benefits of utilizing holistic modalities for self and clients. *Holistic Nursing Practice, 22*(1), 15–24. doi: 10.1097/01.hnp.0000306324.49332.a4

Statistics Canada. (2015). *2011 Census of Canada: Topic-based tabulations*. Retrieved from http://www12.statcan.gc.ca/census-recensement/2011/dp-pd/tbt-tt/Index-eng.cfm

Tajfel, H. (1978). *The Social Psychology of Minorities*. Sacramento, CA: Minority Rights Group.

Tajfel, H., & Turner, J. C. (1986). The social identity theory of intergroup behavior. In W.G. Austin & S. Worchel (Eds.). *Psychology of Intergroup Relations* (pp. 7–24). Chicago, IL: Nelson-Hall.

Wagner, E. H., Austin, B. T., Davis, C., Hindmarsh, M., Schaefer, J., & Bonomi, A. (2001). Improving chronic illness care: Translating evidence into action. *Health Affairs, 20*(6), 64–78. doi:10.1377/hlthaff.20.6.64

Wagner, E. H., Austin, B. T., & Korff, M. V. (1996). Organizing care for patients with chronic illness. *The Milbank Quarterly, 74*(4), 511–544. doi:10.2307/3350391

Offering Health Services in French: Between Obstacles and Favourable Factors in Anglophone Hospital Settings[1]

Éric Forgues, *Canadian Institute for Research on Minority Linguistics*,
Boniface Bahi, *University of Alberta*,
and Jacques Michaud, *independent researcher*

Abstract

This chapter highlights the social and organizational factors encouraging the active offer of French-language health services by professionals working in predominantly Anglophone health facilities. We present a sociological perspective inviting people to consider the complexity of the socio-organizational environment in which health professionals work. Their language abilities seem to be insufficient to ensure services are provided in both languages. The commitment of the administrators and managers, the management of services and human resources, labour relations, the availability of bilingual staff, and the legal and political context must be considered if we are to understand the delivery of French-language health services in all its facets. In a broader perspective, these factors inevitably reflect the social relations that exist between Anglophones and Francophones.

Key Words: health services, socio-organizational environment, language rights, health professionals.

Introduction

The access to French-language health services has attracted a great deal of attention on the part of Francophone actors, especially since the crisis provoked by plans to close the Hôpital Montfort in 1997 (Vézina, 2007). This conflict provided an opportunity for Francophones, politicians, and decision-makers in the public sector to become more deeply aware of inequalities rooted in the provision of health services in the two languages. It also provided an opportunity to take note of the crucial role language plays in the safety and quality of care (Comité consultatif des communautés francophones en situation minoritaire, 2001).

In the period following the crisis, a number of events took place. The *Société Santé en français* (SSF) and its network in the provinces were formed, as was the *Consortium national de formation en santé* (CNFS), in order to encourage wider availability of French-language health services and better access to them through networking and partnership, the development of services offered in French, the promotion of existing services, the expansion of French-language professional training in health and medical disciplines, and research on issues and challenges in French-language health care (Bouchard & Leis, 2008). The shortage of health professionals who speak French is often viewed as the main obstacle to efforts to offer French-language health services (Gagnon-Arpin, Bouchard, Leis, & Bélanger, 2014). This barrier has proven to be fairly significant, more or less so depending on the province concerned. A link seems to be made between the presence of professionals who can speak French and the provision of health services. However, the reality is much more complex. The fact that there are health professionals available who can speak French does not in any way guarantee that services will be offered in this language. The social, political, and legal environment, as well as the organization of labour, staffing, and service delivery, shapes language practices and the construction of language in practice. The language used in the provision of health services depends on, among other factors, the commitment of the administration towards delivering services in French, the perceptions of health professionals, and, more generally, on the legal, political, or social context.

This is the reason we feel it is necessary to adopt a conceptual framework drawing from sociological theories to examine the actions of health professionals in their organizational context and their social environment. We wanted to know which factors, in predominantly Anglophone hospital environments, encourage or facilitate the provision of French-language services for Francophone users. What barriers have to be overcome and what conditions have to be put in place to enable health professionals to offer services in French? This chapter presents the major results of our study.[2] To answer these questions, we decided to conduct case studies in predominantly Anglophone health facilities in four provinces: New Brunswick, Nova Scotia, Ontario, and Manitoba.

Problem and Theoretical Perspectives

Our study considers the social, institutional, and organizational factors that have an influence on the provision of French-language services in predominantly Anglophone hospital settings where there is a proportion of Francophone users. Drawing from the work of Bélanger and Lévesque (1991), we adopt a theoretical perspective that positions the actions of health professionals within the organization where they work. The organization, in turn, is positioned within an institutional (political, legal, and regulatory) context, in a larger system in which social relations among different groups are crystallized.

In the case interesting us, our focus is the linguistic aspect of health practices, the organization of labour, employment, and services, the institutional context, and social relations. Social relations between Anglophones and Francophones can translate on a legal level into laws and public policies in which the needs of Francophones are taken into consideration by protecting the right to use French as the language of service. These relations are not identical in every Canadian province. The demographic weight of Francophones, the importance of their institutions, the historical legacy, and the commitment to language among Francophones in the provinces model the linguistic social relations. As Michel Doucet concludes: "Therefore, because they appear in different contexts and are shaped by a combination of distinct historical, social, and political factors, language rights can only be asymmetrical, in their conception as in their application" (Doucet, 2014).[3]

This phenomenon is reflected in the existence (or non-existence) of laws and policies mandating or inciting public services, including health care services, to offer services in both official languages.

Figure 1. Health Professionals and the Organization

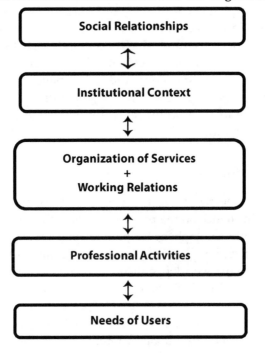

In a health facility, besides Anglophone/Francophone social relations, there are at least two other types of relations that weigh just as heavily on the organization of health services: labour and employment relations, which link employees to their employer, and consumer relations, which link users to service providers. Drawing from regulation theory (Aglietta, 1976; Boyer, 1986; Boyer & Saillard, 2002), Bélanger & Lévesque (1991) propose the concept of consumer relations that helps explain how social relations between service providers and users are regulated. In their opinion, this relationship can be transformed when consumers, as social actors, make a claim or create a demand for services (Bélanger & Lévesque, 1991, p. 25). In this perspective, social demands made by users can certainly exert an influence on the way services are organized.

It is reasonable to conclude that the periodic efforts of Francophones since the end of the 1960s to mobilize, advocate for, and protect their rights demonstrate a strong collective will to have their rights recognized. Their aim has been to transform the existing social relations in order to counter the domination of Francophones by Anglophones and to establish equality in their social relations (Behiels,

2005; Martel & Pâquet, 2010). Claiming their right to services in French and mobilizing for action on this issue testify to the willingness of Francophone actors to transform the effects of inequality in social relations between the two groups. This transformation requires the intervention of the federal and provincial governments which, by establishing the equality of the status of Anglophones and Francophones and recognizing their language rights, would correct the inequality experienced by the latter. The intervention of the government does more than allow individual rights to be protected; it also enhances the cultural vitality of the Francophone minority. "The State, by agreeing to confer rights on the minority group, acknowledges that it has an obligation to act in a way that protects the language and culture of the minority, which generally finds itself in a vulnerable position in relation to the language of the majority" (Doucet, 2014).

Nationally, the equality of status of Francophones and Anglophones was progressively affirmed by the first *Official Languages Act*, enacted in 1969 and replaced by a new *Act* in 1988, and the *Constitution Act, 1982*. The legislation reflected a political consensus, or at least a compromise "politically, recognizing the principle of the equality of the official language and the equality of official language communities is the expression of a fundamental choice arising from a social contract" (Doucet, 2014).

The diagram below illustrates the link between social relations, the struggle to transform them, language debates in public space, political decisions regarding language, and the development and application of rules of law, relevant regulations, and public policies.

Language rights are intended to promote the equality of French and English in Canada's institutions:

> 16. (1) English and French are the official languages of Canada and have equality of status and equal rights and privileges as to their use in all institutions of the Parliament and government of Canada.

As far as New Brunswick is concerned, the *Constitution Act, 1982* promotes equality in the social relations of Anglophone and Francophone communities:

> 16.1 (1) The English linguistic community and the French linguistic community in New Brunswick have equality of status and equal rights and privileges, including the right to distinct

educational institutions and such distinct cultural institutions as are necessary for the preservation and promotion of those communities.[4]

Figure 2. Social Relations, Linguistic Debates, and Political Decisions in Linguistic Matters

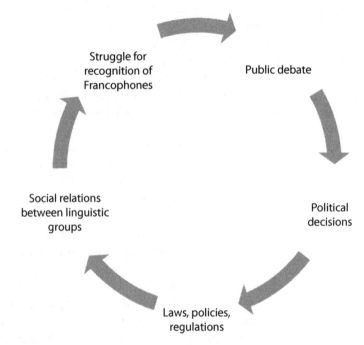

On the level of individual rights, the *Official Languages Act* of New Brunswick affirms the equality of French and English in the public institutions of the Province.[5] In other words, the minority status of the Francophone population should not influence the language of service in these institutions.

On a collective level, the two linguistic communities have a right to their own cultural institutions to support their vitality. Even if legislation and case law do not stipulate that health facilities are included in this category of institutions, the work and struggle of Francophones to protect their right to govern Francophone health facilities should be understood in this perspective. It is a matter of not only meeting the requirements of quality of services, but also of meeting requirements to protect French language and culture in the province.

As well as relying on legal foundations, which legitimize their claims for French-language services, this type of movement can also generate new rights or new language policies. This has been part of the history of Francophones in official language minority communities, in particular in the Hôpital Montfort affair, which served as a springboard for the Canadian Francophone population as a whole at the beginning of the millennium. Francophones in minority communities across Canada formed a movement to ensure better access to French-language health services (Comité consultatif des communautés francophones en situation minoritaire, 2001; Vézina, 2007).

The law can, in certain contexts, mediate the social relations between Anglophones and Francophones. It serves as a counterweight that tips the balance in the direction of the minority, allowing its voice to be heard and its needs to be recognized. Outside the realm of its application, minorities are more likely to be subject to power struggles with Anglophones. However, even within its realm, as we will see, the law does not have a perfect record in balancing the power of Anglophones and Francophones.

The Legal and Regulatory Context of the Language of Service in Four Provinces

In New Brunswick, under the jurisdiction of the *Official Languages Act* and the *Regional Health Authorities Act*, hospitals have a legal obligation to actively offer health services in the official language of the patient's choice.[6] As for Ontario, the *French Language Services Act*, enacted in 1988, "guarantees an individual's right to receive services in French from Government of Ontario ministries and agencies in 26 designated areas." It provides for certain health facilities to be designated to offer particular services in French, and provides for consultations with the Francophone community regarding the organization of French-language health services.[7] Moreover, some health facilities are designated bilingual and must, by virtue of this designation, offer French-language services to the Francophone population. In Nova Scotia, the purpose of the *Act Respecting the Delivery of French-language Services by the Public Service* is "to provide for the delivery of French-language services by designated departments, offices, agencies of Government, Crown corporations and public institutions to the Acadian and francophone community."[8] The French-language Services Regulations (2006), which govern the application of the *Act*, stipulate the obligations of designated departments and services, including the obligation of health authorities to develop French-language service plans based on consultations with the Acadian community.

In Manitoba, the French Language Services Policy was enacted in 1989, and revised in 1999. In it the Government committed to the following: "The services provided by the Government of Manitoba are offered, to the extent possible, in both official languages in [designated] areas where the French-speaking population is concentrated."[9] In 2016, the Government adopted *The Francophone Community Enhancement and Support Act*, affirming "The active offer concept is the cornerstone for the provision of French language services."[10] In the health sector, *The Regional Health Authorities Act* confers on the Lieutenant–Governor in Council the power to make regulations "respecting the obligations of regional health authorities in relation to the provision of health services in the French language, including without limitation, the designation of those regional health authorities which must fulfil the obligations . . ."[11] The *French Language Services Regulation* made under *The Regional Health Authorities Act* provides that the designated hospitals in the province must develop French-language services plans (Southern Health – Santé Sud, n.d.) in consultation with, among other actors, the Francophone communities in their region. According to this provincial regulation, seven regional health offices must offer services in French.

Regarding the way services in the official languages are to be provided, we should note that, in New Brunswick, the two regional health authorities must actively offer health services in both official languages. This is how the health authorities are to apply legislation to active offer:

> [Government institutions] . . . must take appropriate measures to inform the public that services are available in English and French—the official language of their choice. An "active offer" includes answering the telephone or greeting someone in both official languages. They must clearly place the official languages symbol and all correspondence and documents of greeting must be in the language chosen by the client. (Government of New Brunswick, 2005)

In Manitoba, at the time our data were collected, the *French Language Services Policy* stipulated that services must be actively offered in the designated areas, which include some health care services (de Moissac, de Rocquigny, Roch-Gagné, & Giasson, 2011). In Ontario, active offer is subject to guidelines established by the Government, which serve solely as advice, although the Office of the French Language Services Commissioner has recommended that it be made a mandatory directive (Office of the French Language Services Commissioner, 2013). In Nova Scotia, active offer is not mentioned.

It is reasonable to believe that the active offer of health services would create better conditions for Francophone users to receive services in their own language. Ontario's Ontario French Language Service Commissioner, who has long advocated for services in French to be actively offered, explains that supply and demand are reversed in a minority setting:

> In a minority language community, the roles of supply and demand are reversed. Generally, in a majority language community, if there is a demand, it is met. In the case of French-language services, these services first have to be offered in order for the demand from them to emerge. Thus, instead of just a sign that reads "English/French", service providers need to be able to effectively offer high-quality French-language services. The person behind the counter must be able to actively offer these services. (Office of the French Language Services Commissioner, 2008)

The legal and regulatory context must be kept in mind when analyzing the results of this study. As we will see in the next section where we present the theoretical framework, the legal context is a dimension of the social context helping us to understand how language comes into play in the organization of health services.

The Internal Organizational Environment

Aside from the external political and legal environment, a health facility must also deal with internal circumstances, notably the language abilities of its employments, its resources (human, financial, and material), and the management model guiding its operations.

In provinces where external legal requirements ensuring the delivery of French-language health services are rather weak, or nonexistent, internal pressures to respond to a demand may determine how and which services are offered in French. Having a Francophone clientele may encourage managers to put measures into place to meet a particular need. In this context, legal approaches are confronted with management approaches, and negotiate with or surrender to them.

The interest that managers and service providers in the health sector show in having their organization acquire language skills and cultural competence attests to this need to define the conditions needed to best serve a multicultural and multilingual population. Most of the studies on this subject are found in American research. A review of the literature published by Aucoin in 2008 for the *Société santé en français* shows that Francophone organizations have discovered a new interest in research in this area. The study leads to a distinction between two types of responsibilities, that of health professionals and that of health organizations: it is the responsibility of health professionals to develop attitudes, behaviours, and knowledge that allow them to create a quality therapeutic relationship with a patient who has a different language and culture; it is the responsibility of health care systems and organizations to create an environment, policies, resources, and learning opportunities where they can offer services adapted to the language and culture of their patients (Aucoin, 2008, p. 9).

Referring to the National Center for Cultural Competence (Georgetown University, Washington, D.C.), Aucoin also distinguishes between cultural competence and linguistic competence. While cultural competence is the ability to provide care that is responsive to diverse cultural sensibilities and different value systems, linguistic competence is the "capacity of an organization and its staff to communicate effectively, and to convey information in a way that is easily understood by its diverse clients, including persons who have a limited understanding of the majority language, those who have low literacy skills or are not literate" (Aucoin, 2008, p. 9). In his review of the literature, this author points out that there is no accepted theoretical framework used by researchers to study cultural or linguistic competence, but that a conceptual framework is being developed to examine their relationship to the quality of health care.

Drawing from the work of Betancourt (2006) and Beach, Somnat, and Cooper (2006), Aucoin focuses on three conceptual dimensions for his analysis: (1) the clinical dimension (relationship and communication between the health professional and the patient); (2) the organizational dimension (the leadership of the board of directors and the senior management team, strategic priorities, service planning, allocation of human and financial resources, implementation of care plans, etc.); and (3) the systemic dimension (covering the entire health system, public policies, and the social system) (Aucoin, 2008, pp. 14–15). Aucoin gives us a promising path to explore as we develop a conceptual framework in order to continue our research.

After looking at the contributions to the field made by research into the linguistic and cultural competence of health organizations, we developed the conceptual diagrams reproduced here. They are designed to illustrate the external and internal factors likely to influence the provision of health services in French.

Among external factors are financial resources provided by the government, the legal or regulatory framework and provincial policies, the demand for services from Francophone individuals and organizations, professional associations, and the existence or intervention of a commissioner or ombudsperson. It is also important to note that the Francophone population and its representative organizations may themselves contribute to deciding on what French-language services will be offered by promoting an "active demand" of such services, as we have seen in the actions of the *Assemblée de la francophonie de l'Ontario* (*L'Express*, 2009, May 19–25). Thus, Francophone actors keep the issue of French-language services on the radar by actively demanding services in the official language they have chosen to use.

Among the internal factors, we can identify the willingness and commitment of the administration, resources (human, material, and financial), the existence of an internal policy and an action plan on language of service, the management of services and human resources, the linguistic capacity of health professionals and their perceptions about language of service, collective agreements in effect, and the expectations of patients. The way that provision of services in both official languages is defined is undoubtedly of great importance in determining how effective the actual offer will be.

Conceptual Diagrams

Our research provides an overview of some of the elements likely to have an influence on the provision of French-language health services, illustrating the points of view expressed by the respondents in our interviews and our survey, as well as findings from the literature we reviewed.

Figure 3. External Factors for Offer of Services in French

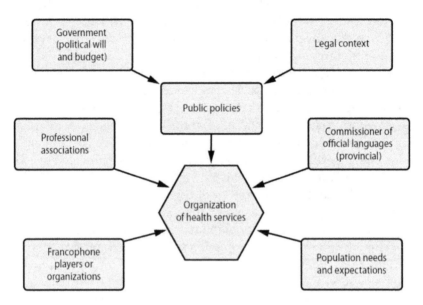

Figure 4. Internal Factors for Offer of Services in French

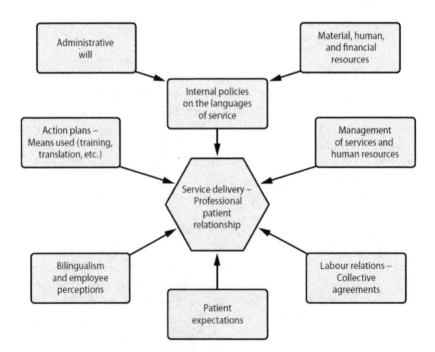

Methodology[12]

The theoretical framework allowed us to develop an analytical grid that included the various factors that influence the provision of services in the two official languages. This analytical grid developed out of a working definition of the concepts that allowed us to break the concepts down into dimensions, indicators and variables (Van Campenhoudt & Quivy, 2011). The following are the themes on which we collected data, using an interview protocol or questionnaire:

- Respondent's background
- Language of patients
- Linguistic skills of respondent
- Language of service
- Health care facility's commitment
- Respondent's perceptions and opinions
- Assessment of linguistic skills and language training in health facilities
- Factors influencing the offer of services in French
- Working language

In the winter of 2010–2011, an electronic questionnaire was published online in both official languages. It was sent to health professionals and employees in each hospital we studied, via an internal electronic messaging system. The study looked at the following hospitals: Yarmouth Regional Hospital in Nova Scotia, located in a region that is 21.4% Francophone; four hospitals in Horizon Health Network in New Brunswick,[13] located in Moncton (a city with a 35.0% Francophone population), Fredericton (7.1%), Saint John (4.8%), and Miramichi (8.5%); Sudbury Regional Hospital in Ontario, situated in a city that is 28.2% Francophone; and Saint-Boniface General Hospital in Saint-Boniface, Manitoba, where 4.1% of the population is Francophone. All the facilities we studied must, to different extents, offer services in the official language of the user's choice.

If we count only the people who completed at least 30% of the questions, 902 respondents took part in the questionnaire (see Table 1).[14] The data analysis is descriptive in nature. In it, we both examine the current state of affairs in the provision of services and strive to understand the factors that may influence the situation.

Table 1. Distribution of Survey Respondents by Health Authority

		Indicate the health authority you work for				Total (%)
		Yarmouth Regional Hospital	Horizon Health Network	Sudbury Regional Hospital	Saint-Boniface Regional Hospital	
Total	Number	96	435	156	215	902
(%)	%	100	100	100	100	100

Besides the survey, 56 semi-structured interviews were conducted during the same period. We interviewed managers at different ranks in the institution's hierarchies and distributed among the health facilities studied, in order to determine the degree to which language is taken into consideration in the organization of health services, and *how* this is done.

We also conducted a review of the literature, analyzing documents dealing with language policies in health care, and strategies and action plans to promote services offered in French (identified through a search of websites and contacts in health facilities). The data we collected helped us to clarify how the legal context, the commitment of senior management, the allocation of resources, and the perceptions of employees influence the provision of French-language services in Francophone minority communities.

Results

Administrative Will

The hospitals we studied have implemented plans to ensure that services are offered in both official languages. Horizon Health Network did so for the first time during the period of our research. Our findings tend to suggest that hospital administrators are committed to a certain degree to offering services in both official languages. A proportion of 65% of respondents reported that their hospital administration assigns considerable importance to services in French. If we break this proportion down by the respondents' language, 56.6% of Francophones and 72.7% of Anglophones shared this opinion. In other words, Francophones are less likely than Anglophones to agree their administration places importance on offering services in French. Furthermore, 67% of respondents feel that their hospital administration displays, to a large extent or to a very large extent, a bilingual corporate image. Finally, 37% of respondents state that the administrators in their hospital commit themselves to offering services in French through their leadership, to a large extent or a very large extent.

Here are other data related to their perception about the commitment of the hospital administration:

- According to 36% of respondents, hospital directors and administrators ask employees, to a large or very large extent, to extend an active offer of service in both official languages;
- According to 35% of respondents, they (hospital directors and administrators) ensure, to a large or very large extent, the presence of bilingual or Francophone staff in the department when organizing work;
- According to 41%, they hire, to a large extent or a very large extent, employees who are able to express themselves in French;
- According to 65%, they provide, to a large extent or a very large extent, written information (brochures, patient information) to patients in both official languages;
- According to 45%, they make health care professionals aware, to a large extent or a very large extent, of the active offer of services in French;
- According to 30%, the hospital directors and administrators consider language skills, to a large extent or a very large extent, in the case of promotions and relocation of staff internally.[15]

Management of Services and Human Resources

The commitment of managers and administrators to active offer varies among facilities. In some hospitals, particularly those in Winnipeg and Sudbury, managers have targeted specific units and departments to offer French-language services (Emergency and the Mother-Child Unit, for example). Human resources departments are also managed in a way that places high value on hiring bilingual employees, making and maintaining a list of bilingual employees who can be asked to work during each shift, and ensuring bilingual communications, in both writing and speaking. However, these arrangements vary depending on the hospital and its departments. Overall, reception services are the most likely to offer French-language services, but beyond the front desk, services in French are, as a general rule, hard to find. Nearly a quarter of respondents rate the measures taken by their departmental managers to offer services in French to Francophone patients as none, very little, or little, while 54.5% rate them as good or very good.

Table 2. Measures Taken by Managers of Facilities to Offer French Language Service to Francophone Patients

			Indicate the health authority you work for				Total (%)
			Yarmouth Regional Hospital	Horizon Health Network	Sudbury Regional Hospital	Saint-Boniface Regional Hospital	
To your knowledge, how do you rate the measures taken by your departmental managers to offer services in French to Francophone patients?	None	Number	5	9	10	14	38
		%	6.6	2.5	7.6	7.8	5.1
	Very little	Number	11	19	10	24	64
		%	14.5	5.3	7.6	13.3	8.6
	Little	Number	10	33	15	25	83
		%	13.2	9.2	11.4	13.9	11.1
	Good	Number	18	78	31	39	166
		%	23.7	21.8	23.5	21.7	22.3
	Very good	Number	17	148	41	34	240
		%	22.4	41.3	31.1	18.9	32.2
	I don't know	Number	15	71	25	44	1.155
		%	19.7	19.8	18.9	24.4	20.8
Total (%)		Number	76	358	132	180	746
		%	100	100	100	100	100

Resources

To offer French-language services, certain resources must be acquired. Among those that need to be available are bilingual employees, language training, and, to a certain extent, the services of interpreters. On the subject of hiring bilingual employees, several people mentioned how hard it is to recruit health professionals. Adding a language requirement increases the difficulty. In our interviews, respondents also pointed out unions are resistant to the designation of positions as bilingual. The language requirement is thought to supersede other requirements, such as technical skills or seniority. Some respondents were afraid to see a requirement or preference for bilingualism supplant other aspects of professional competence: [original: English] "It would be wonderful if we were all bi or trilingual, but I think it is more important to have qualified staff to perform their job, than less skilled people who speak both languages" (Horizon). Linguistic competence is not seen as one of the skills required for providing quality services: [original: English] "If a person can do the job, that is what counts, not which language they can do it in" (Sudbury). Respondents make clear distinctions between technical and language skills: [original: English] "Staff get promoted by seniority, so the language you speak has nothing to do with your job" (Saint-Boniface).

The issue of cost is often raised in the comments. According to some respondents, a choice must be made between quality of care and language: [original: English] "People have to decide if they want their health or their language because the province cannot afford both" (Horizon). Language requirements are thought to be too costly: [original: English] "Too many tax dollars wasted on this issue!" (Horizon). An injustice is perceived when bilingual candidates are required or preferred for certain positions: [original: English] "It seems very unfair from the perspective of an English-speaking Canadian not to mention an enormous financial burden for the province to carry the title of 'Bilingual Province'" (Horizon). This type of language requirement is perceived as a job offer for Francophones, more of whom are bilingual than are Anglophones.

In general, the union position on language of service is a delicate subject. Employees are less comfortable expressing their opinions on this issue. The right of Francophone patients to be served in their own language seems to be in conflict with certain rights of workers. For some respondents, there is a way to resolve the dispute: the administration must work in cooperation with the union to clarify these two types of rights.

Providing language training so employees will become bilingual is one solution to encourage the provision of French services.

However, there are limits to its feasibility. Our data show that language training has *no* or a *low* impact on the provision of French-language services, in the experience of nearly three-quarters of the respondents. Moreover, many respondents stated in our interviews that access to language training is limited and is complicated by schedules that do not always suit employees. Training does not, in any case, seem to make employees more likely to offer services in French and to be comfortable doing so. Many also mention the inadequacy of this method, if classroom training is not supplemented by social activities in French to maintain the learner's proficiency.

Language Environment

In some areas, as respondents noted, the Anglo-dominant context pushes them to use English when communicating with colleagues and patients. It is a fact that most Francophones can speak English. Several people affirmed in interviews or in their comments on the questionnaire that few Francophone clients ask to be served in French. Nearly half of our respondents said that less than 10% of their clientele request such service.

> [original: English] Almost all of my Francophone patients speak perfect English so not a common request. (Sudbury)

> [original: English] If patient speaks français-anglais and asks if you speak French, they don't understand the correct terminology in French and automatically switch to English. (Horizon)

This situation has led respondents to the conclusion that services in French do not represent an actual need; this makes health professionals feel more comfortable about their choice not to serve Francophones in their own language. According to several service providers, the fact that most Francophone patients are bilingual and can speak English diminishes the importance of offering services in French.

Many respondents noted the Anglo-dominant context, in order to justify their own resistance towards language of service.

> [original: English] Saint John is mostly an English-speaking city and I feel far too many of our already scarce resources are being

wasted to appease a small portion of the population. I have met very few Francophones who cannot speak English. I do feel that interpretive services should be available at all times. (Horizon)

[original: English] Once again, you need to look at the city where the hospital is, go into any stores our first language is English, those that cannot speak English are a very low minority. I feel that every department has French-speaking individuals should one not be able to communicate with a visitor or patient. I have worked here for several years and this has not once been an issue. (Sudbury)

People may conceal their concerns with the language of health services under the predominantly Anglophone context, in which Francophones are bilingual. Given this Anglo-dominant context, it might appear to be simpler and more logical for unilingual Francophones to learn English than to provide resources for the provision of French-language services.

When expressed by a bilingual patient, the need for services in French is perceived as a political action. This perception reveals the power relations between Anglophones and Francophones: [original: English] "I do not agree with a Francophone patient who is completely bilingual INSISTING on Service in French and allowing a totally unilingual Anglophone to fumble and stutter . . . I have no tolerance for people 'making a point'" (Horizon).

This comment was made by an employee of a hospital that, nonetheless, has an obligation to offer services in the official language of the patient's choice.

The data from our interviews show that employees feel pressured to speak to each other in English, thereby limiting their opportunities to maintain their proficiency in French. Any professional and administrative communication, written or oral, must be in English. Informal communications can take place in French but if Anglophones are present or nearby, Francophones feel obligated to speak English among themselves, so that the norm of communication becomes English.

The pressure towards English promotes the marginalization of the French fact in hospitals, as some respondents point out. It can happen that Francophone patients and employees communicate in English without realizing they are Francophones. As a result,

respondents are very often unaware that there are Francophone colleagues or patients in the hospital.

The Multicultural Context

From the perspective of several managers and health professionals,
the multicultural nature of the region, the province, or the country
seems to indicate that the need to offer French-language services is
of relative or even little importance.

> [original: English] French is not the only other language spoken
> in NB. We are becoming a melting pot of cultures and I do not
> feel it is fair to only stress French as a second language. (Horizon)

> [original: English] Yes, all languages are important to be acces-
> sible to pts [patients] not just French. (Sudbury)

One respondent thinks that being proficient in Italian is more important to communicate with patients who are seniors: [original: English]
"What about the rights of other nationalities . . . You can't be considered bilingual unless the other language is French . . . In Sudbury,
Italian is a better asset to have in communicating with the elderly
population" (Sudbury).

Other respondents mention the importance of other language
groups:

> [original: English] I feel that the hospitals should offer all lan-
> guages that are dominant in geographical area, not just for French,
> but also in this area, i.e., Ukrainian, Finnish, Italian, etc. (Sudbury)

> [original: English] Well, in the region that I serve, there are just
> as many or more immigrants that speak languages other than
> French that we also have to treat, assist and serve equally.
> (Saint-Boniface)

Some respondents question the fact that employees who speak French
are hired, because of the multicultural context:

> [original: English] Most patients I serve speak anything but
> French. The work area that I am in has a guide of how many
> French-speaking employees they must hire. This is not necessary

for the reason above. If this is what the government wants, why is it just St-Boniface Hospital that has this policy. We are a multi-cultural country. (Saint-Boniface)

Contradicting a widespread perception, one respondent claims that it is not a problem to find staff members who speak French, but that facilities should concentrate on other languages: "It is never a problem to find staff who speak French. It is very hard to find staff who speak Chinese, Japanese, Filipino [Tagalog], Mandarin, Aboriginal languages. That is what this hospital should be concentrating on, not French" (Saint-Boniface).

Other respondents concur:

[original: English] As much as I believe that offering French is important to the French-speaking patients, it is just as important to address the other languages in our specific area. I strongly believe that they are forgotten. (Sudbury)

[original: English] Our patient population is largely Aboriginal—many nurses on our unit have commented that it would be more beneficial to have staff who speaks Aboriginal languages (Ojibwa, Cree, Oji-Cree) than French. (Saint-Boniface)

The affirmation of the multicultural reality is made simultaneously with that of the Anglophone majority:

[original: English] We are a multicultural society. Not only do we have French-speaking people, we also have Ukrainians, Asians, Filipinos, Italians, Germans, East Indians and so on. . . . We must consider the other groups and not make them feel that they are not as special as the French. Singling one group out is very unfair, unrealistic and unprofessional. English is the international language and most people understand it. Let's not rock the boat and play favourites. (Sudbury)

Another comment juxtaposes the multicultural reality with the reality of an Anglophone majority this way:

[original: English] I feel you are putting more relevance on French speaking patients over any other foreign language. What makes them so special? We get just as many Spanish, Filipino, German patients. Should we all have to learn those languages too? This is Winnipeg, Canada. We speak ENGLISH here. (Saint-Boniface)

In the opinion of these respondents, Francophones receive special treatment compared to other minority groups. There should be no difference, they feel, between Francophones and groups of immigrant origin. In the end, all should be assimilated into the Anglophone majority. Another respondent suggests the same thing: [original: English] "Canada is a country of many nations. French should not receive special services." (Saint-Boniface)

When referring to Canada's multicultural context, Anglophones dilute the rights of Francophones in the area of language of service by equating the official language minority with all other ethnic minorities: the right of immigrants is placed on an equal footing with that of Francophones. The management perspective on this matter tends to consider it only in terms of the influence of the language of communication on the quality of care offered. Therefore, no distinction can be made between the Francophone patient and the newcomer who speaks any language other than English. Only one comment by an Anglophone mentions the existence of the two official languages of Canada: [original: English] "French is our second official language in Canada—all health care should be provided in this language because we live in Canada. To not have it available is unacceptable." (Saint-Boniface). However, the vision of the majority of Anglophone respondents is of a multicultural country rather than a country where there are two official languages and the equal rights of Anglophones and Francophones are recognized.

Perceptions of Employees

The data from this study show that 58.3% of respondents totally or partially recognize the right of Francophones to receive services in the language of their choice. The percentage climbs to 90.7% among Francophone respondents, and falls to 43.9% among Anglophones. When French-speaking patients who speak English well ask to be served in French, 40% of respondents agree totally or strongly that they have the right to receive services in French. There again, Francophone respondents are much more inclined to agree that they have the right to be served in French (67.5%) than do Anglophones (26.6%).

In the opinion of the majority of respondents (72.6%), the hospital should assign very great importance or great importance to services in French. The proportion is higher among Francophones (94.4%) than among Anglophones (64.5%). However, somewhat fewer than half of respondents (51.2%) feel their hospital should not make any more effort or should make a little more effort to offer services in French. The proportion of Anglophones (65.3%) who are of this opinion is greater than the proportion of Francophones (20.7%). On the other hand, the majority of respondents (73.0%) state they are willing to make more effort to offer services in French; Anglophones seem less willing to do so than Francophones (65.3% as compared to 92.4%).

When asked about having to offer services in the official language of the patient, several respondents said during the interview that they do not dare to actively offer these services, because they are not bilingual. They are afraid that if the patient speaks French they will be unable to understand or to continue the conversation. This would seem to indicate they are unfamiliar with the measures to take in this situation, or perhaps that they do not want to take them.

Perceived Barriers

We asked respondents to tell us to what extent certain elements of the organization of services could be considered barriers. Looking at the respondents who perceive that the following factors are an average, significant, or major barrier, we find that for 66% of respondents, the insufficient **linguistic skills** of health care professionals is one of the barriers; for 42%, it is **professionals who feel it unnecessary or unimportant** to offer services in French that is a barrier; for 23%, it is **hiring practices** that favour the unilingual Anglophone staff; for 19%, it is **professional promotions** that favour the unilingual Anglophone staff; for 19%, it is the **perceptions of senior hospital administrators** (who feel it unnecessary or unimportant to offer services in French); for 27%, it is the fact that **senior administrators fail to implement systems** aimed at assisting professionals in offering services in French; for 18%, it is the **collective agreement** between the professional association and the employer. Generally speaking, each of these barriers is considered more significant by Francophones than by Anglophones.

The Language in Which Services Are Offered

The interviews revealed that a significant proportion of Francophones do not receive health services in French. The table below shows that, according to 31.6% of respondents, fewer than 30% of Francophone users receive their services in French.

Table 3. Proportion of Francophone Patients Who Receive Services in Their Language (by Health Authority)

Proportion of Francophone patients who receive services in their language (as a %)	Yarmouth Regional Hospital	Horizon Health Network	Sudbury Regional Hospital	Saint-Boniface Regional Hospital	Total (%) (263)
0 – 9.9	5.7	16.2	14.8	29.7	16.4
10 – 19.9	17.1	3.9	8.2	16.2	8.4
20 – 29.9	17.1	3.9	8.2	5.4	6.8
30 – 39.9	8.6	2.3	1.6	8.1	3.8
40 – 49.9	0.0	1.5	8.2	2.7	3.0
50 – 59.9	17.1	8.5	16.4	5.4	11.0
60 – 69.9	0.0	1.5	0.0	5.4	1.5
70 – 79.9	8.6	7.7	8.2	5.4	7.6
80 – 89.9	8.6	13.9	11.5	5.4	11.4
90 – 100	17.1	40.8	23.0	16.2	30.0
Total (%)	100	100	100	100	100

Interviews also helped us to identify the fact that greetings and reception are the main services provided in both official languages. Some departments that serve higher proportions of Francophones (because they provide specialized services, for example) or are designated or prioritized (as they may be in Ontario or Manitoba) also provide more services in both official languages. As for whether these services are *actively* offered in both official languages, the data in the table below indicate that the active offer of service in both official languages is quite marginal (1.6%), while 68% of respondents speak to users in English at their first visit, 16.8% in French, and 13.6% say they speak to them in their language. In the last case, information about the patient's language may be found in his or her medical records (the family name might be a hint), or may be indicated by the colour of the bracelet the patient is wearing (the method used at Saint-Boniface Hospital at the time of this study).

Table 4. Language Used During Patients' Initial Visit

			Health Authorities				Total (%)
			Yarmouth Regional Hospital	Horizon Health Network	Sudbury Regional Hospital	Saint-Boniface Regional Hospital	
In which language do you address your patients upon the initial visit?	Always or more often in English	Number	64	206	84	155	509
		%	72.7	60.2	60.4	86.1	68.0
	In English and French	Number	4	2	4	2	12
		%	4.5	0.6	2.9	1.1	1.6
	More often in French	Number	5	87	23	11	126
		%	5.7	25.4	16.5	6.1	16.8
	In the patient's language	Number	15	47	28	12	102
		%	17.0	13.7	20.1	6.7	13.6
Total		Number	88	342	139	180	749
(%)		%	100	100	100	100	100

We wanted to find out if respondents provided services in French when a user spoke to them in French. A quarter of respondents (25.5%) said they sometimes, rarely, or never reply in French (see Table 5). We asked them what they did when a patient spoke to them in French (see Table 6). Most respondents said they asked if she or he spoke English, and, if so, continued the conversation in English. They may also seek the help of a Francophone colleague to translate or refer the patient to a Francophone colleague. A proportion of respondents will ask if someone accompanying the patient can translate.

Table 5. Language Used by the Patient and Language Used by the Health Professional

			Indicate the health authority you work for				Total (%)
			Yarmouth Regional Hospital	Horizon Health Network	Sudbury Regional Hospital	Saint-Boniface Regional Hospital	
If the patient speaks to you in French, do you serve him/her in French?	Always	Number	39	144	72	37	292
		%	53.4	56.9	64.3	35.9	54.0
	Often	Number	5	29	9	14	57
		%	6.8	11.5	8.0	13.6	10.5
	Sometimes	Number	6	18	9	8	41
		%	8.2	7.1	8.0	7.8	7.6
	Rarely	Number	8	30	11	15	64
		%	11.0	11.9	9.8	14.6	11.8
	Never	Number	15	32	11	29	87
		%	20.5	12.6	9.8	28.2	16.1
Total (%)		Number	73	253	112	103	541
		%	100	100	100	100	100

Table 6. Actions of Professionals When Patient Speaks French

What measures do you take to serve a French patient?	Always – Often (%)
I ask the patient if he/she speaks English and, if so, I continue in English.	36.1
I seek the help of an equally qualified Francophone colleague to translate.	27.0
I refer the patient to a Francophone colleague.	19.6
I seek the help of a Francophone employee, regardless of his/her professional qualifications.	186
I ask the patient if someone accompanying him/her can translate.	18.2
I use the services of the hospital interpreter.	4.2

The majority of employees (79.2%) said that, in their opinion, the hospital where they work is required to offer services in French. Except for the hospitals that belong to the Horizon Health Network in New Brunswick, those in this study have prioritized which departments offer services in French.[16] It is startling to realize that a significant proportion of employees who replied to our questionnaire (48.7%) say they were not informed of the working language, or the language in which they should offer services at their hospital. What is more, 35.4% stated they were never informed of resources available to assist them in offering services in French.

Discussion of Results

The data from this study show that despite the existence of a legal context requiring or inciting hospitals to offer French-language health services, facilities are confronted with several barriers when they try to implement measures for this purpose. Taking language into account in the organization of services depends on factors external to health facilities and on which administrators and managers have little influence. At this level it is political (governments, political parties, ombudsperson), social (Francophone and Anglophone populations), and professional actors who have an influence on the context. These actors can encourage or mandate that language be considered in the organization of health services. Within the health facilities themselves, decision-makers and managers can influence the provision of French-language health services in various ways, starting with the administrators' own commitment and willingness to make offering services in French a core part of the way services are organized. Nonetheless, the actions of these actors are framed by the social relations between Anglophones and Francophones. This means that Anglophone managers and health professionals perceive the situation differently than Francophones. Based on their perceptions, which we have presented, Anglophones tend to minimize the importance of language rights, mainly because of the predominantly Anglophone context to which Francophones have to conform, and the multicultural and multilingual context that dilutes the language rights of the majority. This also minimizes the significance of the rights which, as Michel Doucet reminds us, are aimed at promoting the vitality and the social and cultural development of minorities (Doucet, 2014[17]). Because they see language as a simple tool of communication, Anglophones do not fully understand why a bilingual Francophone would ask to be served in French. "Once a language is no longer considered a social necessary, language rights represent at best a type of accommodation, enabling an individual to communicate, in specific conditions, with the State" (Doucet, 2014).

By stripping a language of its function in constructing and maintaining identity and of its role in the survival of the community, the objective of protecting it in order to ensure the survival of a linguistic and cultural community in an Anglo-dominant context disappears from view. "Politically, the recognition of the principle of the equality of the official languages and the equality of the official language communities is the expression of a fundamental choice rooted in the social contract" (Doucet, 2014).

The principle of equality is also aimed at countering the tendency, in an Anglo-dominant context, to use English as the language of communication. Instead, it should motivate the decision-makers and health professionals to promote the use of French.

The Anglo-dominant context undoubtedly explains the low demand for services in French. A study by Deveau, Landry, and Allard (2009) examining the factors that prompt Francophones to use French-language public services reports that, when the offer of services is made actively in both official languages, there is an increased probability that users will seek services in their own language. In other words, if the offer of services is made in English, Francophones are less likely to ask to be served in French; this applies especially in settings where the minority is very small and Francophones have already become accustomed to the fact that public life and activities happen in English (Landry, Allard, & Deveau, 2011, pp. 38–39). Meanwhile, when bilingual Francophones ask for services in French, it may be perceived as a political act (Charbonneau, 2011). Besides these factors, hospitalization places patients in a vulnerable situation, and they generally feel they are in a weak position to ask for services in their language, even if their situation accentuates their need for them (Bernier, 2009; Boudreau, 1999). At the same time, we know that when communication is hampered by misunderstandings or a lack of understanding, there is a real risk that the quality of care will be affected (Bowen, 2001).

The demand for services in French can arise from other sources, notably from Francophone community organizations that are very well placed to raise the awareness of decision-makers and hospital administrators regarding the importance of offering services in French. The goal is to make it clearly understood that an Anglophone context has an influence on the low rate of demand for services in French. Increasing the awareness of managers also leads to the introduction of measures that will help Francophone patients to feel truly comfortable about choosing French as the language for their health services (Office of the French Language Services Commissioner, 2015).

Conclusion

From our analysis, we can see that despite the existence of a legal context that requires or incites health facilities to offer their services in both official languages, several other factors have to be considered in order for language to be considered a core part of the provision of health services. These factors cannot be viewed independently of the social relations existing between Anglophones and Francophones. The persistence of power relations between the two language groups explains, in part, the barriers that arise on the road toward providing services in both official languages. How and to what extent language is taken into account in the organization of services is a reflection of the state of these relations. Consequently, the way language rights play out in reality is the result of a complex process in which several factors interact. These include social factors stemming from the process of socialization and internalization of certain norms, framing the use of French in particular contexts; economic factors through which material, human, and financial resources are brought into a context where they are limited; cultural factors rooted in the values, beliefs, and perceptions about an individual's identity and of the status and legitimacy of language and language rights; and political factors that play out in relations and balances of force, influence, and power.

The fact that a legal framework has been established does not make it any less necessary to have a strong political commitment, if language rights are to be fully respected. In the opinion of Joseph Yvon Thériault, when language rights exist, this can lead to the impression that the results the community is striving for have already been achieved, and diminishes the motivation and the political will to protect the interests of Francophones or to work for the recognition of the reality of the minority in general. This is one of the effects of what can be called the "juridification of the minority fact,"[18] and which sets aside

> the question of language minorities from public debate on the political stage. Parliaments, the political class of the majority and of the minority, now has permission to spare themselves the need to act—and that accounts largely for what has happened over the last few years . . . The judges will look after it. (Thériault, 2009, p. 53)

Thériault believes that the juridification of the minority fact "has the effect of masking the power relations at play. It brings the language community out of a political relationship in order to define it as a community of rights-holders" (ibid., p. 53). But this process goes further yet. Still in Thériault's words:

> Juridification proceeds from a sort of levelling-off or a flattening that, ultimately, has the effect of emptying the social content from the political and historical contents that gave social action substance and depth. Juridification is, then, the unbounded expansion of the logic of modern law. (ibid., p. 52)

This thesis, in itself, needs to be validated in the field, especially in the case concerning us here, the health field. It is true that Francophone organizations working in the health sector (*Consortium national de formation en santé, Société santé en français* and its affiliated networks), in spite of being born out of protests and claims by Francophone actors, refuse to exert an advocacy role in the health field (Forgues & Mouyabi Mampoumbou, 2014). Even if they are not lobbying organizations, they owe it to themselves to develop strategies to move services in French forward in *legal and political* contexts that may or may not be favourable towards progress, depending on the province.

Even when they are recognized, language rights cannot manage to hide or entirely eliminate the power relations. Despite the fact that they can, to a certain extent, mask the power imbalance, our analysis shows their decisive effect on the application of language rights. Although they need to deal with language rights, power relations continue to create barriers for integrating language needs in the organization of services. They determine how language will play out in the way health services are organized, and the extent to which they will be taken into consideration in the organization of services for Francophone patients, at all levels of organization.

Language rights do not suffice to counter, or even reverse, the domination of the Anglophone majority group towards the Francophone minority. Francophone actors need to understand that the progress made in the area of language of service can be attributed to the mobilization of Francophone and Acadian communities who have engaged on the political level (federal and provincial governments) in advocating for measures to be applied to improve the provision of French-language health services. For language rights to be applied and for political decisions to be respected, organizations and actors must remain vigilant and, if necessary, lead whatever political and legal campaigns are necessary to ensure their rights are respected.

Notes

1. This chapter is based on research funded jointly by the *Consortium national de formation en santé* and the New Brunswick Department of Health, and which has been published as a report (Forgues, Bahi, & Michaud, 2011). We thank everyone who has contributed, even indirectly, to this study.

2. Readers may also be interested in reading the report, which presents the theoretical framework, the methodology, and the results of our analysis in more detail (Forgues, Bahi, & Michaud, 2011).

3. Document published in Kindle format, not paginated.

4. The *Constitution Act, 1982*, Schedule B to the *Canada Act 1982* (UK), 1982, c 11. *Institut canadien d'information juridique*. Retrieved from: https://www.canlii.org/en/ca/laws/stat/schedule-b-to-the-canada-act-1982-uk-1982-c-11/latest/schedule-b-to-the-canada-act-1982-uk-1982-c-11.html. Retrieved February 13, 2017.

5. *Official Languages Act*. Government of New Brunswick, Legislative Assembly. Retrieved from https://www.gnb.ca/legis/bill/editform-e.asp?ID=134&legi=54&num=0&page= Retrieved February 13, 2017.

6. *Official Languages Act*, enacted on June 7, 2001, sanctioned June 7, 2002. *Official Languages Act*. Government of New Brunswick, Legislative Assembly. Retrieved from https://www.gnb.ca/legis/bill/editform-e.asp?ID=134&legi=54 &num=0&page=. *Regional Health Authorities Act*, enacted on January 11, 2001. *Institut canadien d'information juridique* [online]: https://www.canlii.org/en/nb/laws/stat/rsnb-2011-c-217/latest/rsnb-2011-c-217.html. Both retrieved February 13, 2017.

7. Government of Ontario website. Retrieved from https://www.ontario.ca/laws/statute/90f32. Retrieved February 13, 2017.

8. Chapter 26 of the Acts of 2004, amended 2011, c. 9, ss. 17–22, *An Act Respecting the Delivery of French-language Services by the Public Service*. Retrieved from http://nslegislature.ca/legc/statutes/frenchla.htm. The French-language Services Regulations made under Section 10 of the *French-language Services Act*. Retrieved fromhttps://novascotia.ca/just/regulations/regs/flsregs.html. Both retrieved February 15, 2017.

9. French Language Services Policy, March 1999. Government of Manitoba website. Retrieved fromhttp://www.gov.mb.ca/fls-slf/pdf/fls_policy.pdf. Retrieved February 13, 2017.

10. *The Francophone Community Enhancement and Support Act*. Legislative Assembly of Manitoba website. Retrieved from https://web2.gov.mb.ca/bills/41-1/pdf/b005.pdf. Retrieved February 13, 2017. It is important to note that at the time of our study, the *Act* had not yet been adopted.

11. *The Regional Health Authorities Act*, C.C.S.M., c. R34, enacted on November 19, 1996, version in effect since November 9, 2012. Government of Manitoba website. Retrieved from http://web2.gov.mb.ca/laws/statutes/ccsm/_pdf.php?cap=r34. Retrieved February 13, 2017.

12. Our study received approval from the ethics committee of the Université de Moncton as well as ethics committees at the health facilities involved in the study.

13. We received additional funding to include four New Brunswick hospitals in our study.

14. According to the data we obtained on the number of employees in the hospitals we have studied, this figure represents a participation rate of approximately 8% for Yarmouth Regional Hospital, 3% for the Horizon Health network, 4% for Sudbury Regional Hospital, and 5.5% for Saint-Boniface General Hospital. The fact that some groups of employees did not have access to a computer at their workplace should be taken into consideration. Several respondents stated that the questionnaire was too long.

15. Due to the limitations of space, we have not included all the data tables we produced. They are available in the full report (Forgues, Bahi, & Michaud, 2011).

16. At the time of the study, Sudbury Regional Hospital undertook steps to become designated as a fully bilingual hospital facility.

17. We are referring to the Kindle version of the book, which is not paginated.

18. In Thériault's opinion, "juridification" is aimed at "describing a general process through which the judicial sphere comes to be an exemplary site for political organizations and for defining standards and norms in contemporary societies—the government of judges . . ." (p. 51). Thus, a substitution of the legal for the political takes place.

References

Aglietta, M. (1976). *Régulation et crises du capitalisme*. Paris, France: Calmann-Lévy.

Aucoin, L. (2008). *Compétences linguistiques et culturelles des organisations de santé: Analyse critique de la littérature*. Ottawa, ON: La Société Santé en français.

Beach, M. C., Somnat, S., & Cooper, L. A. (2006). The role and relationship of cultural competence and patient-centeredness in health care quality. New York: The Commonwealth Fund.

Behiels, M. D. (2005). *La francophonie canadienne. Renouveau constitutionnel et gouvernance scolaire*. Ottawa, Ontario: Les Presses de l'Université d'Ottawa, *Amérique française* series, 12.

Bélanger, P. R., & Lévesque, B. (1991). La "théorie" de la régulation, du rapport salarial au rapport de consommation. Un point de vue sociologique." *Cahiers de recherche sociologique*, (17), 17–51.

Bernier, C. (2009). Citoyens de deuxième classe? Perceptions de la santé et du système de soins chez les francophones du nord-est de l'Ontario. *Francophonies d'Amérique*, (28), 115–138.

Betancourt, J. R. (2006). *Improving quality and achieving equity: The role of cultural competence in reducing racial and ethnic disparities in health care*. New York: The Commonwealth Fund.

Bouchard, L., & Leis, A. (2008). La santé en français. In J. Y. Thériault, A. Gilbert, & L. Cardinal (Eds.). *L'espace francophone en milieu minoritaire au Canada: Nouveaux enjeux, nouvelles mobilisations* (pp. 351–381). Montréal, QC: Fides.

Boudreau, F. (1999). Langue minoritaire et services de santé mentale en l'an 2000: droits et besoins des francophones de Toronto. *Reflets: Revue d'intervention sociale et communautaire*, 5(2), 123–154.

Bowen, S. (2001). *Language Barriers in Access to Health Care*. Health Canada. Retrieved from http://www.hc-sc.gc.ca/hcs-sss/pubs/acces/2001-lang-acces/index-eng.php. Accessed February 16, 2017.

Boyer, R. (1986). *La théorie de la régulation: Une analyse critique*. Paris, France: La Découverte.

Boyer, R., & Saillard, Y. (Eds.). (2002). *Théorie de la régulation. L'état des savoirs*. Paris, France: La Découverte.

Charbonneau, F. (2011). Dans la langue officielle de son choix: la loi canadienne sur les langues officielles et la notion de "choix" en matière de services publics, *Lien social et Politiques*, 66(Fall), 39–63.

Comité consultatif des communautés francophones en situation minoritaire. (2001). *Rapport au ministre fédéral de la Santé*. Ottawa, Ontario: Santé Canada. Note: A discussion of this report in English is available online: https://sencanada.ca/content/sen/committee/372/soci/rep/rep07dec02-e.pdf. Accessed February 15, 2017.

de Moissac, D., de Rocquigny, J., Roch-Gagné, M., & Giasson, F. (2011). *Disponibilité et accessibilité des services de santé en français au Manitoba, Rapport final*. Université de Saint-Boniface / Institut franco-ontarien de l'Université Laurentienne. Retrieved from http://ustboniface.ca/cnfs/document.doc?id=695

Deveau, K., Landry, R., & Allard, R. (2009). *Services gouvernementaux de langue française en Nouvelle-Écosse: Étude de certains facteurs sociostructuraux, sociolangagiers et psycholangagiers associés à l'utilisation des services en français*. Moncton, NB: Institut canadien de recherche sur les minorités linguistiques.

Doucet, M. (2014). Les droits linguistiques, la démocratie et la judiciarisation. In L. Arrighi & M. Leblanc (Eds.). *La francophonie en Acadie, Dynamiques sociales et langagières, Textes en hommage à Louise Péronnet*. Sudbury, ON: Prise de parole. Document published in Kindle format, not paginated.

Forgues, É., Bahi, B., & Michaud, J. (2011). *L'offre de services de santé en français en contexte minoritaire* (Research report). Institut canadien de recherche sur les minorités linguistiques. Retrieved from http://www.icrml.ca/fr/recherches-et-publications/publications-de-l-icrml/item/8489-l-offre-de-services-de-sante-en-francais-en-contexte-minoritaire

Forgues, É., & Mouyabi Mampoumbou, O. N. J. (2014). La collaboration interorganisationnelle au sein de la gouvernance communautaire en Acadie au Nouveau-Brunswick. In L. Cardinal & É. Forgues (Eds.), *Innovation et gouvernance francophone au Canada* (pp. 97–120). Sainte-Foy, QC: Presses de l'Université Laval.

Gagnon-Arpin, I., Bouchard, L., Leis, A., & Bélanger, M. (2014). Accès et utilisation des services de santé en langue minoritaire. In R. Landry (Ed.). *La vie dans une langue officielle minoritaire au Canada* (pp. 195–221). Sainte-Foy, QC: Presses de l'Université Laval.

Government of New Brunswick. (2005). *Official Languages—Your Rights in New Brunswick*. Fredericton, NB: Public Legal Education and Information Service.

Landry, R., Allard, R., & Deveau, K. (2011). *École et autonomie culturelle. Enquête pancanadienne en milieu scolaire francophone minoritaire*. Gatineau, Québec: Patrimoine canadien et Institut canadien de recherche sur les minorités linguistiques. Nouvelles perspectives canadiennes.

L'Express (2009, May 19–25). Les services en français de l'Ontario, servez-vous en! À offre active, demande active. *L'Express de Toronto*. Retrieved from https://l-express.ca/les-services-en-francais-de-lontario-servez-vous-en/

Martel, M., & Pâquet, M. (2010). *Langue et politique au Canada et au Québec. Une synthèse historique*. Montréal, QC: Boréal.

Office of the French Language Services Commisioner. (2008). Annual Report 2007–2008: Paving the Way. Retrieved from http://csfontario.ca/en/rapport-annuel-2007-2008-ouvrir-la-voie-3. Accessed February 13, 2017.

Office of the French Language Services Commisioner. (2013). *Annual Report 2012–2013: A New Approach*. Toronto, ON: Queen's Printer for Ontario. Retrieved from http://csfontario.ca/en/articles/4136. Accessed February 16, 2017.

Office of the French Language Services Commisioner. (2015). *Annual Report 2014–2015: A Voice for the Voiceless*. Toronto: Queen's Printer for Ontario. Retrieved from http://csfontario.ca/fr/articles/5475. Accessed February 16, 2017.

Southern Health – Santé Sud (n.d.). *French Language Services Strategic Plan*. Retrieved from https://www.southernhealth.ca/assets/AnnualReports/FLS-Strategic-Plan-2013-16.pdf

Thériault, J. Y. (2009). Les langues méritent-elles une protection législative et constitutionnelle? *Revue de la Common Law en français*, 11, 45–54.

Van Campenhoudt, L., & Quivy, R. (2011). *Manuel de recherche en sciences sociales*, (4th ed.). Paris, France: Dunod.

Vézina, S. (Ed.). (2007). *Gouvernance, santé et minorités francophones*. Moncton, NB: Les Éditions de la Francophonie.

PART IV

BILINGUALISM AND THE ACTIVE OFFER OF FRENCH-LANGUAGE SERVICES

Issues and Challenges in Providing Services in the Minority Language: The Experience of Bilingual Professionals in the Health and Social Service Network[1]

Danielle de Moissac, *Université de Saint-Boniface*
and Marie Drolet, *University of Ottawa*, in collaboration with
Jacinthe Savard, Sébastien Savard, Florette Giasson, Josée Benoît,
Isabelle Arcand, Josée Lagacé, and Claire-Jehanne Dubouloz

Abstract

This chapter explores the experience of bilingual professionals with the provision of health and social services in the official language of minority communities in Canada. Seventy-two professionals from Manitoba and eastern Ontario describe the main issues associated with language access, and the challenges with which they are faced in their day-to-day responsibilities with the active offer of these services. Professionals reported challenges such as shortage of bilingual professionals and services, and difficulty identifying clients who wish for services in the official language of the minority and finding bilingual professionals, as well as lack of organizational support to actively offer services in the minority language in health facilities. Some suggestions to better support the practice of active offer are provided.

Key Words: active offer, health and social services, official language, minority communities, professionals.

Introduction

It has become increasingly clear that in order to ensure effective communication between a service provider and a person needing services, both need to "speak the same language". Language concordance is recognized by health systems as being of fundamental importance in the provision of client-centred care (Bowen, 2015; Ohtani *et al.*, 2015; Schwei *et al.*, 2015). A review of the international literature shows that language barriers have a significant impact on accessibility of care, patient safety, and quality and outcome of care, and may incur additional costs due to readmission or prolonged hospitalization (Bowen, 2015). The direct provision of services by a bilingual service provider is the preferred method to ensure language concordance. Professional training programs in the minority official language (Consortium national de formation en santé, 2015), and opportunities integrated into professional practice to further develop linguistic competencies (Betancourt *et al.*, 2003), make it possible for professionals to provide safe and quality services in the service user's official language of choice. The question we need to ask ourselves is whether the presence of bilingual staff is sufficient to ensure that an active offer of services in the minority official language is made regularly and continually. What language issues should be considered? Are there challenges within social service and health facilities making it difficult for a professional to offer services in the service user' official language of choice? A better understanding of the experience of providers is needed to identify the realities and challenges involved in actively offering services in the official language of the minority.

This chapter presents the results reported in two exploratory qualitative studies, one conducted in Manitoba and the other in eastern Ontario. The objective of both was to learn about the experience of bilingual health and social service professionals, whether Francophone or Anglophone fluent-in-French, regarding the offer of services in the minority official language, in this case French language services in two communities outside Quebec. Although these studies were independent and took place in two different minority language contexts, their common objectives, similar research methodologies and comparable sampling make it possible to identify common themes. The legal context regarding language and services in both provinces will be presented, as well as barriers reported in the literature on service provision in the minority language. The methodology used for data collection and qualitative analysis of results will follow. Findings will be categorized in relation to themes emerging from discussions with the participants, more specifically issues and challenges associated with service provision in the minority language. Current practices promoting language access will then be highlighted. Finally, recommendations will be proposed, suggesting helpful strategies to address barriers to the provision of services in official language minority communities.

Minority Language Context in Two Central Canadian Provinces

Although the two provinces where these exploratory studies took place are neighbours, their legal contexts framing language rights and policies are distinct. In Ontario, the *French Language Services Act*, 1986 (Office of the French Language Services Commissioner, 2009) guarantees the right of the public to receive French-language services from Government of Ontario ministries and agencies in 26 designated regions, including the Champlain region in eastern Ontario where the study was conducted. However, services mandated and partially or fully funded by public funds, such as hospitals, children's aid societies, and long-term care facilities are not automatically subjected to the *French Language Services Act*; these organizations can voluntarily request a designation. Their designation may be full or partial (that is, it may apply to certain services or programs and not others within the organization). In particular circumstances, facilities may be urged to request a designation by the Local Health Integration Network (LHIN) and the French Language Health Planning Entity in their region. The latter is responsible for advising the LHIN on the organization of French-language health services in its region (Ontario Ministry of Health and Long-Term Care, 2012), while the LHIN is responsible for improving the coordination and engagement of communities in Ontario's health system.

In Manitoba, a *French Language Services Policy* allows French-speaking Manitobans and facilities that serve them to benefit from comparable government services in the language of the laws of Manitoba (that is, English and French in designated regions, where the French-speaking population is concentrated (Francophone Affairs Secretariat, 1999). Designated regions include three districts in the city of Winnipeg and several rural Francophone communities, mainly in the south of the province (Francophone Affairs Secretariat, 1999). The policy applies to several sectors: in health and social services, it applies to facilities and regional health authorities (RHAs) designated as bilingual (that is, 4 of the 5 RHAs). The *Regional Health Authorities Act* (Government of Manitoba, n.d.) requires bilingual-designated RHAs to submit a French-Language Services plan and have it approved every five years. In addition, the *Santé en français* organization, which is the official voice of the Francophone community in matters of health and social services, advocates for Francophones with governmental, institutional, and professional bodies to improve access to quality services in French throughout Manitoba (Santé en français, 2017).

Barriers to Service Provision in the Minority Language

Besides the language barrier, which can hamper effective communication, other organizational challenges influence institutional capacities related to language access services. International studies on ethnolinguistic minorities have identified some of these challenges: difficulty matching providers and clients with language concordance; limited access to assessment tools and resources in the client's language of choice; and lack of language provisions in organizational policies are among them (Attard *et al.*, 2015; Hudelson & Vilpert, 2009; Mygind *et al.*, 2016). In linguistic minority communities in Canada, gaps in service provision and lack of visibility of bilingual professionals have been identified as important obstacles (Fédération des communautés francophones et acadiennes du Canada [FCFA], 2001). A recent study conducted in hospitals in four Canadian provinces revealed that despite consideration for the language of the minority when planning service delivery, human resources management, and written and oral communications, access to services in French appears to be coincidental (Forgues *et al.*, 2011). Among factors that contribute to the near-absence of active offer are: a lack of recognition on the part of employees and managers alike of the importance or necessity of providing services in the minority language; management practices that favour hiring unilingual Anglophone staff; and lack of commitment from senior management regarding language access provision (Forgues *et al.*, 2011).

Recently, a number of resources have been developed to increase the professionals' capacity to respond to their clients' linguistic needs. Interpreter services and translated documents, such as assessment forms and health-related documents, have been made available

(Bischoff & Hudelson, 2010; Bowen 2004; Semansky *et al.*, 2009). However, interpretation is often provided by volunteers or family members despite reported risks associated with using *ad hoc*, untrained interpreters (Flores *et al.*, 2012; Kilian *et al.*, 2014). Bilingual professionals themselves are often called on by co-workers to act as interpreters (Johnson *et al.*, 1999) or to translate workplace tools (Verdinelli & Biever, 2009). Invariably, these tasks create an additional workload that is neither recognized nor supported systematically (Bouchard & Vézina, 2009; Drolet *et al.*, 2014; Engstrom, Piedra, & Won Min, 2009; Mygind *et al.*, 2016). Organizational support becomes an essential means of helping bilingual professionals, who have a direct influence on access to services for linguistic minority populations.

Study Objectives

These two exploratory studies were designed to better understand the experience of bilingual professionals in terms of challenges associated with providing healthcare and social services in the language of the official minority. The primary objectives were to: (1) describe the challenges professionals face in the provision of services in the minority official language; (2) identify practices that facilitate provision of services in the minority official language in their facility; (3) assess whether professionals have access to tools needed to adequately serve clients in the official minority language; and (4) determine if teamwork or networking among bilingual professionals paves the way for the provision of these services.

Methodology

A qualitative approach was used in order to allow bilingual professionals to express themselves freely regarding their experience of working in health or social services in a linguistic minority setting. With the approval of the ethics committees at both the Université de Saint-Boniface and the University of Ottawa, and voluntary and informed consent from the participants, semi-structured interviews were conducted with groups of professionals. The latter were recruited through personal invitations from members of the research team or through organizations providing social and health services in both official languages. In total, 72 professionals shared their experiences about the challenges of providing services in the language of the minority in their respective settings.

In Manitoba, five focus groups with a total of 29 participants were held in the fall of 2010. Three discussions took place in urban settings and had seven participants each, while the eight other participants, divided into two groups, met in rural communities in the southern part of the province. Professions include audiology, chiropractic, dentistry, nutrition, occupational therapy, dental hygiene, medicine, nursing, optometry, pharmacy, physiotherapy, midwifery, and social work. In eastern Ontario, 43 professionals took part in the study; 21 worked in health care and 22 in social services. Eight focus groups were held in the fall of 2012. Participants came from settings offering services to children, youth, or seniors. Professions represented were occupational therapy, social work, nursing, nutrition, psychology, and service management.

Discussions ranged in length from 90 to 120 minutes, and were recorded for transcription purposes. The transcriptions were imported into NVivo v.9 (QSR International) software for content analysis. Data were coded independently by two members of the research team in each of the universities. A first reading allowed identification of emerging themes that were ranked first in the hierarchy; categories were determined according to the primary themes discussed in the focus groups. For each of these categories, secondary nodes were identified inductively. The analytical protocol was developed and validated by several members of the research team, who were from different health and social professions; an inter-rater and consensus method was used. Results were thus analyzed deductively and inductively through inter-group comparisons (Huberman & Miles, 1991). Finally, content analysis of the various codes was used to describe and regroup them. Data saturation was reached for the urban settings in Manitoba and for eastern Ontario. Given the unique geographical, social, and political characteristics of each of the settings studied, theoretical generalizations would be difficult to make. However, the validity of the data remains significant, as the participants' comments reflected a high level of consensus both in Manitoba and eastern Ontario, and also supported the findings of previous research on this subject (Laperrière, 1997).

Results

Working in a bilingual setting, professionals have to overcome obstacles daily and find ways to better respond to the needs of clients from the linguistic minority. In presenting the comments made by participants, issues and challenges professionals face in the provision of these services will be the primary focus. Concrete examples from specific vulnerable populations will be used to illustrate certain realities. Issues brought forth are mostly client-based and of linguistic and social nature. Challenges, on the other hand, appear to be organizational: insufficient services in the minority language, difficulty identifying clients who wish French-language services, insufficient number of bilingual professionals, and insufficient services available in French, and lack of support for service delivery in both official languages are the main concerns. Practices that professionals adopt to improve minority language access in their workplace will also be presented.

Linguistic and Social Issues

Bilingual professionals spoke about the importance of clients receiving services in the minority language. For some, anxiety increases when language concordance is not possible; this is even more evident where children and seniors, with their families, as well as immigrants, are concerned. As for mental health, service providers in psychology and social work report that clients prefer to communicate in their mother tongue, as they can better express their emotions, feelings, and problems, and can analyze situations in more depth: [original: French] "It's hard to find the right words . . . You're not talking about the weather, here, you're talking about your emotions, your relationships, sensitive and emotional subjects." (O-J3). Professionals also report that clients are more inclined to become aggressive when a service provider speaks a different language, or in a crisis situation involving a child or adolescent. Whether it be a routine appointment or a complex health incident, participants recognize that language concordance is an integral part of care provision.

Issues associated with language variations in both official languages were also reported by participants: several observed extremely variable levels of language, often depending on the client's education level. Some participants pointed out that certain clients, particularly seniors, are unable to read and write easily and hesitate to communicate in their everyday French, which they feel is not the "professional French" they should use at a medical appointment. Furthermore, certain regional expressions, such as "il a du front" (he has a lot of gall) or "j'ai mal au cœur" (which can mean a stomach ache as well as heart pain) are not always understood and can lead to misunderstandings. For other Francophones, medical terminology is easier to understand when it is in English: this is particularly true for seniors, who are more likely to have been educated in English schools and are accustomed to navigating the health system in the majority language. The level of language used by different clients can vary considerably.

To deal with this linguistic diversity, professionals admit that they have to be flexible to accommodate their clients' needs: [original: French] "It's important to be able to adjust to the person's level and explain things in their language, so they will understand." (O-A2). Shifting from one official language to the other is often necessary, to ensure clients understand instructions, according to participants.

Other situations arise when use of both languages is necessary, such as when family members who speak different languages (exogamous families) are present. Professionals sometimes notice a tendency towards assimilation into the majority language, and some clients avoid requesting services in French just to please either Anglophone staff or their family members, especially if the latter only speak English: [original: French] "Well, my daughter-in-law speaks English. My son is with me . . . We'll do all this in English." (O-A1). One participant stressed the importance of having a solid knowledge of both official languages.

Being a member of a minority group also seems to have an impact on the clients' confidence when they speak their mother tongue, particularly in Manitoba. One participant reported: [original: French] "I think we have a minority mindset . . . We think there is a 'proper French' that is better than what we speak." (W-2.1). Another participant felt that this adds to the clients' hesitation to ask for services in the minority language. Often, a professional has to encourage clients to insist on their right to services in their own language, even in designated bilingual facilities. This professional recounted a conversation with a client being treated in a hospital setting:

[original: French] He said that he hated speaking English. I told him, "OK, so ask . . . We're designated bilingual, so if you want a Francophone [nurse], you ask, and we'll try to find one for you." So he said, "OK, that's what I want!" (W-2.4)

Sociodemographic characteristics of vulnerable Francophones may also have a negative effect on access to services in French, as heard in Ontario. Some participants reported that clients with a modest income and limited resources tend to isolate themselves socially, which limits their access to available services. Others notice reluctance, especially among seniors, to reveal their financial situation in order to obtain free services; the tendency to want to maintain confidentiality about economic difficulties discourages them from accessing services to which they are entitled. The socio-economic status of clients in the linguistic minority therefore has to be considered, according to participants, as active offer of services in the minority language is even more vital for this clientele.

Respondents also report that without support in their language of choice, clients are less likely to participate in their care, especially in a group situation. Active offer of services in their mother tongue is more likely to provide the full benefit of care and integration: [original: French] "They are Francophones, they feel like they're a minority, they feel isolated . . . They often need to have someone with them so they'll feel safer there." (O-J3). Language barriers increase the client's dependence on professionals and reduce benefits of care. Participants point out that this situation means that the professional has to spend more time managing a health situation that has become complex because of the language barrier; he or she is then less available to help other clients or potential clients.

Challenges in Service Delivery in the Minority Official Language

According to the participants, bilingual professionals face numerous challenges when providing services in the minority language. Besides shortage of human resources and bilingual services, participants report difficulty identifying which service users want to receive service in the minority language. They also cite problems in finding a bilingual professional among their colleagues to whom they may refer such a service user, and speak of a lack of organizational support for offering services in the minority language, even within a bilingual work setting. These challenges are described in detail below.

Shortage of Bilingual Professionals and Services

According to participants, the main challenge in providing services in the minority official language is a shortage of bilingual professionals and services. As one participant described: [original: French] "When I close a file, I often think, OK, I've made my recommendations, but the resources don't exist. 'Good luck!' . . . I have no choice, and that's what's hardest." (O-J1). Participants report that a shortage of bilingual professionals means that unilingual Anglophone staff members are hired, even in designated bilingual positions. A shortage of professionals and services is significant in rural areas, but participants also report such problems in urban settings, where one would expect greater access to a wider range of services in both official languages.

Identification of Client's Official Language of Choice

Many participants reported difficulty identifying their client's language of choice. In the past, family names were good indications of mother tongue, but that is no longer the case. One participant said that this new reality supports the need for active offer, for in its absence "on manque le bateau" ("we miss the boat"). In order to distinguish Francophone clients, the majority of professionals report using space provided in the client's medical records to document their language preference. Others make a habit of writing the client's language of choice at the top of the file folder as a reminder for future appointments and for co-workers who follow up with this client. On the other hand, nearly half the participants say the language variable is not collected and recorded at all times, and often is not considered as important.

Finding Bilingual Co-Workers, Professionals, and Services

The challenge of finding co-workers able to provide services in the minority language is, according to participants, linked to the fact that not all professionals disclose their bilingualism. As one professional said: [original: French] "It's not everybody who wants to display the fact they're Francophone, you know . . . They were hired because they could speak French, but they don't use it instinctively." (W-3.1). Hesitancy in declaring competencies in both official language stems from many sources, as illustrated below.

Participants from both provinces reported that some professionals are afraid of increased workload due to their ability to communicate in both official languages. They are often asked to interpret or translate for clients or co-workers. Others highlight the fact that their bilingualism makes them more easily identifiable and may endanger their personal safety; for example, one participant shared the experience of a professional who had to deal with a difficult situation in child protection services. Naturally, this person did not want to be recognized by members of the community for fear of negative repercussions. Finally, some participants pointed out that bilingual professionals who have limited second language skills may not feel comfortable identifying themselves as bilingual. Actively offering services is not as common a practice as hoped, several participants have found, and public awareness of services provided in the minority language is limited, which in turn reduces access to these services.

Limited awareness of available bilingual human resources also proves to be a significant barrier in the continuity of care in the minority official language. According to participants, bilingual professionals who want to refer their clients to a specialist or another bilingual professional find this difficult, unless they personally know of such professionals. Moreover, participants mentioned that with time, close connections have been formed with other non-bilingual professionals to whom they currently refer their clients. In this case, a health or social service worker will not seek to develop contacts with bilingual co-workers or specialists. Continuity of care in the client's language of choice is, then, not being fostered.

Lack of Support for Language Access

In a bilingual workplace, several barriers to service in the official language of the minority exist. In a field where communication between clients, members of the care team, and various specialists is vital, the language used is predominantly that of the majority. Since health records are written entirely in English, participants stated that a good knowledge of the majority language is necessary. Those from Ontario emphasized that the policy of access to records, whereby clients have access to records in their own language at their request, is not respected. As one participant specified, professionals have to act as interpreters when linguistic minority clients wish to consult their medical records. Several participants suggested that language proficiency in both official languages should thus be a job requirement, even in facilities designated as exclusively Francophone.

Furthermore, professionals who can function in both official languages are perceived as rare resources and are called upon to perform additional tasks linked to their language skills: translation, interpretation, adaptation of assessment tools, and treatments. When with Francophone clients, bilingual professionals have the choice of conversing in the minority language, but will have to document the consultation in the majority language. Some professionals decide to proceed in the minority language, but others avoid this situation:

> [original: French] Even if I'm bilingual and I can speak French with the person, I have to speak English because if I don't, I don't have the time to re-translate the whole consultation for everyone who's English-speaking here. (W-2.7)

Being bilingual thus represents an increased workload: as one participant stated [original: French] "It's a lot of work for us. You may be lucky enough to have a manager who understands you and everything, but in the long run . . . That doesn't stop your own work from accumulating." (O-A2). Participants feel they get little recognition for this extra work, and, as mentioned above, hesitate to disclose their bilingualism.

Lack of educational and assessment materials in the minority official language was also noted. Although a large number of participants have access to certain resources in the minority official language, the majority of them found these on their own, either from their professional association, private companies, or organizations in Quebec or France. Without bilingual forms, as is the case with most governmental forms in Manitoba, professionals have to simultaneously translate during the consultation or speak in the majority language with the client. Additionally, a social worker in Ontario pointed out that this affects clients' empowerment and autonomy. Due to the lack of appropriate tools in the minority language, social workers are forced to take responsibility for this task when it is normally done by the client. A participant mentioned that being unable to provide a complete range of services in the client's language, throughout the continuum of care, undermines the scope, the quality, and the benefits of a professional's actions.

Participants also observed that in their bilingual workplace, they are not allowed to show preference for clients based on linguistic needs. Staff must provide services to all clients in an equitable fashion. The exception seems to be when services are required by an agency that requests and pays for them to be provided for in a specific language, such as the military, the federal government, or a school district. In addition, participants emphasize the fact that a bilingual professional is not obligated to provide a service in the official language of the minority, unless she or he holds a designated bilingual position. Logistics surrounding service delivery in both official languages and referring Francophone clients to bilingual professionals is extremely complex, acknowledged a participant. Matching resources and needs related to language does not seem to be done systematically, but is rather based on the personal initiative of certain individuals, she added.

Maintaining language proficiency in both official languages was also mentioned by participants as being an obstacle. Since a large number of bilingual professionals attended professional programs in the language of the majority, terminology in the minority language is not always easy to learn or remember unless a sustained effort is made to do so. As for professional training, it is not rare for clinical instruction to be supervised by a preceptor in the majority language. In Manitoba, some participants at the beginning of their career as health professionals had completed their studies in French but clinical placements or internships were in English-speaking workplaces. They were therefore unfamiliar with the English terminology currently used in their field. This is a significant challenge, particularly for professionals whose official language is French and who learn English as a second language: [original: French] "In the setting I found myself in, well, I'd taken all my courses in French, I spoke French, but the people I worked with were all Anglophones" (W-2.6). Furthermore, some participants stated that few professional development education opportunities are available in the minority language outside of Quebec, and limited resources are available to help with travel costs. As some participants said, maintaining proficiency in both official languages is difficult, especially where specific terminology related to their field is concerned.

Practices That Encourage Service Provision in the Language of the Minority

To overcome the challenges described above, bilingual professionals find different ways to facilitate the provision of services in the minority language. First, participants highlighted sincere commitment of many bilingual professionals who try to meet the needs of their clients in their language of choice. Being sensitive to the reality of being part of a minority and to the linguistic insecurity often related to it, professionals adapt their vocabulary, tools, and written information to make them fully accessible to speakers of the minority language. Bilingual service providers also mention developing complicity with their clients, a "real connection" or trusting relationship based on common cultural references that professionals know and reflect. It may also be the case that being a member of a minority brings out a stronger feeling of Francophone identity and sense of belonging for both providers and clients.

Some participants find ways to side-step restrictions imposed on employees in a bilingual workplace. Some may agree to help co-workers "as a favour," add duties to their regular workload, translate documents, act as interpreters, and encourage clients to ask for services in the language of their choice. Others feel supported by their employer, who recognizes the importance of providing services to the Francophone population in the minority official language and makes additional efforts to harmonize professional competencies with the needs of this population.

Researchers also felt a strong spirit of cooperation among co-workers in the workplace, as well as with professionals in other organizations and members of related professions, particularly in Ontario. Professionals said that teamwork and cooperation are essential if they are to serve the population in both languages. Service providers describe their contacts with bilingual colleagues as informal, more personal, and effective. Several attribute this affinity to belonging to a minority. In Manitoba, there is also a sense of commitment, beyond the professional context, such as the case of professionals who volunteer for fundraising activities to maintain language access programs in their region. Participants explained that bilingual professionals generally have a strong desire to support and improve existing services in the minority official language.

Bilingual professionals admit that some organizational initiatives have had a positive effect on access to services in the minority official language. This is especially true in Manitoba. Several participants noted that active offer of French-language services in their workplace is provided at first contact, whether in person or by phone. They recognize the importance of this practice, which involves more than wearing a "Bonjour/Hello" pin. Active offer begins by greeting clients in the minority language and continuing in the language they prefer, if possible. [original: French] "That's why I take the risk of starting off in French, because if you don't start in French, no one will speak to you in French" (W-5.3).

Bilingual signage is also recognized as being beneficial, whether in the professional's office, outside the building, on business cards, in emails, and on websites. Some participants indicated that documents in both official languages are available. Others, however, reported this with caution: in some cases, greeting clients or posting signs in the minority language does not necessarily mean that French-language services are available, even in facilities that are designated bilingual: [original: French] "When the receptionist is bilingual, it gives you an impression, 'Hey . . . Great! They must have bilingual services here,' but it's not him or her [the receptionist] who is providing the actual service" (W-2.1). One participant summarized the situation: Bilingual signs do not necessarily mean bilingual services.

Discussion

The purpose of this chapter is to describe the issues and challenges associated with service provision in the official language of the minority population, as experienced by healthcare and social service providers. A series of focus groups with 72 professionals in Manitoba and eastern Ontario revealed language and social issues for clients at times related to their being members of a minority. The comments made by respondents about challenges of working in a bilingual setting confirm previous findings on this subject. Bilingual professionals make additional efforts in their day-to-day tasks to ensure that quality service trajectories are adapted to meet the needs of Francophones. This calls on the professionals' qualities of perseverance and resourcefulness and a strong sense of collegiality and cooperation.

For access to social services and healthcare for minority populations, language and social barriers cannot be ignored. The Francophone minority population's socio-demographic profile shows higher rates of aging, lower average family income, and an overall lower level of education as compared to the majority group (Bouchard *et al.*, 2009). In addition, participants noted that the minority status contributes to a lack of assertiveness on the part of clients who hesitate to ask for services in French. Studies have shown that members of a minority group are less likely to ask for services in their own language and prefer to "go along" with the norms of the majority group (Allaire, 2007; Drolet *et al.*, Chapter 6 in this collection; Hogg & Abrams, 2004). This is reported more frequently in Manitoba, a province with no law calling for French-language services. It is possible that legal support may have a positive influence on access to care for linguistic minorities; more research on the subject would be valuable.

Since service user have a range of language proficiencies, professionals have learned to adjust their vocabulary in order to be understood. Some use regional expressions or alternate between French and English. Participants confirm the importance of active offer for all service users, as it enables identification of language of choice and improves the chances that referral to bilingual services is possible. Furthermore, professionals recognize that language concordance nurtures a stronger relationship between service user and provider. The quality of the relationship with the service user and the sense of trust are stronger, as language and sense of belonging to the same group are shared. This complicity, according to Santiago-Rivera and her colleagues (2009), increases effectiveness of care. The feeling of belonging also promotes engagement and interest among bilingual professionals in cooperating with their bilingual colleagues and better serving the official linguistic minority population in their community.

Challenges identified by bilingual professionals in terms of access to services in the minority language are related to the low availability of such services and lack of support; these factors influence the way professionals work and their ability to offer services on a continuum, including specialized services and continuity of care in the minority language. Bilingual professionals are perceived as a rare resource to whom all requests for language access services are directed. Because of the bilingual context and the minority nature of the language used by the service user, tasks such as translating material, interpreting for co-workers and families, and working more closely with clients result in an increased workload for bilingual professionals; in turn, they may hesitate to identify themselves as bilingual since they receive little support and recognition for the extra duties they are required to perform. As described by Engstrom and colleagues (2009), inadequate recognition given for additional efforts needed to serve clients can lead to difficulties in staff retention, thus increasing the shortage of qualified bilingual professionals. Organizational adjustments are needed to recognize additional duties inherent to bilingual staff in a bilingual workplace in a minority environment.

Limited knowledge of bilingual staff and resources available in the community is a barrier, as it may contribute to a perception of shortage of services in the minority language. Thus, existing services may not be utilized to their full potential. This is of concern, as the availability of bilingual professionals is limited. Statistics Canada has reported challenges in listing bilingual professionals in most provinces and territories because of limited data in the census (Bouchard *et al.*, 2009). Initiatives such as the Observatory of Minority Health,[2] which aims to fill these knowledge gaps and to improve access to bilingual health professionals and services for the Francophone population of Ontario, are useful tools in this regard. With increased knowledge of bilingual professionals' availability and geographic distribution of official linguistic minority populations, service provision can be adjusted accordingly. To do so, the language variable is needed as an integral component in administrative databases.

Furthermore, participants suggest adding language competencies to annual membership renewal forms requested by their professional association. Greater awareness of the importance of this variable and the added value of providing this information is needed, both by members and management of professional associations or orders. If the language variable of both clients and professionals is collected regularly, an observatory for all provinces and territories might facilitate service organization at the local and provincial levels, based on the needs of minority language communities and available resources.

Networking between bilingual professionals has also been suggested as a means of increasing their visibility and providing them the opportunity to share experiences, best practices, and bilingual workplace tools. Professionals would gain from increased peer support and cooperation with co-workers and members of their profession (Savard *et al.*, 2013; Verdinelli & Biever, 2009). For new professionals or students, meeting other bilingual professionals working in minority settings, as well as visiting bilingual workplaces that would be suitable for an internship or work placement, would be advantageous. The benefits of networking, especially in a minority context, are numerous.

Professionals acknowledge the difficulty of maintaining client-centred care on a continuum in the official minority language, especially if service organization does not encourage identification of clients' official language of choice or the practice of active offer. Some professionals suggest adopting a model of centralized or integrated services (Hébert, Tourigny, & Gagnon, 2004; Lafortune, Béland, &

Bergman, 2011). Integrated services could promote access to services in the minority language, notably through the establishment of a single-entry system whereby clients could be directed to a team of primary and multidisciplinary social services, healthcare, and community services in their official language of choice. Such a model is currently being explored in Manitoba and Ontario for Francophone seniors, among other populations.

In conclusion, these studies have provided an opportunity to document challenges of working in a bilingual workplace in a linguistic minority setting, as well as strategies that bilingual social service and health professionals currently use to provide services in the official minority language. Access to services in the language of the minority must not, however, rest solely on the shoulders of bilingual professionals. Organizational measures to improve language access services need to be integrated into the system through concrete, positive, and measurable actions that support professionals and their clients in accessing services in their language of choice and in their community.

Notes

1. Our research was supported by the *Consortium national de formation en santé*. We would like to thank *Action Marguerite* and its staff members, as well as the research team from the University of Ottawa, for a pleasant and productive partnership, and Janelle Delorme for her collaboration in this research.
2. http://www.obs-minorityhealth.ca/#english

References

Allaire, G. (2007). From "Nouvelle-France" to "Francophonie Canadienne": A historical survey. *International Journal of the Sociology of Language, 185*, 25–52.

Attard, M., McArthur, A., Riitano, D., Aromataris, E., Bollen, C., & Pearson, A. (2015). Improving communication between health-care professionals and patients with limited English proficiency in the general practice setting. *Australian Journal of Primary Health, 21*(1), 96–101.

Betancourt, J. R., Green, A. R., Carrillo, J. E., & Ananeh-Firempong, O. (2003). Defining cultural competence: A practical framework for addressing racial/ethnic disparities in health and health care. *Public Health Reports, 118*, 293–301.

Bischoff, A., & Hudelson, P. (2010). Access to healthcare interpreter services: Where are we and where do we need to go? *International Journal of Environmental Research and Public Health, 7*(7), 2838–2844.

Bouchard, L., Gaboury, I., Chomienne, M.-H., & Gagnon-Arpin, I. (2009). *Profil santé des communautés francophones minoritaires du Canada / Health profile of French-speaking minority communities in Canada.* Ottawa, ON: Santé Canada and Réseau de recherche interdisciplinaire sur la santé en contexte minoritaire au Canada.

Bouchard, P., & Vezina, S. (2009). *L'outillage des étudiants et des nouveaux professionnels: Un levier essentiel à l'amélioration des services de santé en français.* Ottawa: Consortium national de formation en santé.

Bowen, S. (2004). *Language Barriers Within the Winnipeg Regional Health Authority: Evidence and Implications.* Winnipeg, MB: Winnipeg Regional Health Authority.

Bowen, S. (2015). *The Impact of Language Barriers on Patient Safety and Quality of Care.* Ottawa: Société Santé en français. Retrieved from https://sante francais.ca/wp-content/uploads/SSF-Bowen-S.-Language-Barriers-Study.pdf Accessed January 7, 2017.

Consortium national de formation en santé. (2015). *Étudier en français en santé, des carrières qui font du bien!* Ottawa, ON: Association des collèges et universités de la francophonie canadienne (ACUFC). Retrieved from http://cnfs.net/ Accessed August 18, 2015.

Drolet, M., Savard, J., Savard, S., Benoît J., Arcand I., Lagacé J., Lauzon S., & Dubouloz, C-J. (2014). Health services for linguistic minorities in a bilingual setting: Challenges for bilingual professionals. *Qualitative Health Research, 24*(3), 295–305.

Engstrom, D. W., Piedra, L. M., & Won Min, J. (2009). Bilingual social workers: Language and service complexities. *Administration in Social Work, 33,* 167–185.

Fédération des communautés francophones et acadiennes du Canada (FCFA). (2001). *Improving Access to French-Language Health Services.* Ottawa, ON: Fédération des communautés franocphones et acadiennes. Retrieved from http://www.fcfa.ca/user_files/users/40/Media/Pour%20un%20 meilleur%20acc%C3%A8s%20%C3%A0%20des%20services%20de%20 sant%C3%A9%20en%20fran%C3%A7ais%20-%20EN.pdf. Accessed February 27, 2017.

Flores, G., Abreu, M., Barone, C. P., Bachur, R., & Lin, H. (2010). Errors of medical interpretation and their potential clinical consequences: A comparison of professional versus ad hoc versus no interpreters. *Annals of Emergency Medicine, 60*(5), 545–553.

Forgues, É., Bahi, B., Michaud, J., Deveau, K., Boudreau, J., & St-Onge, S. (2011). *L'offre de services de santé en français en contexte francophone minoritaire*. Moncton, NB: Institut canadien de recherche sur les minorités linguistiques.

Francophone Affairs Secretariat. (1999). *French Language Services Policy*. Winnipeg, MB: Government of Manitoba. Retrieved from http://www.gov.mb.ca/fls-slf/pdf/fls_policy.pdf. Accessed February 27, 2017.

Government of Manitoba (n.d.). *The Regional Health Authorities Act*. Winnipeg, Government of Manitoba. Retrieved from http://web2.gov.mb.ca/laws/statutes/ccsm/_pdf.php?cap=r34. Accessed February 27, 2017.

Hébert, R., Tourigny, A., & Gagnon, M. (2004). *Intégrer les services pour le maintien de l'autonomie des personnes*. Montréal: Éditions EDISEM.

Hogg, M. A., Abrams, C., Otten, S., & Hinkle, S. (2004). The social identity perspective: intergroup relations, self-conception, and small groups. *Small Group Research*, 35, 246–276.

Huberman, M. A., & Miles, M. B. (1991). *Analyse des données qualitatives: Recueil de nouvelles méthodes*. Brussels, Belgium: de Boeck-Wesmael.

Hudelson, P., & Vilpert, S. (2009). Overcoming language barriers with foreign-language speaking patients: A survey to investigate intra-hospital variation in attitudes and practices. *BMC Health Services Research*, 15(9), 187.

Johnson, M., Noble, C., Mathews, C., & Aguilar, N. (1999). Bilingual communicators within the health care setting. *Qualitative Health Research*, 9, 329–343.

Kilian, S., Swartz, L., Dowling, T., Dlali, M., & Chiliza, B. (2014). The potential consequences of informal interpreting practices for assessment of patients in a South African psychiatric hospital. *Social Science and Medicine*, 106, 159–167.

Lafortune, L., Béland, F., & Bergman, H. (2011). Le vieillissement et les services de santé: Une réorientation des pratiques cliniques plutôt qu'un défi économique. *Revue vie économique*, 3(1), 1–13.

Laperrière, A. (1997). Les critères de scientificité des méthodes qualitatives. In J. Pouprat *et al.*, (Eds.), *La recherche qualitative: Enjeux épistémologiques et méthodologiques* (pp. 365–389). Montréal, QC: Gaétan Morin.

Ministère de la Santé et des Soins de longue durée de l'Ontario (2012). *Entités de planification des services de santé en français*. Toronto: Imprimeur de la Reine pour l'Ontario. Retrieved from www.health.gov.on.ca/french/publicf/programf/flhsf/health_planning_entitiesf.html. Accessed January 30, 2017.

Mygind, A., Norgaard, L.S., Traulsen, J.M., El-Souri, M., & Kristiansen, M. (2016). Drawing on healthcare professionals' ethnicity: Lessons learned from a Danish community pharmacy intervention for ethnic minorities. *Scandinavian Journal of Public Health*. [Epub preceding print at the time of writing]

Office of the French Language Services Commissioner. (2009). 2008–2009 *Annual Report: One Voice, Many Changes.* Toronto: Queen's Printer for Ontario: Commissariat aux services en français. (2009). *Rapport 2008-2009: Une voix, des changements.* Toronto: Imprimeur de la Reine pour l'Ontario. English version.

Ohtani, A., Suzuki, T., Takeuchi, H., & Uchida, H. (2015). Language barriers and access to psychiatric care: A systematic review. *Psychiatric Services,* 66(8), 798–805.

Ontario Ministry of Health and Long-Term Care. (2012). *French Language Health Planning Entities under the* Local Health System Integration Act, 2006 *and Regulation 515/09.* Retrieved from http://www.health.gov.on.ca/en/public/programs/flhs/planning.aspx. Accessed February 27, 2017.

Santiago-Rivera, A. L., Altarriba, J., Poll, N., Gonzalez-Miller, N., & Cragun, C. (2009). Therapist's views on working with bilingual Spanish-English clients: A qualitative investigation. *Professional Psychology, Research and Practice,* 20, 436–443.

Santé en français (2017). *Vision, mandat, champs d'activités et axes stratégiques.* Winnipeg, MB: Santé en français. Retrieved from https://santeenfrancais.com/qui-nous-sommes/mandat. Accessed January 17, 2017.

Savard, S., Arcand, I., Drolet, M., Benoît, J., Savard, J., & Lagacée, J. (2013). Les professionnels de la santé et des services sociaux intervenant auprès des francophones minoritaires: L'enjeu du capital social. *Francophonies d'Amérique,* 36, pp. 113–133.

Schwei, R. J., Del Pozo, S., Agger-Gupta, N., Alvarado-Little, W., Bagchi, A., Chen, A. H., & Jacobs, E. A. (2016). Changes in research on language barriers in health care since 2003: A cross-sectional review study. *International Journal of Nursing Studies,* 54, 36–44.

Semansky, R. M., Altshul, D., Sommerfield, D., Hough, R., & Willging, C. E. (2009). Capacity for delivering culturally competent mental health services in New Mexico: Results of a statewide agency survey. *Administration and Policy in Mental Health,* 36, 289–301.

Verdinelli, S., & Biever, J. L. (2009). Spanish-English bilingual psychotherapists: Personal and professional language development and use. *Diversity and Ethnic Minority Psychology,* 15, 230–242.

CHAPTER 9

Recruitment and Retention of Bilingual Health and Social Service Professionals in Francophone Minority Communities in Winnipeg and Ottawa[1]

Sébastien Savard, *University of Ottawa*, Danielle de Moissac, *Université de Saint-Boniface*, Josée Benoît, *University of Ottawa*, Halimatou Ba, *Université de Saint-Boniface*, Faïçal Zellama, *Université de Saint-Boniface*, Florette Giasson, *Université de Saint-Boniface*, and Marie Drolet, *University of Ottawa*

Abstract

The difficulty in recruiting and retaining employees able to work in both official languages has been identified as one of the most significant reasons why Francophone seniors in minority language communities are unable to access social services and health care in French. This chapter presents the findings of a study of 55 professionals interviewed in six focus groups, who worked in bilingual organizations in one of the two regions studied (Winnipeg, Manitoba and Ottawa, Ontario). We hoped to identify the factors that led these employees to work in bilingual organizations and those that had encouraged them to stay in the organizations where they worked. Our findings show that the desire to contribute to the well-being of Francophones and the opportunity to obtain stable positions offering good working conditions are among the most important recruitment factors. The quality of the work environment and the opportunity to work in a diverse and inclusive workplace are retention factors mentioned regularly by the study participants. A greater recognition of the additional workload associated with working in both languages, and the recruitment of senior bilingual management staff, are among the recommendations proposed to improve the recruitment and retention of bilingual staff.

Key Words: Recruitment and retention, social service and health professionals, Francophones in minority language communities.

Introduction

The shortage of bilingual health and social service professionals is a problem with significant consequences for the health of Francophones living in minority language communities in Canada (Bouchard & Vézina, 2009; Drolet *et al.*, 2014; Gauthier, 2011). In fact, the difficulty recruiting these professionals represents one of the greatest barriers to access to services in French. A preference for working in acute-care clinical settings in urban locations and the mobility of professionals make the challenges of recruiting and retaining staff members in certain settings (such as rural and remote areas), and in certain fields (such as long-term care) even more difficult to overcome. In this chapter, we uncover the various elements characterizing the conditions of practice for health and social service professionals working in Francophone minority communities. Through their comments, we also explore the factors encouraging the recruitment of professionals and their desire to remain in a bilingual workplace. The study was conducted in two Canadian cities, Ottawa and Winnipeg, in order to compare the perspective of bilingual professionals in two different minority language contexts.

We will begin by providing a brief background to the study, situating it in the broader context of research on access to social services and health care for Francophones living in minority language communities in Canada, and more specifically on the obstacles or difficulties experienced by this population when attempting to access appropriate services in their language. We will continue with a presentation of our analytical framework based on models developed by other researchers interested in linguistic identity construction and the recruitment and retention of human resources. We will then describe the methodological framework used to conduct this study and present the major results of our research. Some recommendations intended to improve the recruitment and retention of bilingual health and social service professionals in Francophone minority communities will be suggested in the conclusion.

Background

There is no guarantee that all Francophones living in minority language communities who wish to receive social services and health care in French will be able to access them. In Manitoba, we have found that, on average, 25% of Francophones claim to receive care and services from a bilingual professional (de Moissac *et al.*, 2014). This percentage varies depending on the type of professional. For example, the percentage of Francophones who claim to access services in French from nurses is 32% (de Moissac *et al.*, 2014). There is an improvement in the rate of French-language services with regard to general practitioners: the percentage of clients receiving care in their language by their family physician was 14% in 2006 (Corbeil *et al.*, 2006), rising to 28% in 2008–2009 (Chartier *et al.*, 2012). In Ontario, Marmen and Delisle (2003) show that, although the proportion of Francophone family physicians and nurses is higher than that of Francophones in the general population, these doctors still cannot meet the needs of the population. These professionals are not available at all times and do not necessarily practise in the cities and regions where Francophones need access to their services (Marmen & Delisle, 2003). According to the Ontario Ministry of Health and Long-Term Care, a statistical profile of health professions in the province (2012a) indicates 8.5% of health professionals in the province speak French. They are, however, unevenly distributed. For example, in the area served by the Champlain Local Health Integration Network (LHIN), which includes, among other localities, the Greater Ottawa Area, 37.8% of professionals are able to communicate in French, while this proportion falls to 0.8% in northwestern Ontario. Thus, the degree of difficulty Francophones have in finding health professionals who speak French varies greatly between regions.

The identification of barriers in accessing social services and health care in French has been examined in several studies (Drolet *et al.*, 2014; de Moissac *et al.*, 2012a; Forgues *et al.*, 2011); as Part 4 of this book describes, the challenges identified by Francophone health and social service professionals in Manitoba and in Ontario are very similar. The shortage of professionals offering services in French, and the difficulty identifying Francophone clients and employees, are both significant barriers (Drolet *et al.*, 2014; de Moissac *et al.*, 2012a). This is true even though several professionals we met acknowledge a greater awareness to the needs of Francophones and an increase in French-language services in the last few years. Professionals report a lack of knowledge of the human resources available in French and a lack of formal integration and networking for these resources. To bridge these gaps, professionals put informal cooperative partnerships in place with colleagues in their facility or other organizations, so they can benefit from a support network (Savard *et al.*, 2013). Moreover, Bouchard & Leis (2008) emphasize the importance of community networking in structuring an integrated and well-coordinated social service and health care system for Francophones living in minority communities.

A number of studies explore the availability of bilingual human resources in bilingual-designated facilities. Gousseau (2009) describes the current needs and availability of human resources in facilities and agencies designated as bilingual in Manitoba, and reveals the greatest challenge is being able to fill professional positions, in particular those for registered nurses, licensed practical nurses, health care aides, and mental health workers. In a later study, Gauthier (2011) confirms these findings in an exploratory study of language proficiency. The author found "there were various reasons why finding qualified people to fill designated bilingual positions was difficult, including the shortage of trained personnel, inappropriate recruitment methods and the fact that these resources were being lured away by major urban facilities." The shortage of bilingual staff thus seems to disproportionately affect rural and remote areas, as well as long-term health facilities, because new graduates are more interested in working in acute care and in urban settings. It seems that there is no true recruitment strategy adapted to the needs of the Franco-Manitoban community (Gauthier, 2011). Furthermore, managers of social service and health care facilities designated as bilingual recognize that the ethnocultural diversity of the immigrant work force and the linguistic profile of these workers—that is, those with little knowledge of English—represent new challenges for us to consider (de Moissac *et al.*, 2012b).

In a unpublished study funded by the *Société santé en français* (SSF) on the language training needs of health professionals working with Francophone communities, managers surveyed in Ontario mentioned the greatest obstacle to offering services in French lay in the recruitment and retention of bilingual staff; this applied especially (as in Manitoba) in rural and remote areas. The measures introduced to remedy this situation vary, ranging from offering language training, or recruiting in Quebec, to hiring employees who are not yet bilingual with conditions that encourage or require bilingualism to obtain permanent status. This confirms the results of a study conducted a few years earlier (Société santé en français [SSF], 2006) showing that in four regions of Ontario (northern, mid-northern, southeastern and southern) the difficulty in recruiting bilingual professionals was an important, if not *the* most important, cause of limited access to services in French. The other significant factors working against French-language services are the lack of awareness in the population that the services exist and the lack of integration and coordination of existing resources.

A Conceptual Framework for Recruiting and Retaining Bilingual Professionals in a Minority Language Community[2]

Several theoretical frameworks describe the factors influencing the recruitment and retention of employees in their work settings. We propose a conceptual framework adapted to the particular situation of professionals working in a bilingual setting in a minority language community. As Figure 1 illustrates, this framework is based largely on the motivational model created by Dolea and Adams (2005), who argue that environmental and sociocultural (macro) variables influence the language proficiency and the psychological needs of the employee (micro), as well as organizational support in the work setting (meso). Together, these conditions influence the choice of the employee to work in this setting and to remain engaged, satisfied, and motivated to perform her or his job effectively.

On the macro-level, there are variables related to the political, economic, and social context, which have an influence on the vitality of the French language in a community and on the conditions that favour the recruitment of bilingual employees by institutions. In Ontario, for example, a law protects access to services in French for Francophones, while in Manitoba, the rights of Francophones to receive services in their own language are subject only to a policy. This reflects a different positioning of French in the two provinces, and has an impact on the capacity of Francophones to speak their language in daily life, to receive schooling in French, and to work in French. All these elements necessarily influence the language proficiency of employees over the medium to long term. The more opportunities Francophones have to speak their language, the more they feel that French is valued and supported; the more they want their children to attend French schools, the more they will try to work together in French—even if it is the minority language in their community—simply because it makes them feel comfortable. In the long run, this translates into the ability of health and social service facilities to recruit bilingual professionals with greater ease. Laws and policies also influence the way regional health authorities (in Manitoba) and local health integration networks (in Ontario) are able to respond to the needs of the Francophone population to access French-language services. The variables of availability and conditions of access to bilingual jobs are also linked to environmental conditions that influence the recruitment and retention of bilingual staff. In the two provinces studied, job opportunities are very favourable for bilingual employees seeking work in the health sector. The ability to be hired rapidly is particularly important for newcomers, Francophones and Allophones alike. In addition, the working conditions offered can meet both economic and social needs; for instance, they generally make it possible to reach a work/life or work/family balance.

Francophone communities in Manitoba and in Ontario are much more heterogeneous than 20 years ago as newcomers joined the existing Franco-Ontarian and Franco-Manitoban population (Conseil de planification sociale d'Ottawa / Social Planning Council of Ottawa), 2010; Commissariat aux langues officielles / Office of the Commissioner of Official Languages, 2007). This means organizations, as well as employees and service users, have to adapt, especially in situations where the requirement to provide services French is combined with a shortage of bilingual health professionals. The existence of organizations working to improve access to social services and health care in French in a community—such as the SSF and the *Consortium national de formation en santé* (CNFS)—should be considered a factor that can influence the ability of organizations to offer health care and working conditions for bilingual employees in a positive manner.

The model of ethnolinguistic vitality described by Landry and his colleagues (2006) identifies two dynamics—social determinism and self-determination—as influences on the capacity and the motivation of an individual to speak and work in his or her mother tongue in locales where it is the minority official language. Social determinism, which originates in the ideological, legal, and political framework (number, power, status) in which the minority language community is situated, defines the position occupied by the minority language and the tools it possesses to develop. Self-determination, on the other hand, originates in the type of linguistic and cultural socialization that an individual experiences (forexample, a community that values and fosters the vitality of the minority language) and in the individual's psycholinguistic development,[3] which often depends on the position of the minority language in his or her immediate family. These two dynamics also cause the minority language to either become more fragile or to flourish in a given community.

Figure 1. Conceptual Framework for Recruiting and Retaining Bilingual Professionals in Official Language Minority Communities, Based on Dolea and Adams (2005) and Landry *et al.* (2008)

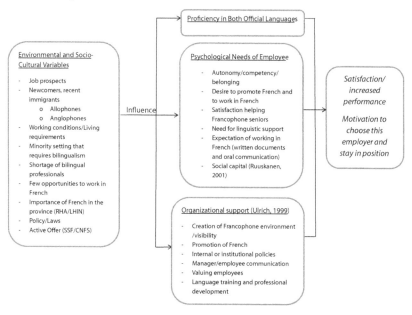

On the micro-level, there are the psychological needs of the employee, which include the values, needs, and expectations that influence his or her motivation to perform well in the workplace (Deci & Ryan, 2002). In other words, is the job (and are the tasks performed) consistent with the professional's values? Does the job enable the employee to meet her or his psychological needs (for belonging, etc.) as well as material needs? Does it meet expectations in terms of tasks, contexts, and outcomes? The framework we have adapted includes among the psychological needs the variables associated with language, such as proficiency in both official languages and the desire to promote French and to work in the employee's mother tongue or the first official language she or he learned. Last, the opportunity for bilingual professionals to be part of a community with a great deal of social capital, as modelled by Ruuskanen (2001), is also a way of meeting a need, increasing the employee's motivation to stay in the job or workplace. As a brief reminder, social capital refers to the resources[4] and privileges that belonging to a community allows an individual to enjoy; the links between the members of the community are numerous and rich, and encourage the creation of relationships of trust and a sense of belonging to the collective.

On the meso-level, factors are associated with organizational support from the bilingual health or social service facility. These factors include internal policies that make bilingualism tangible and facilitate the promotion and use of both official languages in all the day-to-day tasks that affect the client, the client's family, and the employees, as well as in those activities that encourage the greater visibility of a Francophone space in the community. Added to this are the human resource management practices focused on meeting the needs of employees and on fostering their well-being (Ulrich, 1999), such as those encouraging employees to express themselves and managers to listen to their concerns, open communication between managers and employees, and a climate that encourages continuous learning.

With this adapted conceptual framework, we can proceed to developing research questions and analyzing collected data in order to better understand how environmental and sociocultural variables, language proficiency, employees' needs, and organizational practices influence the recruitment and retention of bilingual professionals in a minority language setting.

Research Questions

Better access to health care and social services in French in minority language communities depends, among other things, on the recruitment and retention of bilingual professionals. In a situation where there is a shortage of bilingual health and social service professionals, fundamental questions have to be asked: Which factors facilitate the recruitment and retention of these professionals in a Francophone or bilingual work setting? What are the realities of working in a Francophone or bilingual facility in a minority language community? What challenges do bilingual professionals face in these settings, in terms of practising their profession? Do social support networks, whether formal or informal, exist within the facility or with other organizations in the community? Finally, what strategies should be priorities in order to facilitate the recruitment and retention of bilingual professionals?

We respond to these questions in our study, and pay particular attention to the issues associated with language and requirements for bilingualism that impact the professional lives of health care workers, and also the work environment.

Methodology

We decided qualitative methods were the best choice for our research; this approach makes it possible to become more familiar with the realities of bilingual work settings in the two minority language communities in our study. We conducted focus groups with health professionals in direct contact with seniors. Most were nurses, personal care workers and social workers, but there were also occupational therapists, speech-language pathologists, and recreation specialists working in long-term care facilities or providing services in residences offering assistance and support. In Winnipeg, participants were recruited through a contact person in each setting, who was responsible for circulating a written or electronic invitation among her or his co-workers in the facility. The contact person was not the immediate supervisor of the employees invited to participate, as it was important to avoid a relationship of authority that could influence participation in the study. In Ottawa, one of the discussions took place as the first part of a previously planned meeting of facility employees. Employees could choose whether to participate in the conversation. Those participating in the second focus group were informed of the project by means of a poster inviting them to contact the research associate if they wanted to take part, or by means of an email message sent directly to a list of employees who had taken part in an earlier study and agreed to be re-contacted.

Four focus groups were conducted with employees of the Actionmarguerite organization in Winnipeg, two in the Saint-Boniface area (n=14) and two in Saint-Vital (n=22). In Ottawa, two groups took part in the research, a group from the Montfort Renaissance residence (n=14) and a combined group of Community Care Access Centre (CCAC) and Ottawa General Hospital (n=5) employees. A total of 55 professionals participated in the focus groups. The discussions were facilitated by members of the research team during the fall of 2013 and most were held during participants' working hours.

The data from interviews were coded through a predetermined procedure: initial reading of 20% of the transcriptions for the purpose of identifying the categories (general annotation describing the basic content in the corpus excerpt) and emerging themes (annotation specifying what is discussed in more detail) (Paillé & Mucchielli, 2008); reaching a consensus among team members on the categories and themes; developing a list of codes (abbreviations for categories and themes) and definitions of each; validating the list of codes; coding the data using this list of codes of the three transcriptions and calculating the degree of inter-rater agreement (Huberman & Miles, 2002); and coding the remainder of the data according to the list of codes already identified, while allowing new codes to emerge. This procedure was followed separately in each of the sites (Ottawa and Winnipeg) using the same list of codes. Once the analysis at each site was completed, the observations were compared to discover similarities and differences. The rigorous procedure made it possible to conduct a deeper analysis, discover the meaning of the whole, then extract the excerpts and identify the precise phenomena revealed.

Results

We deal with four major themes in this section: environmental and sociocultural variables; language proficiency; the psychological needs of employees, particularly those related to social capital; and organizational support. These themes are discussed in light of factors encouraging the recruitment and retention of bilingual professionals; quotations supporting the themes are included and statements are noted as RO (respondent from Ottawa) and RW (respondent from Winnipeg).

Environmental and Sociocultural Variables in a Bilingual and Minority Setting

Certain environmental variables explain the context in which professionals in the health and social service sectors carry out their work, and suggest factors that may encourage recruitment and retention. Thus, the results of our study showed that being able to work in a bilingual setting is an attractive factor for recruiting employees. Indeed, nearly all respondents mentioned their desire to work in a bilingual or Francophone setting because they are more comfortable with the French language.

> [original: French] They said the working language here was French; that's why everyone, all of us, chose to come here, because the working language, they said, was French. (RW-1)

Many participants said the language they spoke with residents had a tangible effect on them. Moreover, Francophone residents were more comfortable speaking French and, in the case of dementia, French was the only language of communication. Participants also noted that speaking French with agitated clients has a calming effect.

Residents and families were very grateful for the efforts made by staff offering services in French, and some residents even remembered being so happy when a bilingual attendant returned from a vacation because they could again receive care in French. Clients appreciated being able to communicate more comfortably and to express their needs more easily; this translates into less resistance to treatment. Professionals also appreciated having the opportunity to speak in French with residents and other staff members because they felt more comfortable and could express themselves more freely.

In a long-term care facility designated as bilingual in a minority community, linguistic duality was described as follows by participants: although the language of communication with Francophone residents is more often French, the working language, including that used for spoken communication between members of the care team and for documentation, is English. In a minority community, even in a facility designated as bilingual, English dominates. One participant in Winnipeg even stated that [original: French] "it's as if a Francophone here is not viewed as someone who gets first consideration" (RW-2), while in Ottawa, a participant said:

[original: French] Often, at official meetings or events, we are exposed to a lot of English. Like, everything that is official is done in the English language, like the staff days, official meetings, really it's all in English. (RO-1)

English dominance results from the fact that French is the minority language in the region, even in a designated bilingual setting. Participants stated that numerous employees are not bilingual. Furthermore, in a situation in which outside services need to be involved, a knowledge of English is essential. Every document, including medical records, reports, and health forms, must be completed in English. Participants acknowledge it is necessary to use English since the residents' state of health and records must be understood by all professionals, both inside the facility and outside in the case of emergencies, consultations, or transfers of care to a hospital centre or other services. On the other hand, participants admit this means that every resident or family member who speaks only French will not be able to understand what is written in the records. For the resident who prefers and is entitled to care and services in French, there seems to be a certain disconnect in this regard.

Participants are encouraged to actively offer services in French when speaking to residents and their families. On the other hand, their immediate supervisors may not be bilingual. Moreover, participants raised the point that professional development courses are almost always in English (as evidenced by posters in classrooms where our Winnipeg focus groups took place). This facility, designated bilingual, is not really a space where the French language is alive and well as part of the daily life of employees. Linguistic duality raises certain challenges in terms of the environment and the sociocultural context of the facility. Participants also raised the point that bilingualism in the workplace causes tensions between Francophones and Anglophones. This is particularly germane to Winnipeg, where participants worry about segregation and excluding employees who cannot speak French.

Language Proficiency

Some health care workers note they sometimes have initial difficulty communicating with residents because of language differences or accents in French. All the same, professionals and residents later end up understanding each other merely through exposure to these differences.

> [original: French] It's a different French here (laughter). There are a lot of residents here who have, you know, a Grade 4, 5 education, so there's a lot of jargon, slang. So it's a different French than I was accustomed to. But no, not really. (RW-5)

In terms of communication between employees, some professionals speak to their bilingual co-workers in French because they feel more comfortable doing so. Others take advantage of the opportunity of working with a colleague from their home country to speak in their vernacular, which sometimes makes other colleagues uncomfortable.

> [original: French] Also, because there are a lot of languages here, a lot of nations, two people might speak in the mother tongue. And when you hear them, I don't know what they're saying, you're frustrated, directly. "Is he talking about me or what?" Yeah, there's that. (RW-6)

The origins of employees present another challenge to the diversity of language skills. Several health professionals were immigrants who had recently arrived from countries where French, English, or another language is spoken. These professionals speak French and English with different accents depending on their country of origin, thereby creating a linguistic diversity that can make communication difficult.

> [original: French] A challenge for me, I find, is when there are different types of French, from different countries, so that even me, and I can usually understand French, but the way that certain people speak, I can't understand them. (RW-4)

Besides the variable language skills among Francophones, professionals often face considerable language barriers with some of their unilingual Anglophone colleagues. In Winnipeg, for example, meetings between employees and supervisors are generally conducted in English. Although the workplace is bilingual, most supervisors communicate more often in English. Beyond affirming they are bilingual, they do not actually speak French to employees unless the latter show a real need for it. [original: French] "With my supervisors, they speak to you in English. If you don't understand, then you tell them you didn't understand, and they will speak French to you." (RW-1)

Not using French very often, or preferring to speak English, can create a feeling of linguistic insecurity[5] that contributes to French deficits. The fact that meetings are conducted in English jeopardizes the French-language proficiency of employees. They run the risk of losing their practical use or proficiency in French, which gives way to the English language that is ever-present in bilingual work settings.

> [original: French] You know, I complain a lot, I often say, "Why don't we speak French when there is just one person who speaks English?" Here, everyone speaks French, there is just one person and the meeting automatically switches into English. (RW-1)

One element reported frequently by professionals is translating from French to English in the records, which causes additional work.

> [original: French] I find it hard, when you've done your whole procedure or your family conference in French, and then you go back to your office, and you have to write your report, but in English. It isn't easy, because once again you have to think about it, you have to reflect. But also, the fact you have to interpret everything that you did in another language means it isn't easy. (RO-3)

Respondents' comments speak to the importance of knowing both languages well. Some professionals commit to doing interviews with Francophone clients in French, knowing they will have to translate the information they write in the records, but others prefer English to avoid extra work. Several professionals are frustrated by having to translate, because it requires a solid knowledge of terminology in both languages as well as additional time.

When an organization offers the opportunity to work in both languages, however, this was identified as a factor to make it easier to recruit bilingual health care workers. In fact, for people who have recently arrived in Canada, and who speak French as their second language but do not speak any English (or very little), being able to work mainly in French and having the opportunity to learn or improve their proficiency in English is an undeniable advantage. This reality was observed mainly in Ottawa, where we find organizations where French is truly the language of the workplace. Some professionals from Quebec have chosen to work across the border in Ontario to improve their English. One source of frustration mentioned by several participants in Winnipeg, in particular, is the fact that, while they make considerable efforts to improve their English, their Anglophone colleagues do not show the same motivation to improve their French, despite the fact that they have bilingual positions. It would seem that very little follow-up is done to ensure Anglophones hired in bilingual positions meet the language requirements of their position.

The Psychological Needs of Employees

In this section, we discuss the comments of focus group participants addressing the values, expectations, and needs that can influence the motivation and performance of employees according to Dolea and Adams (2005). Besides language proficiency need, one of the elements related to values participants mentioned as motivating them to apply for bilingual positions, as well as to remain working in an organization that offers French-language services to Francophone minority communities, is their sense of pride in belonging to the Francophone community. Their pride is illustrated by, among other things, their desire to contribute to the development and improvement in French-language services, thereby contributing to the survival and retention of gains in French made by their community.

> [original: French] Well, personally, I find, you know, in Canada as a whole I mean, the two official languages are French and English, I mean, basically, being able to live in those languages in your daily life. For me, it's really important to nurture the language, to nurture Francophone society, not only in Ontario. For me that's really important. (RO-2)

The sense of attachment felt by bilingual professionals is not limited to their connection with the Francophone community; it also connects them to their clientele of seniors. Respondents in Winnipeg and

Ottawa frequently mentioned that their interest in working with seniors led them to apply for a job in the organization where they now work. This interest seems to have transformed into a deep feeling of attachment towards the residents and service users with whom they are in daily or regular contact. The quality of the relationship they have developed with the residents is one of the elements most often mentioned as a source of satisfaction in their workplace.

The factors leading or motivating employees to stay working in a bilingual position are similar to those that led them to apply for their current job. However, a few elements constitute factors that contribute solely to their motivation to remain in their current position. What arises from the study as the most important retention factor is the quality of the work environment. Respondents working in the Winnipeg area and those in the Ottawa area emphasized the quality of their connections with their co-workers and with the residents as one of their primary sources of satisfaction in their current job. The opportunity to work in a bilingual setting with interesting people from diverse cultural and linguistic backgrounds is another reason behind their desire to continue in their position with their current employer.

Social Capital at the Centre of Psychological Needs

At the centre of participants' comments about factors motivating them to apply for a bilingual position and remain in it, we often find elements that suggest to us that for Francophones, working in a bilingual setting makes it possible to gain and use their social capital to its greatest potential. Furthermore, the attraction a bilingual environment holds for them is also associated with the existence of a great amount of social capital within the Francophone minority community itself. We observed that the bilingual professionals participating in our study have a great feeling of belonging toward the Francophone community. In fact, several respondents mentioned having chosen their employer, at least in part, because the job available would enable them to work in French and with Francophones. These respondents care a lot about the well-being of the Francophone minority community and want to contribute to their growing and thriving culture. Among Francophone or bilingual professionals, there is also a level of closeness and trust that does not often exist among their Anglophone colleagues.

[original: French] Well, for us in the hospitals, it's pretty much Anglophone, it's an environment that is really, really, really Anglophone, unfortunately. Francophones stick together. That's what we do. Colleagues get together to chat, at lunch, or on the phone, we really like being together. (RO-3)

This collegiality appears to be more of a reality in Ottawa than in Winnipeg, however. It seems easier in Ottawa to communicate in French with managers who are often bilingual, and employees do not hesitate to communicate in French with co-workers. Conversely, in Winnipeg, professionals cannot always communicate with their supervisors in French because they are often Anglophones. Employees also hesitate to speak French openly with their co-workers, out of a fear of excluding those who are unable to understand or speak French. Even between Francophones, communication is less easy, because the French spoken by Franco-Manitobans and by Francophones born outside Canada is so different that it is sometimes difficult for them to understand each other. The feeling of belonging to a Francophone community in the workplace is, therefore, stronger and easier to maintain in Ottawa than in Winnipeg.

Organizational Support

Certain organizational practices motivate health and social service professionals to apply for and stay in bilingual positions. Not surprisingly, the working conditions offered by the employer represent an important factor. Salary structures, ample opportunities, rapid access to employment after short-term training, and career stability were often mentioned, especially in Winnipeg, as elements influencing the decisions to apply to and remain with their employer. Respondents in Ottawa made special mention of good working conditions such as flexibility in the organization of their work, the diversity of the staff members, and job security.

On the other hand, a bilingual employee's satisfaction may suffer as the result of human resource management practices that are considered irritants. For example, some respondents mentioned it is sometimes difficult to apply for another job in their organization because their employer prefers them to stay in their current position; it is too hard to replace them, due to the shortage of bilingual professionals.

Other irritants can also be attributed to organizational support leaving something to be desired, namely the inability of some Winnipeg participants to communicate in French with their unilingual Anglophones supervisors, and the lack of acknowledgement of the particular contributions and additional work associated with having to work with clients in both official languages.

Conclusion and Recommendations

This study has enabled us to gain a better understanding of the factors influencing the recruitment and retention of bilingual social service and health care professionals working in minority language communities. Referring to the model proposed by Landry *et al.* (2006), we have presented some observations and propose recommendations addressing the two dynamics that influence the vitality of a language in a minority context: social determinism and self-determination. The authors observed that bilingual employees feel pride in their ability to serve the Francophone population, and see themselves as playing an important role in the promotion of French language and Francophone culture and society in their workplace and in their community. Self-determination, therefore, works in favour of promoting French and the rights and interests of Francophones. In fact, being able to work in a bilingual setting is an advantage sought by Francophones wanting to maintain their proficiency in both official languages. Bilingual professionals recognize the importance of the language for their residents or clients, with whom they develop a deep attachment reinforced by the language they share. This contributes to the quality of the environment, and thus to the meso-level in the model of motivation put forward by Dolea and Adams (2005). The attachment also responds to a psychological need, or to the micro-level in the model, because connections with Francophone residents and bilingual co-workers give employees an opportunity to increase their social capital. These connections become a significant source of satisfaction and encourage the retention of employees. A recruitment strategy directed toward professional internships in bilingual workplaces has met with some success in the field of health and social services, because the structure and length of placement programs make it possible to enter the work force rapidly and increase the familiarity of new graduates with bilingual work settings.

The reality of working in a bilingual setting is not without challenges, however, because the predominance of English means that bilingualism is difficult to put into practice. The fact that French is seldom or too seldom used in so-called bilingual settings can threaten the linguistic security of this language. It is difficult to promote the use of French in the absence of an institutional mission and policies ensuring that all employees know the minority language. According to the participants we interviewed, the lack of professional development offerings in French, of bilingual managers, and of follow-up of language training in both languages represent elements that work against the ability to maintain a bilingual workplace. Several employees added there is a lack of recognition of the additional workload generated by tasks required to meet the needs of Francophone clients in a minority language community. This discourages professionals from actively offering services in French. In a minority community, socialization in the minority language by professionals in their work setting and by the aged population in their everyday life contribute to the ethnolinguistic vitality of the community (Gilbert *et al.*, 2005; Landry *et al.*, 2006). This environmental variable on the macro-level has a profound influence on the recruitment and retention of bilingual professionals.

It is possible to formulate recommendations addressing the three groups of primary actors, each of whom has a particular role to play to encourage the recruitment and retention of bilingual staff in facilities offering health and social services in Francophone minority communities. At the micro-level, where the bilingual employees themselves are located, the employees should act as ambassadors of French and the Francophone community in their own workplace, and recognize the importance of actively offering French-language services. An informal network of Francophone and Francophile co-workers encouraging the use of French in units, floors, or departments, as well as outside the workplace, can help develop bilingual social capital that contributes to an overall sense of belonging. All employees must be open to the diverse cultures living together in the global Francophone community.

According to the concept of organizational support proposed by Ulrich (1999), organizations with a mandate to provide bilingual social services and health care are responsible for creating a working environment that encourages, facilitates, and promotes French language and cultures. Employers should see themselves as agents to promote the presence of French and Francophones in the workplace, by making the language and culture visible and ensuring the services offered are actually available in French. This involves hiring a greater number of bilingual professionals, supervisors, and managers. Language training in both official languages must be offered, and follow-up has to be systematic.

Professional development activities in both official languages represent another way of promoting bilingualism within the facility. To encourage the retention of staff members, organizations should make greater efforts to enrich the sense of belonging employees have toward their workplace. The employer must also assume responsibility for connecting Francophones so they can develop a sense of common belonging to the Francophone world, and for raising employee awareness of cultural diversity. The additional workload associated with offering bilingual services and with the efforts made by employees must be acknowledged. A financial bonus for bilingual services might be considered. Facilities for seniors should take advantage of every occasion making contact with future health and social service graduates, thereby promoting the idea of working with this population and to make the advantages of a career in this field more widely known. The authors' findings support the concept of being known as an "employer of choice." In the context of bilingual work settings in minority communities, an employer ought to be recognized as being an employer of choice if the facility: (1) offers a working environment where employees feel comfortable communicating in either official language; (2) supports employees who want to pursue language training in either official language; (3) acknowledges the efforts of bilingual employees who provide services in both languages; and (4) fosters a sense of belonging to the workplace.

The third actor is comprised of regional and national government departments and agencies responsible for funding health care and social services in French. This group can act on the social determinism dynamic in the model presented by Landry et al., (2006). Regional health agencies are included, as are provincial and national organizations such as: Société Santé en français and its branches; the Consortium national de formation en santé, which promotes education and training in French for health and social service professionals; and other associations that promote Francophone language and culture. These organizations must continue to advocate for the rights of Francophones and fight for the entrenchment of French-language service policies into law, especially in Manitoba. Organizations could facilitate language training in both official languages for health professionals, and provide the follow-up necessary for maintaining an adequate level of language proficiency. Agencies could institute an incentive policy to firmly establish respect for bilingual position designations by defining operating rules in designated facilities and units that mandate bilingual practices, and by funding a bilingual bonus program. To give one example, nurses hired in a position designated as bilingual in a Winnipeg facility receive a bonus. This practice should be extended to other groups of professionals. Moreover, a national organization could show leadership by creating an association of bilingual health and social service professionals for the purpose of encouraging mutual support and solidarity among them.

Recruitment strategies for bilingual health and social service professionals should be aimed at the values, needs, and expectations of employees who wish to serve Francophone clients in a minority context. To ensure that these employees remain bilingual, language support in both official languages is necessary. This support will make it possible to maintain and even improve the language skills of employees; as we explained earlier, this is an important factor in recruiting and retaining bilingual professionals in our model. A facility designated as bilingual that is recognized for offering services in French must actually create a work environment where employees, clients, and their families feel comfortable, at all times, communicating in the official language of their choice. Finally, the ability to recruit bilingual staff—and therefore to offer services in their own language to Francophones in minority communities—does not depend solely on commitment, pride, and attachment on the part of the professionals involved. Neither does it depend exclusively on the management practices of health and social service facilities, especially those designated as bilingual. Instead, it depends on the commitment of the entire Francophone community.

Notes

1. Our research has been supported by Health Canada through the Consortium national de formation en santé. We thank Monique Bohémier for her contribution to this study.

2. For a more detailed presentation of the theoretical frameworks on which the one chosen for this study is based, see the research report published by de Moissac, D., *et al.* (2014).

3. Psycholinguistic development corresponds to the attitude and the behaviours a person has developed or adopted in the course of linguistic socialization, and can be seen in his or her desire to integrate, ethnolinguistic identity, linguistic motivation, language proficiency, and linguistic behaviours.

4. Resources can take several forms, such as influence, information, support, assistance, references, and financial and material resources.

5. Linguistic insecurity refers to an employee's feeling regarding her or his ability to communicate effectively in French.

References

Bouchard, L. & Leis, A. (2008). La santé en français. In J. Y. Thériault, A. Gilbert, A. et L. Cardinal, L. (Eds.). *L'espace francophone en milieu minoritaire au Canada: Nouveaux enjeux, nouvelles mobilisations* (pp. 351–381). Montréal, QC: Éditions Fides.

Bouchard, P., & Vézina, S. (2009). *L'outillage des étudiants et des nouveaux professionnels: Un levier essentiel à l'amélioration des services de santé en français.* Ottawa, ON: Consortium national de formation en santé.

Chartier, M., Finlayson, G., Prior, H., McGowan, K.-L., Chen, H., de Rocquigny, J., Walld, R., & Gousseau, M. (2012). *La santé et l'utilisation des services de santé des francophones du Manitoba / Health and healthcare utilization of Francophones in Manitoba.* Winnipeg, MB: Manitoba Centre for Health Policy.

Commissariat aux langues officielles (2007). *Les indicateurs de vitalité des communautés de langue officielle en situation minoritaire 1: les francophones en milieu urbain: La communauté francophone de Winnipeg.* Available in English as: Office of the Commissioner of Official Languages (2007). *Vitality indicators for official language minority communities 1: Francophones in urban settings: The Winnipeg Francophone community.*

Conseil de planification sociale d'Ottawa (2010). *Profil de la communauté francophone à Ottawa.* Ottawa, ON: Author.

Corbeil, J.-P., Grenier, C., & Lafrenière, S. (2006). *Les minorités prennent la parole: Résultats de l'Enquête sur la vitalité des minorités de langue officielle.* Ottawa: Statistique Canada.

Deci, E. L., & Ryan, R. M. (Eds.). (2002). *Handbook of self-determination research.* Rochester, NY: University of Rochester Press.

de Moissac, D., Ba, H., Zellama, F., Benoit, J., Giasson, F., & Drolet, M. (2014). Le recrutement et la rétention des professionnels de la santé et des services sociaux bilingues en situation minoritaire. (Unpublished report).

de Moissac, D., de Rocquigny, J., Giasson, F., Tremblay, C.-L., Aubin, N., Charron, M., & Allaire, G. (2012a). Défis associés à l'offre de services de santé et de services sociaux en français au Manitoba: Perceptions des professionnels. *Reflets: Revue d'intervention sociale et communautaire, 18*(2), 66–100.

de Moissac *et al.* (2014). *Le recrutement et la rétention de professionnels de la santé et des services sociaux bilingues en situation minoritaire.* Université de St-Boniface and Université d'Ottawa. 65 pages. http://ustboniface.ca/file/documents---recherche/Recrutement-et-rtention-des-professionnels-bilingues-2014.pdfh

Dolea, C., & Adams, O. (2005). Motivation of health care workers: Review of theories and empirical evidence. *Cahiers de sociologie et de démographie médicales, 45*(1): 135–61.

Drolet, M., Savard, J., Benoît, J., Arcand, I., Savard, S., Lagacé, J., & Dubouloz, C. (2014). Health services for linguistic minorities in a bilingual setting: Challenges for bilingual professionals. *Qualitative Health Research, 24*(3), 295–305.

Gauthier, H. (2011). *Étude exploratoire sur les compétences linguistiques à l'embauche.* Winnipeg, MB: Conseil communauté en santé du Manitoba.

Gilbert, A., Langlois, A., Landry, R., & Aunger, E. (2005). L'environnement et la vitalité communautaire des minorités francophones: Vers un modèle conceptuel. *Francophonies d'Amérique, 20,* 51–62.

Gousseau, C. (2009). *Étude sur l'état de la situation actuelle et projection d'avenir des professionnels et professionnelles de la santé bilingues.* Winnipeg, MB: Conseil communauté en santé du Manitoba.

Huberman, A. M., & Miles, M. B. (2002). *The qualitative researcher's companion: Classic and contemporary readings.* Thousand Oaks, CA: SAGE Publications.

Landry, R., Allard, R., & Deveau, K. (2006). Revitalisation ethnolinguistique: Un modèle macroscopique. In A. Magord (Ed.), *Innovation et adaptation: Expériences acadiennes contemporaines* (pp. 105–124). Brussels, Belgium: P.I.E.-Peter Lang.

Marmen, L., & Delisle, S. (2003). Les soins de santé en français à l'extérieur du Québec. *Tendances sociales canadiennes, 11,* 27–31.

Paillé, P., & Mucchielli, A. (2008). *L'analyse qualitative en sciences humaines et sociales.* Paris, France: Éditions Armand Colin.

Ruuskanen, P. (2001). *Trust on the border of network economy: Social capital and trust.* Jyväskylä, Finland: Kaj Limonen.

Savard, S., Arcand, I., Drolet, M., Benoît, J., Savard, J., & Lagacé, J. (2013). Les professionnels de la santé et des services sociaux intervenant auprès des francophones minoritaires: L'enjeu du capital social. *Francophonies d'Amérique,* (36), 113–133. doi:10.7202/1029379ar.

Société santé en français (2006). *Préparer le terrain. Soins de santé primaires en français en Ontario. Rapport provincial.* Ottawa: Author.

Ulrich, D. (1999). *Human resource champions: The next agenda for adding value and delivering results.* Boston, MA: Harvard Business School Press.

CHAPTER 10

Active Offer, Bilingualism, and Organizational Culture[1]

Sylvain Vézina, *Université de Moncton*

Abstract

In this chapter, the author approaches active offer from the angle of organizational culture. He presents the results of a survey of health professionals working in Anglophone and Francophone hospital facilities in New Brunswick. The organizational culture of these institutions is discussed in light of research in the sociology of organizations, not as a fate but as a construct, as are the rules of the organizational game (hierarchical relations, job description, collective agreements, and so on). The research reveals the predominance of an organizational culture centred on bilingualism, which leads to a persistent confusion between the notions of active offer and bilingualism. From this point of view, although bilingualism is essential to a high-quality active offer in both official languages, it can also be counter-productive when it comes to introducing a culture that is favourable to active offer. The findings show the emphasis placed on bilingualism is often perceived by unilingual people as a threat to the balance of powers within the system, frequently leading to resistance toward any measure favourable to active offer. Hence, the author suggests the value of a culture of active offer should be articulated in terms of the objectives of safety and high-quality care in the official languages.

Key words: health professionals, hospital facilities, organizational culture, bilingualism, active offer, New Brunswick.

Introduction

It is evident that besides the skills and knowledge related to health professions, the active offer of safe, quality services in both official languages also involves acquiring the notions and tools required to provide it. In the opinion of many, developing a form of leadership among health professionals in order for them to act favourably towards active offer is an important part of this process.

Although the commitment of people working in health care facilities is indispensable to the practice of active offer, they cannot carry all the responsibility alone. The health system, its rules, and the procedures that govern the way organizations operate, must be part of the structure and provide support and guidance to the employees. Several researchers have earlier identified a wide range of organizational factors favourable to active offer (Bouchard, Beaulieu, & Desmeules, 2011; Forgues, Bahi, & Michaud, 2011). Of note are such measures as ensuring that signs and documents are available in both official languages, encouraging people to wear a pin showing the languages they speak, etc. We will come back to these measures as our analysis proceeds.

As part of our study we want to look specifically at organizational culture and, more precisely, at the particular importance of entrenching active offer into the basic values of the health system. What we mean by organizational culture is the shared values, beliefs, and expectations of the people who belong to the organization (Schein, 1991, 1992; Siehl & Martin, 1984). The question at the core of our exploration is the following: What is the influence of the organizational culture on the commitment of health professionals to practising active offer? In order for the practice of active offer to be sustained in their behaviour, we would argue that they not only need to be aware of it and trained in how to deliver it, but also to be supported. This support would come from the recognition that active offer is one of the essential values of our health systems and of the provision of safe, quality care in our health facilities.

Our interest in organizational culture nonetheless requires us to refine our analytical framework, borrowed from the model presented by Crozier and Friedberg (1977). We should acknowledge that these authors were wary of explaining organizational phenomena based on culture; their distrust stems from a desire to remain free of any determinist reasoning. It is true enough that at the time *L'acteur et le système* was published, culture was most often presented as a factor imposed on the will of actors, determining their behaviour within the organization (Geertz, 1964; Parsons & Shils, 1951; Triandis, 1972; among others). This perspective is completely incompatible with the propositions of strategic analysis, which instead places the intentions of the actor at the centre of the model (d'Iribarne, 2005). Nevertheless, Crozier hoped to "reinvent culturalist analysis" by examining not "why" (as a determinist would), but rather "how" (the processes, practices, mechanisms involved) culture is transformed (Crozier, 1971).

It is in this sense that we will approach organizational culture: not fatalistically as a force imposed on actors but, instead, as a construct similar to the organizational rules of the game (hierarchical relations, job description, collective agreements, and so on). Even more important, we do not intend to approach culture as a mechanical object that management operates to manipulate employees but in an interactionist perspective, considering that real change depends on relations between actors that lead to a transformation of values working together to guide action. When it is approached from this angle, we can see that organizational culture depends on the will of employees and managers in the organization, as well as on the prevailing dynamics in the setting, which is understood here as the environment of the organization.

The constituent values of an organizational culture are constraints as much as they are zones of uncertainty, and are thereby able to be used by actors to structure their relations. Thus, culture presents itself as an issue, a source of power that makes it possible to frame relationships among actors, whether conflictual or cooperative, without determining the nature of the relationships (d'Iribarne, 2005; Sainsaulieu, 1983, 1997; Semache, 2009). From our point of view, changing the culture means changing the rules of the game and the modes of regulation used in the health system.

We are keeping this in mind when we state that raising awareness and training health professionals, while essential, are not sufficient. To enable them to act favourably towards active offer in the official language of the user's choice, awareness and training need to be accompanied by favourable modes of management and organization; this calls for an organizational culture that places explicit value on the principles of active offer. This means the actors involved must act to influence the underlying values of work within health facilities.

In other words, since organizational practices and resource management are defined according to the values promoted within it, active offer must be a part of this picture. If this does not happen, managers and staff in the facility will very likely pay little attention to it. For this reason, we will try identifying the predominant values circulating in New Brunswick's hospital facilities regarding language. How much importance is given to language matters? Are these values compatible with active offer? What are the effects of the working language on that in which services are provided? How does the external language environment influence practices related to active offer?

Although the situation of official languages in New Brunswick at first seems quite positive, given the legal provisions[2] in the province, we must recognize that active offer of health services in the language of the user's choice does not generally translate into reality. Too often, individuals in a minority language situation first speak in the language of the majority, believing this will simplify their relationship with staff, that they will be served more quickly, or that the services provided will be of better quality. The spontaneous reaction of the health professional will generally be to continue in the language of the majority, even if she or he speaks the minority official language. We would argue that the organizational culture, understood as a construct in the same way as is the organization, explains a large part of this state of affairs.

Methodology

For our survey, we selected five points of service of health care, all characterized by daily contacts with many patients and located in six regional hospitals in New Brunswick. The points of service we examined were: emergency, admission/reception, outpatient clinics, medical imaging, and phlebotomy/blood tests. Three of the facilities we surveyed are part of the Horizon network (in which the language of operations is English): Miramichi Regional Hospital, Saint John Regional Hospital, and Dr. Everett Chalmers Regional Hospital. In the Vitalité network (where the operations are bilingual), the hospitals studied were: Chaleur Regional Hospital, Dr. Georges L. Dumont University Hospital Centre, and Campbellton Regional Hospital.[3]

We used two data collection methods. The first comprised 35 semi-structured interviews with managers responsible for the units and departments we were studying and for the facility's human resources department. The second was a questionnaire distributed during the same period to employees, including health professionals (physicians, nurses, laboratory technicians, aides) and support staff (in the areas of reception, admissions, and scheduling), all of whom worked in the points of service in the six facilities under study. As well as a sociolinguistic profile, the questionnaire included a series of 58 statements designed to measure the respondents' levels of awareness and training for active offer, the respective roles they thought they played in active offer, and their access to required resources. The questionnaire was available online, in both official languages, through Survey Monkey. Respondents were encouraged to participate by the people responsible for official languages in the regional health authorities and by their immediate supervisor. Of a population estimated at about 1,600 employees, we received 415 completed questionnaires, giving us a proportion of a little under 26%, which we consider excellent.

Profile of Respondents

The data relating to the profile of the survey respondents provided us with the following information: More than 60% were 40 years of age and over, including 32% who were 50 years and over. A very large majority of respondents (91%) were women; this was not a surprising finding, as the jobs in the health sector are recognized as being occupied in large part by women.

Figure 1. Distribution of Respondents by Age Group

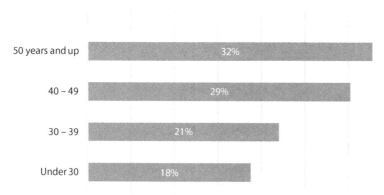

Two elements of linguistic data appear important to include here. First, in terms of the language used with colleagues (working language), only 10% of respondents reported working only in French, while 45% reported working only in English. The same proportion (45%) said they used both official languages.

Figure 2. Language Used with Co-workers

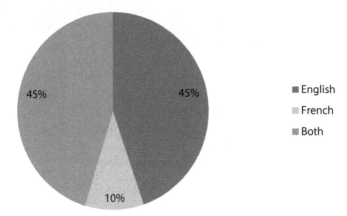

A second element of note is the fact that, when asked in which language they felt comfortable using to serve their patients, we can observe that only 1% of respondents indicated French, 37% English, and a substantial proportion of 62% indicated both.

Figure 3. Language in which I Am Comfortable Serving My Patients

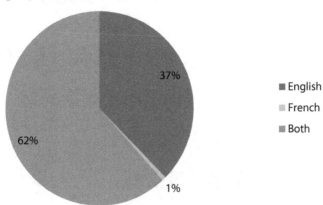

This said, a significant imbalance was observed in the distribution of bilingual staff throughout the regional health authorities. While 89% of respondents from facilities in the Vitalité network state that they are comfortable serving their patients in both official languages, only 26% of those from Horizon network facilities consider they have those skills in both official languages.

Figure 4. Language Proficiency According to Health Network

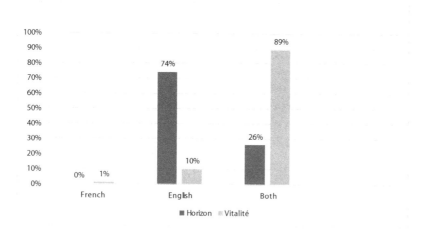

Lastly, out of an identical number of managers visited in each of the facilities, 21 are Anglophone and 14 Francophone. It is also important to specify that the objective of these interviews was, above all, to discover the challenges faced by managers in putting active offer into practice and to identify the tools available to them.

Active Offer of Services in the Official Language of the User's Choice, and Culture of Bilingualism

New Brunswick proudly displays its status as Canada's only officially bilingual province. Various legislative measures and provisions are in place to support this status. A culture of bilingualism like this represents an undeniable asset for offering health services in both official languages, but it seems far from adequate regarding **active** offer. Indeed, the **active** aspect of offering services means that it is not the user's responsibility to demonstrate her or his choice of language of service. The responsibility belongs to the staff of health facilities, who must identify clearly, without speculation or supposition, the official language in which the patient wishes to be served, and to act accordingly.

Our survey clearly indicates there is confusion between the notions of active offer and bilingualism. For example, we collected numerous comments from people working with users emphasizing their inability to practise active offer due to inadequate language skills in one of the two official languages. For example, one person stated: [original: English] "I don't make the active offer because I don't speak French." Others pointed out: [original: French] "Lack of second language education." The discomfort of unilingual staff is clearly noted. One person wrote: [original: English] "Most employees do not feel comfortable in both languages; therefore active offer is not always made." Another stated: [original: English] "People who are not bilingual do not want to give the impression that they are by speaking a few given words in French."

We suggest that the confusion existing between bilingualism and active offer fosters this type of comments, and it is our opinion that every employee—unilingual or bilingual—needs to participate in active offer. In the current context emphasizing bilingualism, a unilingual professional will have trouble subscribing to the practice of active offer, feeling incompetent because of a lack of fluency in one of the official languages. This has the effect of discouraging and demotivating the employee.

In other words, in a setting that places bilingualism as a central value, mastering the official languages becomes an important source of power capable of engendering a state of imbalance in the system unfavourable to unilingual staff. When this happens, the feeling of incompetence in their linguistic abilities becomes a threat to the power balance, and translates into resistance on the part of unilingual employees who are faced with a practice that excludes them.

Related to this idea is the extreme discomfort several unilingual employees expressed about greeting people with "Hello/Bonjour." For them, saying this sends a false message to service users, who mistakenly believe they are talking to a bilingual employee. These respondents consider such a practice unethical because they are unable to continue the conversation in the language of the patient's choice: [original: English] "It's like misleading patients when you're telling them Hello/ Bonjour and in reality, you're not bilingual . . ." They expressed discomfort: [original: English] "I really feel uncomfortable misleading people;" [original: English] "Staff are extremely uncomfortable reciting words in a language they do not speak or understand." They even expressed anxiety: [original: English] "People are sometimes nervous, trying to help patients out thinking they may say the wrong thing to them." This discomfort hides considerable frustration at having to depend on bilingual members of the organization to perform their duties.

Their frustration will also have the effect of engendering a form of denial about the role language plays in the quality and safety of care. We read comments such as: [original: English] "I feel we are here to provide a healthcare service and not a language service" or [original: English] "I feel I can provide as good a service in my language of choice." One person even stated that: [original: English] "I feel that my Health Authority has many more pressing issues to deal with rather than an active offer."

The attitude expressed in these comments, far from being favourable towards active offer, illustrates the resistance of unilingual staff towards the idea. But active offer does not require bilingualism on the part of *all* employees; rather, it is *institutional* bilingualism that is essential. The organization has to be seen as enabling unilingual staff members to contribute in their own way, with assurance and conviction, to active offer in the official language of the user's choice. Employees, both unilingual and bilingual, must be relieved of the individual responsibility for actively offering health services in the language of the user's choice, so this responsibility can be seen as a collective one, in which each person has a role to play.

Furthermore, the confusion between bilingualism and active offer will affect bilingual staff just as much. Surprisingly, bilingual employees will consider themselves free of any obligation to practise active offer, in virtue of their language skills. Indeed, many staff members responded that their point of service practised active offer effortlessly, because the majority possessed the language skills necessary to serve patients in both official languages: [original: French] "Patients are served in the language of their choice, because staff members are bilingual"; [original: French] "All the employees here are bilingual, so active offer does not present any problems." In fact, the majority of respondents from the Vitalité network stated that the practice of active offer did not represent a major challenge. This was not because the network or the facility placed particular importance on it; it was out of necessity. One nurse commented: [original: French]

"As Francophones living in this region, we're bilingual out of necessity." Similarly, another stated: [original: French] "Here there are as many Francophones as Anglophones, which means that we are able to receive and offer bilingual services in our hospital."

We have to acknowledge that knowing both official languages does not guarantee the active nature of the practice—that is, without the user having to ask—; it merely makes it possible to offer services in both official languages. In the course of our research in the health sector, we witnessed dozens of conversations between a service user and health professional in which both spoke English for a long time before they realized they were both Francophones. Evidently, active offer was not practised by the professional, despite being bilingual!

Shortage of Bilingual Human Resources

As stated earlier, there is no doubt having bilingual human resources available is crucial to providing services in both official languages (Forgues *et al.*, 2011). The following comment illustrates this fact very well:

> [original: English] It is not being made because there is not always a bilingual person available to translate and it takes way too much time to go and try and find someone and take them away from their duties to come and translate for me!

Survey respondents said they were not always able to identify a bilingual person available from among their colleagues to help them on the spot. They said they were often forced to go and find help on the floor or in another unit in order to be able to offer adequate care in the chosen language. This procedure is a double loss of time, because both employees will have to suspend their duties temporarily. With this kind of obstacle, the efficiency of the workplace and the quality of services offered to patients are negatively affected because of the delays they cause. Moreover, the additional duties imposed on bilingual employees can be a heavy burden and should therefore be a matter of concern for managers.

The managers we met with usually recognized the necessity of organizing shifts in a way that ensured adequate numbers of bilingual staff. However, putting this into place is often an arduous task, mainly because of the lack of bilingual employees. It is especially so in facilities in the Horizon network. In some of the points of service we studied, it is difficult, if not impossible, to ensure there are bilingual employees on all shifts. In such cases, active offer is simply not practised. Furthermore, only 37% of the respondents believed that work shifts in their unit or department were decided in a way that took the language abilities of every employee into account. As far as we could observe, this is not due to a conscious intention on the part of the managers, but stems simply from the availability or not of bilingual employees.

The survey pointed to several gaps in the area of staffing. Managers indicated that it is a common practice to hire unilingual employees, even when the position is designated bilingual. A manager in a department suffering from a lack of bilingual human resources confirmed that: [original: French] "When we hire, the language criterion isn't really a criterion for us, or it isn't high on the list of hiring procedures, I would say." The reticence of managers to impose language criteria when required is accentuated by the attitude of unions, which frequently denounce the assignment of language criteria to certain positions, believing them to be too numerous or unfounded. In short, both union and institutional culture leave little room for values favourable to active offer in a service organization. Sadly, it seems, making the necessary resources available for active offer to become a reality is rarely—or not at all—an important consideration.

Impact of the Environment on the Practice of Active Offer

The culture of an organization is affected by its external as well as internal environment (McShane, Steen, & Benabou, 2008; Semache, 2009; Zghal 2003). Throughout our study, we noticed the predominance of reactive behaviours on the part of employees towards their patients' language:

> [original: French] The majority of Francophone patients are bilingual, out of necessity, and sometimes speak English spontaneously when they are in contact with the hospital.
>
> Patients are very often bilingual, and want to be served in English: that makes it easier for us!

> The language in which the patient expresses himself first is the language in which services are offered to him. Very often, at the end of the conversation, we realize that a patient who spoke English at the beginning and throughout was actually much more Francophone than Anglophone.
>
> Sometimes Francophone patients don't identify themselves as Francophones when they arrive; they start speaking English right away. Automatically, they get served in English!
>
> Generally we approach the patient in French, and if he indicates he only speaks English, then the staff serves him in English.

Because hospital employees tend to be more reactive than proactive, it is the language used by the patient at first contact that seems most often to determine the language of service. This tendency can be explained, in our opinion, by both the internal environment—the working language used by staff members among themselves—and by the external environment—the dominant language in the community served by the facility.

First, the working language itself conveys the essential values of the organization and creates rules of the game that influence the communicative practices towards users. Most managers we met insisted on reminding us which of the languages was their working language. This expresses a strong attachment to a language and a culture in each network, facility, or point of service. The attachment to an organizational culture founded on a language inhibits the creation of an internal environment conducive to the practice of active offer.

Next, in relation to the external environment, several respondents claimed it was not necessary, in some Francophone or bilingual regions, to promote active offer because it was done automatically. For example, one person stated on the survey: [original: French] "Active offer is automatic! We are Francophone and bilingual out of necessity." Another wrote to us: [original: French] "We are in a bilingual region, so we understand the importance of serving people in their language."

This attitude is not without its consequences for the access to services in the official language of the user's choice. We should remember that the patient in a language minority situation often uses the language of the majority when communicating with health facilities, thus accepting the idea of being served in that language, even if using one's mother tongue is beneficial for one's health and safety.

Other people alluded to the unilingual nature of the community, saying it would be practically useless to actively offer health services in both official languages in their facility. We would even be told, in some settings, that the arrival of a considerable number of tourists or immigrants in the community would make it just as necessary to offer services in foreign languages as in the official languages: [original: English] "In our city, there is great cultural and linguistic diversity (Asian, Spanish, etc.) due to numerous tourists coming in on a cruise, which makes it very difficult to manage different languages." Similarly, another professional stated: [original: English] "We treat patients every day who speak other languages, such as Chinese, Italian, Spanish, etc., and they come with translators and it works fine." This is a well-known strategy. It consists of minimizing the issue of official languages to the maximum degree, as well as minimizing the power of actors who speak both official languages, by diluting the languages in an environment that is supposedly multilingual and multicultural.

The idea we can draw from all these accounts is that the working language and the linguistic practices characterizing the community served seem to impose themselves on the choice of language of communication used with the patient. Determining the language of service appears to be more a matter of habit than of conviction. This leads us to believe that we are still a long way away from a culture of active offer.

Proven Measures from Organizational Culture

We have just established that the prevailing organizational culture in the hospital facilities we studied places bilingualism at the centre of their values, but without actually taking active offer into account. We think it would be opportune to look at some of the concrete methods proposed to support the practice of active offer.

Although the results of our survey show that 76% of respondents said they had been given clear instructions about active offer in their point of service, several of the comments we received seem to indicate the opposite. We frequently read statements such as: [original: French] "The hospital administrators do not place enough importance on active offer;" [original: French] "There is definitely a lack of direction from managers about the language of service." [original: French] A "lack of awareness of the advantages of active offer in both official languages" was noted. One respondent even commented: [original: English] "Inadequate training, lack of interpreters, lack of support." It seems appropriate to add this comment by one of the respondents, illustrating the absence of values related to active offer in the culture of health systems: [original: French] "This survey is the first opportunity I have had to hear about active offer. Raising the awareness of employees about this topic at the time they are hired would be a good idea."

When survey respondents said they were satisfied with the organizational support they received and the clarity of instructions, they were generally making reference to wearing a pin, greeting people with the phrase "Hello/Bonjour," or to bilingualism. As for the managers, those we met generally acknowledged they did not have any clear guidelines to follow, or any effective tools available, to encourage their staff to systematically practise active offer.

In light of these findings, we have made some observations connecting organizational culture to three of the practices of active offer most often promoted: signage and materials in both official languages; listing the official language chosen by the patient in medical and hospital records; and wearing a pin.

Signage and Materials

Bouchard, Beaulieu, and Desmeules (2011) write that having signage and materials available are ways of showing the capacity to practise active offer. On our visits to different sites, we could see numerous bilingual posters and documents had been systematically displayed. Despite this effort, we observed the availability of signage rarely translates into real organizational *will* to practise active offer. In the majority of cases, the presence of bilingual signs and documents seems to serve the primary purpose of showcasing an image the organization is trying to project—being attentive to its obligation to fulfil language requirements—rather than to reflect the reality of actually meeting those obligations. Most often, despite bilingual signage, it is the users who have to adapt to the language of the employees, and not the reverse. But to have a meaningful effect on active offer, both posting signs and making materials available in the two official languages must be framed by a culture of organizational commitment toward active offer. Without this commitment, these measures remain incidental or secondary.

Beyond the posted signs, the nature of the message also merits our attention. In an organization culturally committed to active offer, the message should be geared precisely toward the opportunity to be served in the official language of one's choice, and toward highlighting the advantages to which this leads. The message should translate the existence of solid values and beliefs about active offer. For example, messages like the following are more closely connected to a culture that values active offer:

- French or English: In which language would you like to be served?
- For your safety and ours, ask to receive health services in the official language of your choice!
- Don't forget: Put the official language of your choice in your medical and hospital records, and make sure it's respected!

When we discussed this issue, those responsible told us that signs with this type of message would suggest a commitment the organization is unable to fulfil—a response that says a lot about the level of commitment toward active offer values such as guaranteeing access to services of comparable quality in both official languages, or the importance given to the language of communication to ensure patient safety!

Listing Language in Records: Disparity in Practices

Listing which official language the patient prefers for services in medical and hospital records certainly contributes to an active offer of health services. However, there is a great disparity in the way institutions deal with this matter, and even in the way departments and units in the same institution do so. Although this information is included on labels placed on forms, in records, or on bracelets in some points of service, in others employees do not take the time to write it down. It even happens that errors are made, often inadvertently, when identifying the language. For example, if a Francophone patient speaks English when registering—and this is often the case— there is a high risk that the patient will be identified as Anglophone and this is what will be written in the records. Similarly, a Francophone patient with a name that sounds English runs the risk of being served in English, without anyone's checking the language listed in the records. The dominant value of bilingualism explains, in large part, how such mistakes are made. Since the employees work from the theory that nearly all patients from the minority population speak English fluently, they feel it is pointless to look up their language preference. This is even more true in highly bilingual settings. Requiring or making mandatory the practice of listing the language in records would be no guarantee that the patient would receive services in the language of his or her choice. Neither would it suffice to change long-time habits. It is, therefore, essential for such a measure to be supported by a culture that values active offer, and by practices and operating modes that make the official language of the user's choice a priority for safe, quality care.

Wearing a Pin

Along the lines of the previous two methods, wearing a "bilingual" pin can be considered an element favourable towards active offer. When asked the question: *"Are you in favour of making it mandatory for all bilingual staff members to wear a pin identifying the languages they speak?"* the majority of survey respondents (59%) said they were favourable (31%) or very favourable (28%). However, a significant proportion said they were not very favourable (18%) or unfavourable (17%) to this idea. Surprisingly, 55% of the respondents who said they were not very favourable or unfavourable to this idea also confirmed they were comfortable serving patients in both official languages.

We suggest this finding can be explained, at least in part, by the fact some bilingual employees, afraid of being called on to play the role of interpreters and thus expose themselves to an overload of work that is rarely acknowledged by the employer, prefer to not advertise their bilingualism. In the case of wearing a pin, again, the practice has to be backed by an organizational culture that values language skills and that presents this contribution to staff members as something that is essential for the safety and quality of care, both for the patients and for the staff of the facility or point of service as a whole.

Reinforcing the Value of Active Offer
in the Organizational Culture of Health Facilities

A number of authors concur that organizational culture is strong when the majority of its employees adopt the dominant values of the organization (Bryman, 1989; Hatch, 1993; Martins & Terblanche, 2003; McShane et al., 2008; Parker & Bradley, 2000; Pfeffer, 1981). The challenge, then, is to explicitly insert active offer in the dominant values of the organization and connect it to the collective responsibility for ensuring safe, quality health services in both official languages. An organizational culture favourable to active offer should insist on what unites people (for example, safety and quality of care) rather than what divides them (for example, imposing the "Hello/Bonjour" greeting). It is of primary importance to ensure that leaders have continuing support to be able to help and motivate the greatest possible number of employees to be positive about active offer. The challenges involved in putting this practice in place would be, without a doubt, much easier to identify.

Actors need to be motivated by an operational and detailed definition of active offer, including its advantages for users, health professionals, facilities, and the health system as a whole. It is vital to push beyond good intentions so that entrenching active offer in the values, objectives, mission, and vision of regional health authorities, as well as facilities, is seen as a necessity. An important element of the successful implementation of these measures lies in raising the awareness of staff members, including managers, so that everyone recognizes the virtues of active offer and promotes its underlying principles as a matter of ethics and professional responsibility.

In a context in which employees practise active offer systematically, they would do so freely and would not see it as an extra burden, but rather as an important ability that serves to improve the safety and quality of care. As a manager commented in the survey: [original: French] "I think it's a matter of habit. I don't think that when people are hired they get a good explanation of how important the two official languages are for public services in New Brunswick."

We must therefor make sure all employees understand the system's commitment towards active offer. This means recognizing the importance of meeting standards and the measures that come with it—from the way people are greeted, through communications during the entire process, to monitoring the quality of services. The task consists of informing managers and employers of their legal and professional obligations in the area of language of service, and making sure they have the means to fulfil these obligations.

Furthermore, it would be essential to provide the administration and managers of units and departments with the support necessary to put realistic and appropriate measures in place for active offer. For example, to support the administration and managers, the regional health authorities must clearly define their expectations about active offer so that each facility and point of service is following the same course of action and is accountable. This statement of expectations must be accompanied by concrete tools to develop the skills of the administration, managers, and employees. This should include training sessions, the introduction of a process to mentor or support employees, and the identification of the principles of organizing the services required by active offer.

The development of these management policies would serve not only as an incentive to encourage the staff to systematically practise active offer, but would also make it possible to recognize the contribution each person makes to it.

It is also very important to offer adequate support to professionals who have doubts about their ability to contribute to active offer because of their limited language skills. These professionals need to understand their role and be reassured about the procedures to follow (for example, knowing to whom the patient can be referred in an efficient fashion) so that services could be provided to all users within a comparable timeframe. Processes must be clear, familiar, and easily applied. The contribution of bilingual staff must also be recognized and their workload assigned accordingly. This will deepen their commitment without creating overwork.

Respecting the Value of Active Offer in Staffing

The costs incurred for second language training are generally very high because they include both the costs associated with training as well as those for replacing employees during training sessions. We should add the fact that adults may take years to acquire the language skills they need to be considered bilingual. Consequently, we believe that an adequate recruiting and staffing strategy is the most promising solution. In other words, the language abilities of health care staff should be an important component at the time of hiring, following a rigorous process that respects the values of an organization geared towards active offer.

It is vital to properly determine the language requirements of a position by specifying the nature and the frequency of tasks that must be carried out in French and/or in English. This exercise consists of ensuring that a sufficient number of positions—enough to ensure the safety and quality of care—are designated as bilingual. Next, an appropriate tool must be used to evaluate each applicant's language skills in order to improve and standardize the staffing process for positions designated as bilingual.

To maintain good labour relations in the health sector, it would also be essential to engage a constructive dialogue with union actors around the values associated with active offer, emphasizing workers' professional responsibility, ethics, and safety of care. The factors determining language requirements for certain positions must be clarified and, more significantly, respected. Finally, it is important to fill positions designated as bilingual with bilingual staff by developing an appropriate recruiting and staffing strategy. Once this staffing process has been put in place, measures would have to be taken to give managers access to a complete inventory of the language abilities of their staff, and to enable adequate management in the perspective of active offer.

Conclusion

Our survey enabled us to take stock of the impact of organizational culture on the practice of active offer of services in the two official languages. We would argue that in order for active offer to be achieved, it must be placed at the centre of organizational culture so all staff members understand the choice of an official language is more than a right for the user; it is a professional obligation based on ethics, quality of service and safe care, and it is every employee's responsibility. Active offer would therefore mean mobilizing all actors, both inside and outside the health system, in a transformation of values that will guide the provision of services in both official languages. Beyond bilingualism, inclusive values and principles have to be promoted and upheld to ensure the health system, composed of both unilingual and bilingual staff, is governed by shared objectives related to the quality and safety of care.

Health professionals need to distinguish "active" offer from offer of service, and recognize it is only by offering health services from the initial contact with the patient, in both official languages— without the patient's having to ask for it—that we can ensure equitable access to safe, quality health services. The practice of active offer must not only rely on clearly defined processes known to all employees, but also on human resources management and on organizational principles allowing unilingual as well as bilingual staff members to contribute with conviction to its achievement.

For employees who have been viewing active offer through the lens of bilingualism, it engenders a great deal of stress and frustration. We believe that by implementing the means necessary to fulfill this renewed vision of active offer, we will succeed in reducing tensions and hesitations expressed by a large number of unilingual respondents. In short, the issue of transforming organizational culture has become a necessity if an effective active offer in health care servicesin both official languages is to be achieved. Once they are inspired by shared values that recognize communication as a safety factor and an important aspect of the quality of care, actors will, it seems to us, be more inclined to work together to offer health services in a way that respects both official language communities.

Notes

1. This chapter makes use of some of the major findings from a study conducted during a course in the master's program in health administration at the Université de Moncton. The author would like to thank the Consortium national de formation en santé (Université de Moncton unit) for its support, and to acknowledge the contribution of the following students: André Morneault, Barbara Frigault-Bezeau, Serge Boudreau, Carole Gallant, Francine Gaumont, Jeanne d'Arc Noubissi Cheucheu, Jessica Haché, and Stéphanie Gautreau.

2. *Official Languages of New Brunswick Act; Regional Health Authorities Act; An Act Recognizing the Equality of the Two Official Linguistic Communities in New Brunswick.*

3. In New Brunswick, the name "Health Network" does not correspond to the *Act* governing health care, which refers to "Regional Health Authority A" and "Regional Health Authority B." Thus, Regional Health Authority A corresponds to Vitalité Health Network and Regional Health Authority B corresponds to Horizon Network. In this report, we use both "network" and "regional health authority" interchangeably.

References

American Medical Association. (2006). *An Ethical Force Program Consensus report. Improving communication—improving care, how health care organizations can ensure effective, patient-centered communication with people from diverse populations.* Retrieved from https://accrualnet.cancer.gov/sites/accrualnet.cancer.gov/files/conversation_files/pcc-consensus-report.pdf

Bastarache, M., Braen, A., Didier, E., & Foucher, P. (1986). *Les droits linguistiques au Canada.* Montréal, QC: Les Éditions Yvon Blais Inc.

Bouchard, P., Vézina, S., & Savoie, M. (2010). *Rapport du Dialogue sur l'engagement des étudiants et des futurs professionnels pour de meilleurs services de santé en français dans un contexte minoritaire.* Moncton, NB: CNFS.

Bouchard, L., Beaulieu, M., & Desmeules, M. (2011). L'offre active de services de santé en français en Ontario: Une mesure d'équité. *Reflets: Revue d'intervention sociale et communautaire, 18*(2), 38–65. doi: 10.7202/1013173ar.

Bouchard, P., & Vézina, S. (2009). *L'outillage des étudiants et des nouveaux professionnels: Un levier essentiel pour l'amélioration des services de santé en français. Rapport de recherche présenté au secrétariat national du Consortium national de formation en santé.* Retrieved from http://cnfs.net/fr/-publications-formation.php?publication=658

Bryman, A. (1989). Leadership and culture in organizations. *Public Money & Management, 9*(3), 35–41.

Canadian Heritage. Interdepartmental Coordination Directorate. (2011). *Good Practices. Implementation of Section 41 of the Official Languages Act.* Support to Official-Language Minority Communities and Advancement of English and French. Retrieved from http://www.pch.gc.ca/DAMAssetPub/DAM-pgmLo-olPgm/STAGING/texte-text/llo-ola_1373544654391_eng.pdf?WT.contentAuthority=10.1

Consortium national de formation en santé (CNFS). (2011a). *Analyse comparative de l'offre de formation en santé en anglais et en français: Rapport final.* Raymond Chabot Grant Thornton. Retrieved from http://francophoniecanadienne.ca/wp-content/uploads/2014/11/Analyse-comparative-programmes-formation-postsecondaire-Sommaire-ex--cutif-12-sept-2011.pdf

Consortium national de formation en santé (CNFS). (2011b). *Formation à l'offre active des services de santé en français*. Retrieved from http://cnfs.net/fr/loutillagedesetudiantscnfs.php

Consortium national de formation en santé (CNFS). (2013). *Boîte à outils pour l'offre active*. Retrieved from www.offreactive.com/

Crozier M. (1971). Sentiments, organisations et systèmes. *Revue française de sociologie, 12*, 141–154.

Crozier M., & Friedberg E. (1977). L'acteur et le système. Paris, France: Éditions du Seuil.

Forgues, É., Bahi, B., & Michaud, J. (2011). *L'offre de services de santé en français en contexte minoritaire*. Moncton, NB: Institut canadien de recherche sur les minorités linguistiques. Retrieved from http://francosantesud.ca/wp-content/uploads/a-L%E2%80%99offre-de-services-de-sant%C3%A9-en-fran%C3%A7ais-en-contexte-francophone-minoritaire-ICRML.pdf

Gagnon-Arpin, I., Bouchard, L., & Chen, Y. (2010). *L'accès aux services de santé dans la langue minoritaire: analyse secondaire de l'EVMLO*. 78e Congrès de l'ACFAS, Montréal, QC.

Gauthier, H., & Reid, M-A. (2012). *Compétences linguistiques et qualité de services: Argumentaire pour des services de soins de santé en français de qualité*. Manitoba: Santé en français. Retrieved from http://santeenfrancais.com/sites/ccsmanitoba.ca/files/attachments/argumentaire_version_francaise_maj_avril_2014.pdf

Geertz, C. (1964). Ideology as a cultural system. In D. Apter (Ed.), *Ideology and discontent* (pp. 47–76). New York, NY: Free Press of Glencoe.

Gouvernement du Québec. (2010). *Diversité, gestion, compétitivité, innovation: Cadre de référence en matière de gestion de la diversité ethnoculturelle en entreprise*. Retrieved from http://diversite.gouv.qc.ca/doc/Cadre_Reference_Diversite.pdf

Hatch, M. J. (1993). The dynamics of organizational culture, *Academy of Management Review, 18*(4), 657–663.

d'Iribarne, P. (2005). Analyse stratégique et culture: Un nécessaire retour aux sources. *Revue française de sociologie, 46*(1), 151–170.

Lortie, L., & Lalonde, A. J., in collaboration with Bouchard, P. (2012). *Cadre de référence pour la formation à l'offre active des services de santé en français*. Ottawa, ON: Les sentiers du leadership pour le Consortium national de formation en santé. Retrieved from http://www.design-site-web.com/umoncton/wp-content/uploads/2013/08/6cadre-de-reference-un-incontournable1.pdf

Martins, E. C., & Terblanche, F. (2003). Building organizational culture that stimulates creativity and innovation. *European Journal of Innovation Management, 6*(1), 64–74.

McShane, S. L., Steen, S. L., & Benabou, C. (2008). *Comportement organisationnel*. Montréal, QC: Chenelière/McGraw-Hill.

Office of the Commissioner of Official Languages. (2007). *Performance Report 2006–2007: Atlantic Canada Opportunities* (archived). Retrieved from http://www.ocol.gc.ca/html/acoa_apeca_06_07_e. php

Office of the Commissioner of Official Languages for New Brunswick. (2006). *2005–2006 Annual Report*. Retrieved from http://officiallanguages.nb.ca/sites/default/files /imce/pdfs/ annual_ report_2005-2006.pdf

Office of the Commissioner of Official Languages for New Brunswick. (2012). *From Words to Actions. 2011–2012 Annual Report,* Retrieved from http://officiallanguages.nb.ca/sites / default/files/imce/pdfs/2011-2012_annual_report.pdf

Parker, R., & Bradley, L. (2000). Organizational culture in the public sector: evidence from six organizations. *International Journal of Public Sector Management, 13*(2), 125–141.

Parsons, T., & Shils, E. A. (Eds.). (1951). *Toward a General Theory of Action*. Cambridge, MA: Harvard University Press.

Pfeffer, J. (1981). Management as symbolic action: The creation and maintenance of organizational paradigms. *Research in Organizational Behaviour, 3,* 1–52.

Reflet Salvéo. (2013). *Rapport final: Forum bilingue de développement de capacité pour les fournisseurs de services de santé et services sociaux en français de la RGT*. Retrieved from http://refletsalveo.ca/sante/ images/PDF/rapportannuel/Forum%20French%20 Connection%20mai%202013.pdf

Réseau des services de santé en français de l'Île-du-Prince-Édouard, en collaboration avec la Société santé en français. (2007). *Les répercussions des problèmes de communication sur la prestation de soins de santé de qualité aux communautés et patients de langue minoritaire*. Retrieved from http://santeipe.ca/wp-content/ uploads/Expos_Position_RSSF_FR.pdf

Sainsaulieu, R. (1983). La régulation culturelle des ensembles organisés. *L'année sociologique* (Troisième série), *33,* 195–217.

Sainsaulieu, R. (1997). *Sociologie de l'entreprise: Organisation, culture et déve-loppement* (2nd ed). Paris, France: Dalloz.

Schein, E.H. (1991). What is culture? In P. Frost, L. Moore, M. Louis, C. Lundberg, & J. Martin (Eds.). *Reframing organizational culture* (pp. 243–253). Newbury Park, CA: Sage.

Schein, E.H. (1992). *Organizational culture and leadership* (2nd ed.), San Francisco: Jossey-Bass.

Semache, S. (2009). Le rôle de la culture organisationnelle dans la gestion de la diversité. *Management & avenir, 8*(28), 345–365.

Siehl C., & Martin, J. (1984). The role of symbolic management: How can managers effectively transmit organizational culture? In J. D. Hunt, D. Hosking, C. Schriesheim, & R. Stewards (Eds.). *Leaders and managers: International perspectives on managerial behavior and Leadership* (pp. 227–239). New York, NY: Pergamon.

Société Santé en français (2007). *Santé en français, communautés en santé: Résumé du plan directeur 2008–2013.* Retrieved from http://franco.ca/ssf/documents/ResumePlan2008-2013.pdf

Triandis, H. C. (1972). *The Analysis of Subjective Culture.* New York, NY: Wiley, Inter-Science.

Zghal, R. (2003). Culture et gestion: Gestion de l'harmonie ou gestion des paradoxes? *Gestion, 28*(2), 26–32.

PART V

ISSUES AND STRATEGIES IN EDUCATING FUTURE PROFESSIONALS

CHAPTER 11

Teaching Active Offer: Proposal for an Educational Framework for Professors[1]

Claire-Jehanne Dubouloz, Josée Benoît, Jacinthe Savard, Paulette Guitard, and Kate Bigney, *University of Ottawa*

Abstract

Not only do we need to train health care and social service professionals about active offer, we must also train their trainers (professors). Most professors teaching in health care and social service programs in French have not received training in teaching strategies to prepare future professionals who will one day work in minority Francophone communities. This prompted us to examine the most appropriate type of education for these professors. This chapter explores educational perspectives on andragogy and presents our conceptual framework for education, including the pedagogical setting and types of knowledge needed (content knowledge, skills [know-how], attitudes [soft skills], as well as how to put those into action [knowledge to act]), to prepare professionals to work in the area of active offer. Finally, we offer our thoughts on the particular issues and challenges of teaching active offer, as identified in a pilot project to implement education on active offer.

Key Words: teaching active offer, official language minority communities, health care and social service professionals, pedagogy, andragogy, adult education.

Introduction

In response to studies about training future health care and social service professionals in the active offer of services in the official language of one's choice in official language minority communities (OLMCs),[2] the need to educate professors[3] has also been noted. Thus, this chapter explores educational perspectives and different types of knowledge involved in teaching and learning about active offer, as well as the issues that arise in teaching active offer. It is divided into five sections: (1) description of the context; (2) educational perspectives; (3) educational framework for teaching active offer; (4) thoughts on educating professors about active offer and issues arising in their training; and (5) conclusion.

Context

The first section of this chapter introduces the context of education and training in the active offer of social services and health care in the official language of one's choice in OLMCs.

A number of different methods have been used to augment training for the active offer of French-language social services and health care as a result of the training offered by the *Consortium national de formation en santé* (CNFS) and the development of support materials such as the Toolbox for the Active Offer, published online

Table 1. Demographic Characteristics of Survey Respondents

Mother tongue	
French	90%
English	9%
Other	1%
Work setting	
University	53%
College	47%
Program	
Medicine	20%
Nursing	20%
Social Work or Social Services	13%
Other(rehabilitation, nutrition, physical education, radiology)	47%
Position*	
Professor or instructor	82%
Co-op or clinical placement coordinator	19%
Program director or chair	16%
Other	18%

*Respondents could choose more than one answer, if applicable.

in 2013 (http://www.offreactive.com/). This electronic resource was created by the *Groupe de recherche et d'innovation sur l'organisation des services de santé* (GRIOSS) at the Université de Moncton, in cooperation with the CNFS, and offers many resources and training tools

Table 2. Distribution of Questions (Type and Number) by Questionnaire Sections

Section of questionnaire	Type of questions	Number of questions
1) Demographic characteristics of professors or trainers	Open or multiple choice	11
2) Education received by professors or trainers on 6 themes: needs of Francophones living in minority contexts in terms of social services and health care, health determinants, cultural competency, linguistic competency, and active offer.	Open or multiple choice	For each of the 6 themes, there were 5 questions: education received, education desired, format of education received, content of education received, whether education met needs.
3) Personal beliefs and values of professors or trainers about French-language health and social services	5-point Likert scale (from strongly disagree to strongly agree)	5 Example of question: I believe that preparing future health and social service professionals to work in Francophone minority communities is one of my responsibilities.
4) Contents of courses on Francophone Minority Communities (FMCs) (knowledge, skills, and attitudes) in courses provided by the respondents	5-point Likert scale (from not at all to always)	Knowledge – 10 Example of question: Do you teach your students about the importance of providing services of equal quality in both official languages? Skills – 4 Example of question: Do you teach your students the skills they need to communicate in French in a way that builds a good relationship with a Francophone client in a minority setting? Attitudes – 5 Example of question: Do you teach your students how to be reflective practitioners in a Francophone minority community?
5) Learning material used or available to teach these contents	5-point Likert scale (from not at all to always)	2 Example of question: Do you have access to learning and resource material in French?

**Table 2. Distribution of Questions (Type and Number)
by Questionnaire Sections (*continued*)**

Section of questionnaire	Type of questions	Number of questions
6) Framework in which students learn about the specific characteristics and needs of FMCs	Multiple choice	1 Example of question: The information that **you teach your students** in health and social service programs regarding Francophone minority communities presented as part of...
7) Learning activities on FMCs	Multiple choice	1 Example of question: In my program, I use the following learning activities to teach about Francophone minority communities:
8) Support and commitment of workplace to encourage teaching of FMC content	5-point Likert scale (from not at all to always)	4 Example of question: In respect to the content I teach to enable students to work in Francophone minority communities . . . I my teaching unit encourages faculty engagement and professional development

related to active offer (Chapter 2). Other research has been conducted to better understand the needs of educational institutions and, in particular, the needs of professors in the teaching of active offer.

An in-depth exploratory study was carried out in 2012 to examine pedagogical approaches and content used to teach active offer of French-language services in health and social work programs in minority settings. A 29-question survey was sent to professors in the 11 member institutions of the CNFS. Of the potential participants (n = 1,673), 123 responses were received, for a response rate of 7%.

The results describe trends (expressed in averages or percentages) discovered in the various themes considered in the questionnaire. Our findings show that respondents do not feel very well equipped to teach about active offer in their classes (Benoît *et al.*, 2015). Indeed, when they were asked about which aspects of active offer they been instructed in, more than half reported they had not been given any information about: determinants of health of Francophones in a linguistic minority situation (55%); specific social service and health care needs among Francophones in minority communities (61%); language proficiency (76%); cultural competence (61%); specific elements of the active offer of French-language services (69%); and teaching strategies to prepare future professionals who will be called to work in minority Francophone communities (71%). The last figure is very significant, and prompted us to look more closely at the type of training or education in active offer that would be most appropriate for professors in these programs.

Moreover, some respondents noted they would like to be taught about the different survey themes to raise their awareness about Francophones in minority settings, as well as to improve how they teach students on this subject. Other respondents, however, pointed out obstacles such as the lack of time, the fact they do not already teach this content in class, or their own perception that they are already sufficiently competent. One last point of interest is that 86% of respondents "agreed completely" that it is important to educate faculty members on this subject. The survey clearly demonstrated a lack of knowledge about active offer among professors in health and social work programs.

The Cultural Context of Active Offer

According to Betancourt and Green (2010), becoming aware of and meeting the needs of a diverse population requires learning a variety of skills. Ensuring that service providers can offer care and services effectively requires a culturally competent staff (Coutu-Wakulczyk, 2003). Culturally competent care providers recognize that a client's culture encompasses many elements, such as beliefs, attitudes, and values, which influence care and services as well as communication (Health Canada, 2001). Cultural competence in health care is the "provision of health care that responds effectively to the needs of patients and their families, recognizing the racial, cultural, linguistic, educational and socio-economic backgrounds within the community" (Masi, 2000, p.8, quoted in Health Canada, 2001, p. 229). We believe active offer is closely associated with the recognition of the culture of the minority. Professors who teach members of the minority language community in health and social work programs must be conscious of culture, which in turn influences the design of education for future health care and social service professionals.

Having laid out the context of education on active offer, as well as some of the elements of cultural competence in health care, we will now provide an analysis of issues relating to potential education on active offer as they relate to professors.

Educational Perspectives

In this section, we present certain educational theories underlying issues in active offer teaching: (1) the pedagogical setting presented by Legendre (1983, 2005); (2) definitions of three basic types of knowledge needed to develop professional competence identified by Boudreault (2002); and (3) andragogic concepts for adult education, and the critical paradigm.

Pedagogical Setting of Active Offer

We will explore the act of teaching active offer in minority language settings by using the theoretical model of the pedagogical setting presented by Legendre (1983, 2005) and adapting it to professional development. The pedagogical setting is composed of four inter-related subsystems, namely the Subject, the Object, the Agent, and the Environment. The Subject designates the person or persons in the learning situation (the learner or student); Object corresponds to the objectives the Subject wants to attain and the knowledge the Subject wants to integrate; Agent refers to the resources that assist and facilitate the Subject's learning, including people, approaches, and processes; Environment represents the context in which the Subject, the Object, and the Agent interact, and includes everyone involved in the learning situation (teachers, administrators, other students), operations that contribute to learning (enrolment, evaluation, curriculum development, administration), and equipment and facilities that contribute to the learning process (rooms, equipment, teaching resources, finances).

The Subject, the Object, and the Agent interact in relationships which Legendre (1983, 2005) calls pedagogical relationships. There is a didactic relationship between the Agent and the Object, a teaching relationship between the Agent and the Subject, and a learning relationship between the Subject and the Object. In examining the pedagogical setting around education about active offer, we are particularly interested in the teaching relationship.

The Three Basic Types of Knowledge to Develop Professional Competence

In discussing continuing education for teaching professors of professional programs, Boudreault (2002) describes interrelations among three different types of knowledge involved in professional competence. Boudreault explores the rationale behind developing different combinations of these types of knowledge: the interrelation between knowledge and attitude makes professionals knowledgeable, the interrelation between attitudes and skills produces adaptability, and the interrelation between skills and knowledge creates productivity.

Boudreault (2002) defines "knowledge" as knowing or possessing systematic or organized knowledge; "knowing how to be" as a grouping of attitudes and soft skills[4] that includes outlooks, perceptions, and values that are generally connected to a context; and "skills" as know-how or the abilities that come with experience working in a profession. The diagram presented in Figure 1 illustrates these types of knowledge and the interactions between the combinations. He also shows that education that does not include practical skill development will only create a knowledgeable professional, training that does not include knowledge will only produce an implementer, and education that does not include the development of soft skills could only produce a performer. Therefore, Boudreault (2002) defines professional competence as:

> The consequence of a simultaneous relationship of attitudes, knowledge, and skills, where each one of these elements is connected to the others and exerts an influence on the others in relation to the context of the social groups towards whom the individual's education is geared. (p. 26)

Figure 1. Development of Professional Competencies According to Boudreault (2002)

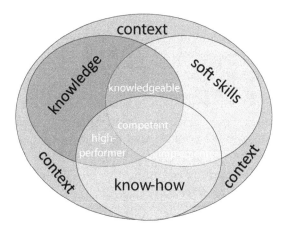

Andragogy and Its Perspectives on Adult Education

The work of several key authors in the field of education will be discussed in this section. Their ideas will help us create a vision of the type of education for active offer that could be made available in the future to professors who are, in every other way, experts in their disciplines. Educating professors requires us to use an andragogical framework. Andragogy is defined by Legendre as "the science that examines all aspects of the theory and practice of teaching adapted to adults" (Legendre, 2005, p. 76). It is important to remember two basic principles: the learner is an autonomous, self-directed person, and the educator is a facilitator of learning rather than a transmitter of knowledge. Hypotheses underlying andragogy describe adult learners as individuals with independent self-concepts directing their own learning who have varied experiences in their personal and professional lives and who solve problems daily. Adult learners engage in inquiry for and through "doing" and have a special interest in learning that is connected to their professional activities (Knowles, 1980). Our educational program for professors in health and social service programs will be designed with these characteristics of adult learners in mind.

Adult educators play a variety of roles. Sometimes they are content specialists and facilitators helping adults learn the content (Kolb, 1984); at other times they are artists and critical analysts (Brookfield, 1990). Adult educators create a learning environment linked to action or practice (Knox, 1986) that enables them to critically analyze their own teaching (Apps, 1991), and promoting critical thinking in learners (Mezirow, 1994). Although they act with a certain degree of professional authority, their main tasks are to motivate and guide the learners with whom they are working (Grow, 1991).

Pratt (2005) provides a synthesis of five perspectives in adult education,[5] bringing together the various roles reminiscent of the educational framework outlined in Legendre's pedagogical setting. Pratt emphasizes that each perspective has its own advantages for the professor, the educational content, and the environment, and that each is connected with different teaching strategies. We have chosen to look at three of these perspectives: transmission of content, apprenticeship and learning based on real situations, and teaching as a vector of social change or critical perspective. These seem particularly important for framing learning objectives related to knowledge, skills, and attitudes in active offer.

Active offer can be taught from a perspective of "transmission," focusing on the effective delivery of the content: the concepts, definitions, and research data that describe the challenges of accessing care and services in the minority official language.

Teaching skills (or know-how) is similar to "apprenticeship" or learning in a real situation. It may take the form of modelling during internships in a health or social service setting, where the preceptor or clinical instructor actively offers services, or of role play in the classroom, using complex teaching or simulated professional scenarios to role play situations the future professionals may face. This perspective is intended to develop a community of learners and enable the professor to become the means by which content is produced, which Pratt (2005) represents by the fusion of the Agent and the Object.

Developing the attitudes and soft skills related to active offer fits very well into a perspective of social reform or critical thinking, an approach helping students discover their own values and beliefs as reflected by their attitudes in a given society. For example, before introducing the subject of active offer into the course, professors would first examine their personal beliefs and values about asking for and offering services in the official language of their choice, in order to give meaning to the content they will teach and to demonstrate the importance of active offer in their behaviour. As they are teaching, professors would also encourage students to reflect on their own beliefs and actions when they are requiring or receiving health or social services, and on the use of their language of choice.

In his writing about the reflective practitioner, Schön (1994) explores how to guide learning about soft skills and attitudes. According to this theorist, professors need to demonstrate reflection in-action (professors reflect on and change their behaviour or teaching method as it is happening, in the actual classroom situation) and reflection on-action (professors take a step back from their day-to-day practice, and think about the content and their reasons for teaching the way they do). We believe this kind of reflective practice is an essential part of teaching active offer to professors. It allows them to position themselves in their actions and behaviours regarding active offer, hence to understand how they can adapt teaching methods to include this type of self-awareness and inquiry in their classroom practice. Reflective practice thus becomes a catalyst and spurs the creation of future reflective practitioners.

Educational Framework for Teaching Active Offer

The theoretical perspectives described above guided us as we developed a conceptual framework for education. In the sections that follow we will define knowledge, skills, and attitudes related to active offer. Acquiring all of these types of knowledge should lead to professional competence and skills that will make it easier for professionals to actively offer services in official language minority settings. We will then examine the two-fold role of the professor in teaching active offer, and will present a synthesis of the framework proposed.

The Three Types of Knowledge as They Relate to Teaching Active Offer: Guidelines

We explored the three types of knowledge (knowledge, skills, and attitudes) through the survey of professors in member institutions of the CFNS (Benoît *et al.*, 2015) and through an extensive compilation of literature on the subject. The results enabled us to make an inventory of the different elements of knowledge necessary for an effective active offer of French-language services. The results were then validated by groups of experts. The elements of knowledge were published in the *Lignes directrices pour la formation à l'offre active des futurs professionnels en santé et en service social œuvrant en situation francophone minoritaire* (Dubouloz *et al.*, 2014) and are summarized in Table 3. These elements of knowledge for teaching active offer apply to students as well as professors, and are organized around the needs of the learner-student in professional programs and around the professor in educational programs for students in OLMCs.

These guidelines will be used in our objectives for education and training, to formulate recommendations for action in the area of teaching for university and college professors.

Professional Competence or Knowledge to Act

Our guidelines are based on the three types of basic knowledge leading to professional competence. Legendre (2005) integrates knowledge, skills, behaviours, and attitudes in what he calls *savoir-agir*, which means knowing how to act or the "ability to put a wide range of resources, both internal and external, in particular the knowledge and experiences acquired in the school setting and those arising out of everyday life, into action" (p. 1203). According to the CNFS, the knowledge to act in the area of active offer is the outcome of a variety of

Table 3. The Three Types of Knowledge in Education on Active Offer (Based on Bouchard & Vézina, 2010, and the Consortium national de formation en santé [CNFS], 2012.)

Knowledge: Information linked to active offer

- Know the specific characteristics of FMCs (statistics, customs, particular needs, and other traits);
- Know the details of active offer, such as its definition, behaviours that promote active offer, and determinants of active offer;
- Know the importance of active offer to the health of FMCs (for example, patient safety);
- Know the basic principles of cultural competency;
- Know the fundamental principles of linguistic competency;
- Know Canada's language laws.

Skills: Competencies linked to active offer

- Convey the importance of actively offering services;
- Demonstrate leadership skills related to active offer;
- Recognize and participate in the development of a network to encourage active offer.

For professors/trainers:
- Use the tools available to teach active offer.

For students:
- Use the tools available to make active offer.

Attitudes: Values and attitudes linked to active offer

- Have a positive attitude towards active offer;
- Demonstrate professional ethics regarding diversity;
- Be conscious of own values and beliefs towards people from other cultures;
- Be sensitive to the needs of FMCs in order to support active offer;
- Be aware of own capacity and feelings about linguistic competency;
- Be aware of own capacity and feelings about cultural competency.

For professors/trainers:
- Demonstrate these attitudes when interacting with students from Francophone minority communities.

For students:
- Demonstrate these attitudes when interacting with clients from Francophone minority communities.

learning experiences leading to knowledge, skills, and attitudes related to active offer. Knowledge to act can evolve into "ethical leadership"[6] through which a health or social service professional can highlight the importance of the active offer of French-language services in her or his workplace, thus becoming a catalyst for change and innovation (Consortium national de formation en santé [CNFS], 2012). Within the framework of educating professors, this ethical leadership can also be a trigger for social change—in this case begun in the classroom by the professor who has new knowledge about active offer to share.

The Two-Fold Role of Professors in Teaching Active Offer

First of all, it is important to clearly understand the educational value of the professor in this pedagogical setting. The value lies in being both a teacher of active offer and an actor in active offer. In their role as teachers, professors teach students the essential elements of knowledge, including the knowledge base (for example, the characteristics of OLMCs), skills (for example, the behaviours that promote the active offer of services in official language minority communities; see Chapter 12), and attitudes (for example, attitudes towards active offer to be applied in their future professional practice in OLMCs) related to active offer.

In their role as actors, professors demonstrate these elements of knowledge, including their knowledge base (the social, political, cultural and health reality of OLMCs), their skill in actively offering services (demonstrated through their own behaviours and actions in the classroom with students from OLMCs), and their own attitudes and values toward their learners and community. The behaviour and attitudes of the professor must take into account the linguistic insecurity (Boudreau & Dubois, 2008; Desabrais, 2010) that frequently arises in minority settings, and the natural tendency of code switching or translanguaging (Cook, 2001; Otheguy, García, & Reid, 2015; Poplack, 1980). For example, in FMCs, to facilitate the development of language proficiency necessary for actively offering French-language services, the professor should promote the use of French in the classroom. However, if a professor insists that students from FMCs use standard French, she or he runs the risk of discouraging them from pursuing their studies in French (Landry, Allard, & Deveau, 2010). Meanwhile, learners from communities where French is spoken by the majority will not become aware of, or be sensitive to, the linguistic insecurity of others: their classmates, or their future clients who may be embarrassed to address a professional in French because they do not feel competent or comfortable in standard French (Deveau, Landry, & Allard, 2009). Furthermore, Allard, Landry, & Deveau (2005) suggest people can become more conscious of, and sensitive to, the challenges of language and culture in an official language minority community if they have positive experiences or if they can observe ethnolinguistic models demonstrating their commitment to this community. Professors serve, then, as role models for their students. Their soft skills and the commitment they show to OLMCs will have a significant impact on building their students' awareness in respect to active offer.

Synthesis of the Conceptual Framework for Teaching Active Offer

Figure 2 is a synthesis of different types of knowledge and learning, all of which can be helpful for professors developing teaching practices to use in academic programs preparing students to work in health care and social services in OLMCs. We can see the category of skills is considered to be the most important type of knowledge in the teaching relationship, ranking before the other two types. Knowledge to act is depicted here as an outcome of all the components in the framework.

Figure 2. Types of Knowledge Demonstrated by Competent Educators in Their Teaching Practices

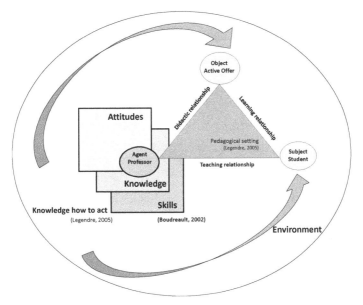

Thoughts on Issues in Teaching Active Offer

Particular issues arise when active offer is taught in minority language settings. A pilot project in 2014–2015 on introducing education on active offer to students in Bachelor of Social Work and Master in Occupational Therapy programs gave us some insight into the kind of issues and challenges involved.

Both programs in the pilot project had a mission to prepare students to work in Francophone minority communities. The project was intended, first of all, to document the strategies and mechanisms used by the program directors and professors to insert active offer into the curriculum. Second, the project gave us the opportunity to document the teaching strategies used and their impact on the students' learning experiences. The thoughts provided below were inspired by the comments of the five professors who took part in the pilot project; their comments were collected during group interviews at the end of the academic term when they taught their course. The interview questions were based on the analysis and evaluation of program implementation in Champagne *et al.* (2009).

Table 4. Professors Participating in Pilot Project

Program	Professor Partner	Year-Level
Occupational Therapy	Prof1	1st year, Master's
	Prof2	2nd year, Master's
	Prof3	2nd year, Master's
Social Work	Prof1	2nd year, Bachelor's
	Prof2	3rd year, Bachelor's

Issues in Teaching the Knowledge Base

Professors who teach in Francophone health and social service programs in universities and colleges outside Québec, and who need to contribute to developing educational content on the active offer of French-language services in OLMCs, are hired for their expertise in their discipline or field. Although faculty members at universities and colleges having a particular mission towards OLMCs may come from anywhere in the world, they are rarely expected to be familiar with the characteristics of the different Francophone student populations in their classes and they do not receive any preparatory training about OLMCs or about active offer. On the other hand, proficiency in French and the ability to teach in French are essential qualifications for hiring or tenure at most of these universities and colleges with a Francophone mission.

The professor-participants in the pilot project reported prior to the project that they were unaware of what their students needed to know about active offer. Instead, they assumed they were simply teaching in French and would prepare the future professionals in their classes to work with members of OLMCs. Since they had not been raised in an environment where French was a minority language, they were unfamiliar with the exact characteristics of OLMCs and were unaware of the scope and extent of the challenges involved in offering care and services in these settings.

Issues in Teaching the Skills

Professional development for professors in colleges and universities is generally done on a voluntary basis and depends on individual needs. The training most frequently offered is to develop teaching skills, but it is optional. In their professional development and mentorship program for college-level faculty, St-Pierre and Lison (2009, p. 26) note that:

> Teachers in the college system are hired as specialists in the discipline they teach or in the profession targeted by the program of study in which they work. They are not required to have an academic background that qualifies them in teaching, nor to enrol in credit courses in professional development.

This is also true of university settings.

Another problem arises when university programs establishing the guidelines for faculty professional development compartmentalize planning. This causes an additional challenge for developing different types of knowledge related to a common concept such as active offer, which is to be taught in a range of health and social service disciplines. Thus, another obstacle in the planning process occurs when we offer continuing education opportunities for active offer in official language minority communities in an interprofessional or interdisciplinary framework.

The professors taking part in the pilot project sometimes felt stressed by the idea of offering this new element; they were not sure how to present it in their disciplinary context. It was also stressful to think their students might react negatively to perceptions this was an important concept in their professional program. For some of them, the concept of active offer was new: they had to familiarize themselves with the idea and, at the same time, decide on appropriate pedagogical strategies. One mentioned she was taking a "risk" by adding a new element and adopting a different pedagogical approach. However, most of the professors appreciated the experience of adding this content to their course and said they would do it again.

The majority of the professors chose and adapted materials in the Tool Box (http://www.offreactive.com/) and said they greatly appreciated this resource. They said the Tool Box is a good resource for a professor and an attractive reference to share with their students. However, the Tool Box is not a standalone curriculum for learning about active offer. Participants indicated professors using it need to have a solid knowledge of pedagogy and an advanced level of teaching skills to succeed in teaching it to their students.

Some professors also called on experts in the field—for example, a representative of CNFS or employees of Francophone organizations—either to offer a basic education in active offer or to take part in a round table. This way, they were able to draw on resource people to develop their skills base. Professors in the social work program also said they appreciated the help of a research assistant working on the project as they prepared their material. They felt they could communicate with her and contact her when they had questions or wanted feedback. Based on their comments, we feel that having access to a mentor may be beneficial for the professors when they are learning about active offer.

Issues in Teaching Attitudes

None of the professors taking part in the pilot project had grown up in a community where French was a minority language. They admitted that, before starting work at the university, they were not very familiar with the reality of Francophone minority communities. For them, receiving or asking for services in French, their mother tongue, had never been a problem. They confirmed they had become more and more aware of the particular characteristics of Francophones who live in minority settings, and more attuned to their role as professors or placement coordinators in preparing their future graduates to work with members of OLMCs in health care and social work settings.

In conclusion, the observations of professor-participants in education on active offer are very positive. They believe the learning in their courses should be reinforced by a placement or internship in a Francophone minority setting, and that other learning experiences during their academic program could contribute to a greater awareness about active offer on the part of their students.

Conclusion

This chapter started with an introduction to active offer in the social services and health care sector in official language minority communities by contextualizing education on active offer and the cultural aspect, which takes the diversity of OLMCs into consideration. In the context of a pedagogical setting (Legendre, 1983, 2005), we determined which three types of basic knowledge contribute most to professional competence in an andragogical perspective. We then applied these theoretical perspectives by proposing more specific definitions of the knowledge base, skills, and attitudes involved in active offer, and suggested that the acquisition and interaction of these three types of knowledge leads to knowledge to act. This led to a synthesis of our conceptual framework in which we locate the position of the professor/agent who integrates and teaches the three types of knowledge, thereby demonstrating her or his knowledge to act on active offer. Finally, in the last part of the chapter, we presented some thoughts on the particular issues involved in teaching active offer, as identified in a pilot project that introduced an educational component on active offer into professional courses.

Our proposal for an educational framework on teaching active offer meets professors' needs, revealed in first study, to have a solid foundation in the knowledge, skills, and attitudes involved in teaching active offer. With this foundation, professors can develop the knowledge to act that will give them confidence in their role as catalysts or agents of social change. Indeed, our findings suggest that professors feel a certain amount of insecurity about introducing this new concept into courses in their disciplines.

We suggest this type of preparation for teaching active offer should be delivered through an experiential approach that fosters a reflective practice, as presented by Schön (1994). The preparation would initially serve to raise the professors' awareness of the issues related to accessing services in the official language of one's choice in a minority setting, and of the importance of active offer in OLMCs. Next, pedagogical resources would be suggested; professors could use this material in their subsequent teaching. Materials would include the Tool Box for the Active Offer, the *Mesure des comportements de l'offre active* (Chapter 12), and an observation protocol for active offer behaviours (article in preparation). This education would act as a mechanism for improving resources as knowledge on active offer evolves. Indeed, the concept of active offer as a means to promote access to services in the official language of one's choice in a minority setting is relatively new. Research currently under way will no doubt generate new ideas about best practices in active offer, teaching approaches and assessment methods, and changes in the practice of health and social service professionals who have benefited from education on this subject.

To support professors as they plan and prepare courses that include education on active offer, it would be helpful to appoint a resource person in educational institutions. This person's mission would be the education of health and social service professionals. He or she would have a solid knowledge of active offer and of the tools and resources available, as well as a sound understanding of university pedagogy, and would be available to answer the professors' questions, provide them with materials and ideas, and guide or mentor them, depending on their needs.

Finally, it would also be beneficial to establish an active offer community of practice. A community of practice (Wenger, 1998) consists of a group of people working together to create local solutions to problems they face in their professional practices. After a certain time, and as these people share their knowledge and expertise, they develop a common foundation of learning. A community of practice on active offer might include professors from a range of disciplines, someone from the CNFS as an expert in the concept of active offer, and perhaps a person who is specialized in university teaching. This community of practice could play a leadership role in active offer in the educational institution.

The active offer of services in the official language of one's choice is a key lever ensuring a professional relationship that is safer and more respectful of the rights of users in health care and social service facilities. Educating professors about active offer would help them, in turn, educate future professionals who have integrity, are competent, and work from a client-centred approach. In essence, they will be better able to comply with the ethics codes of their professions.

Notes

1. We wish to thank the CNFS for its financial support for this initiative to educate professors in health and social service programs about active

offer, which allowed us, in the first phase of our research, to situate this education in the conceptual framework outlined in this chapter.

2. This need has been well researched by such authors as P. Bouchard and her colleagues, in Chapter 2 of this book.

3. We use the term "professor" in this chapter to refer to instructors, trainers, and teachers in various programs of medicine, health care, social work, and social and human services at both the college and university levels.

4. Following a discussion in 2017 with Professor Renald Legendre from the Université du Québec in Montreal, who is the author of the *Dictionnaire actuel de l'éducation,* we have chosen the term "pedagogical setting" in English as the closest term to the French model now well ingrained in education theories in Québec of the "Situation pédagogique." It encapsulates the three components in interrelation during a teaching/learning situation, i.e., the Subject, the Object, the Agent, and the Environment as key elements that influence this situation. Other terms seem to be used in English that refer to the "Situation pédagogique," namely: pedagogical, situation, environment, surrounding(s), ecosystem, and context.

5. Pratt (2005) labels his five perspectives Transmission (of content), Apprenticeship (in which the learner learns by performing authentic tasks and/or in real settings), Developmental (based on cognitive stages), Nurturing (caring for learners and facilitating their personal growth), and Social Reform (teaching as a vector of social change).

6. The CNFS identifies behaviours of ethical leadership that are connected to personal, social, and cultural values and promote the active offer of services in the minority language (CNFS, 2012, p.22).

7. Boudreault's diagram was developed in French; the authors of the current chapter communicated with him in order to discuss possible English translations. The French term "savoir-être" is usually translated as "people skills" but professor Boudreault's definition of "savoir-être" is larger; Boudreault therefore preferred the term "soft skills", defined by *The Collins English Dictionary* as "desirable qualities for certain forms of employment that do not depend on acquired knowledge: they include common sense, the ability to deal with people, and a positive flexible attitude."

References

Allard, R., Landry, R., & Deveau, K. (2005). Conscientisation ethnolangagière et comportement langagier en milieu minoritaire. *Francophonies d'Amérique, 20,* 95–109.

Apps, J. (1991). *Mastering the teaching of adults.* Malabar, FL: Krieger.

Benoît, J., Dubouloz, C-J., Guitard, P., Brosseau, L, Kubina, L-A., & Drolet, M. (2015). La formation à l'offre de services en français dans les programmes de santé et de service social en milieu minoritaire francophone au Canada. *Minorités linguistiques et société, 6,* 104–130.

Betancourt, J. R., & Green, A. R. (2010). Commentary: Linking cultural competence training to improved health outcomes: Perspectives from the field. *Academic Medicine, 85*(4), 583–585. doi:10.1097/acm.0b013e3181d2b2f3.

Boudreau, A., & Dubois, L. (2008). Représentations, sécurité/insécurité linguistique et éducation en milieu minoritaire. In P. Dalley, & S. Roy. (eds.), *Francophonie, minorités et pédagogie* (pp. 145–176). Ottawa, ON: University of Ottawa Press.

Boudreault, H. (2002). *Conception dynamique d'un modèle de formation en didactique pour les enseignants du secteur professionnel* (Doctoral dissertation). Université de Montréal, Montréal, QC.

Brookfield, S.D. (1990). Using critical incidents to explore learners' assumptions. In J. Mezirow (Ed), *Fostering critical reflection in adulthood* (pp. 177–193). San Francisco: Jossey-Bass.

Champagne, F., Brousselle, A., Hartz, Z., Contandriopoulos, A-P., & Denis, J-L. (2011). L'analyse de l'implantation. In A. Brousselle *et al.* (Eds.), *L'évaluation: concepts et méthodes* (pp. 229–230). Montreal, QC: Les Presses de l'Université de Montréal.

Consortium national de formation en santé (CNSF). (2012). *Cadre de référence pour la formation à l'offre active des services de santé en français.* Ottawa, ON: Consortium national de formation en santé.

Cook, V. (2001). Using the first language in the classroom. *Canadian Modern Language Review, 57*(3), 402–423. doi: http://dx.doi.org/10.3138/cmlr.57.3.402

Coutu-Wakulczyk, G. (2003). Pour des soins culturellement compétents: le modèle transculturel de Purnell. *Recherche en Soins Infirmiers, 72,* 34–47.

Desabrais, T. (2010). L'influence de l'insécurité linguistique sur le parcours doctoral d'une jeune femme acadienne: une expérience teintée de la double minorisation. *Reflets: Revue d'intervention sociale et communautaire, 16*(2), 57–89. doi:10.7202

Deveau, K., Landry, R., & Allard, R. (2009). *Utilisation des services gouvernementaux de langue française: Une étude auprès des Acadiens et francophones de la Nouvelle-Écosse sur les facteurs associés à l'utilisation des services gouvernementaux en français.* Moncton (NB): Institut canadien de recherche sur les minorités linguistiques.

Dubouloz, C-J., Benoît, J., Guitard, P., Brosseau, L., Kubina, L-A, Savard, J., & Drolet, M. (2014). Proposition de lignes directrices pour la formation à l'offre active des futurs professionnelles et professionnels en santé et en service social œuvrant en situation francophone minoritaire. *Reflets: Revue d'intervention sociale et communautaire*, 20(2), 123–151. doi:10.7202/1027588ar.

Grow, G. O. (1991). Teaching learners to be self-directed. *Adult Education Quarterly*, 41(3), 125–149.

Health Canada. (2017). *"Certain circumstances" Equity in and responsiveness of the health care system to the needs of minority and marginalized populations.* Ottawa, ON: Health Canada. Retrieved from http://www.hc-sc.gc.ca/hcs-sss/alt_formats/hpb-dgps/pdf/pubs/2001-certain-equit-acces/2001-certain-equit-acces-eng.pdf. Accessed February 10, 2017.

Knowles, M. S. (1980). *The modern practice of adult education: From pedagogy to andragogy.* Englewood Cliffs, NJ: Prentice Hall/Cambridge.

Knox, A. (1986). *Helping adults learn.* San Francisco, CA: Jossey-Bass.

Kolb, D. A. (1984). *Experiential learning: Experience as the source of learning and development.* Englewood Cliffs, NJ: Prentice Hall.

Landry, R., Allard, R., & Deveau, K. (2010). *École et autonomie culturelle. Enquête pancanadienne en milieu scolaire francophone minoritaire.* Moncton, NB, and Ottawa, ON: Institut canadien de recherche sur les minorités linguistiques et Patrimoine canadien.

Legendre, R. (1983). *L'éducation totale.* Montreal, QC: Éditions Ville-Marie.

Legendre, R. (2005). *Dictionnaire actuel de l'éducation* (3rd ed.). Montreal, QC: Guérin.

Mezirow, J. (1994). Understanding transformation theory. *Adult Education Quarterly*, 44(4), 222–232.

Otheguy, R., García, O., & Reid, W. (2015). Clarifying translanguaging and deconstructing named languages: A perspective from linguistics. *Applied Linguistics Review*, 6(3), 281–307. doi:10.1515/applirev-2015-0014.

Poplack, S. (1980). Sometimes I'll start a sentence in Spanish y termino en español: Toward a typology of code-switching. *Linguistics, 18*(7-8), 581–618.

Pratt, D. D. (2005). *Five Perspectives on Teaching in Adult and Higher Education.* Malabar, FL: Krieger.

Schön, D. A. (1994). *Le praticien réflexif: À la recherche du savoir caché dans l'agir professionnel.* Montréal (QC): Les éditions logiques.

St-Pierre, L., & Lison, C. (2009). *Une formation continue à mon image. Étude de caractéristiques des enseignantes et enseignants des collèges francophones membres de PERFORMA en relation avec la formation continue.* Research report. Sherbrooke, QC: Université de Sherbrooke/Secteur PERFORMA.

Wenger E. (1998). *Communities of practice: learning, meaning, and identity.* Cambridge, England: Cambridge University Press.

CHAPTER 12

Behaviours Demonstrating Active Offer: Identification, Measurement, and Determinants[1]

Jacinthe Savard, *University of Ottawa* and *Institut du savoir Montfort*,
Lynn Casimiro, *Collège La Cité* and *Institut du savoir Montfort*,
Pier Bouchard, *Université de Moncton*, and Josée Benoît, *University of Ottawa*

Abstract

In this chapter, we present the behaviours we have identified encouraging and demonstrating the active offer (AO) of social services and health care in French in minority settings, how we measured them, and how we used these measurements to identify the determinants of AO. We will discuss the tools we developed to measure individual AO behaviours, individual perception of organizational support for AO, and personal characteristics that influence AO behaviours (determinants). Various quantitative methods were used to reach our objectives. The results demonstrate that organizational support is the most important determinant of individual AO behaviours. Once controlled for, additional factors included three personal characteristics that increase propensity to demonstrate AO behaviour: education about AO, affirmation of Francophone identity, and competency in French. The sense of competency in English, on the other hand, has a negative association with AO of French-language service. A better understanding of these determinants enables us to refine our strategies to improve the awareness and education of future health and social service professionals on AO.

Key Words: active offer behaviours, measurement, determinants, organizational support, individual behaviours, quantitative research.

Introduction

In previous chapters, we examined the importance and challenges of actively offering social services and health care in the official language of the user's choice in official language minority communities (OLMCs). We also looked at the challenges of preparing the next generation of health and social service professionals capable of taking concrete actions to support AO. We will review some of these topics in order to better explain the process used to develop our OA measurement tools.

There are several definitions of AO (Bouchard & Desmeules, 2011) and we have selected this one for its simplicity and clarity: "Active offer can be considered as an invitation, verbal or written, for people to use the official language of their choice when accessing services. This invitation must precede their service request" (translated from Bouchard, Beaulieu, & Desmeules, 2012, p. 46). Several authors emphasize the importance of actively offering a service[2] in French in Francophone minority communities (FMCs) before the user[3] asks for it: the sense of linguistic insecurity regarding the user's own language skills in French (Desabrais, 2010; Deveau, Landry, & Allard, 2009); the historical and current lack of services in French (Lortie & Lalonde, 2012) that leads to the conviction it will be impossible to receive them (Société Santé en français, 2007); the fear of not receiving these services quickly (Bouchard *et al.*, 2012; Drolet *et al.*, 2014; Lortie & Lalonde, 2012); the belief that services in French will potentially be of lower quality (Drolet *et al.*, 2014); the internalization of a minority identity (Tajfel, 1978; Tajfel & Turner, 1986), which may result in the user having difficulty asserting his or her right to services in the language of the minority (Drolet *et al.*, in Chapter 6); the sense that it is easier to speak in English rather than listen to a professional[4] struggling to speak in French (Deveau *et al.*, 2009); the lack of French vocabulary when speaking about health issues, which may lead the user to wonder if spoken or written information will be harder to understand in French than in English (Bouchard, Vézina, & Savoie, 2010; Deveau *et al.*, 2009).

Because of these characteristics, the user may not ask to receive services in French and service providers will most often spontaneously offer services in the dominant language (de Moissac *et al.*, 2012; Forgues, Bahi, & Michaud, 2011). Thus, AO means more than simply posting a sign offering services in both languages; it entails taking culturally appropriate and sensitive actions so all users will feel comfortable receiving health services in their own language.

Why Measure Active Offer and its Determinants?

Research by Bouchard and her colleagues (Bouchard & Vézina, 2009; Bouchard, Vézina, Cormier, & Laforge, in Chapter 2) in communities across Canada suggests that even people who have been educated in French and who live in a Francophone minority community are underprepared when it comes to recognizing issues connected to the active offer of services in French and taking action to improve the comfort level of people requesting these services. Since educational efforts have recently been invested to better equip service providers to understand the concept of AO and its application to social services and health care, it is important to find ways to evaluate the results of these efforts. Several evaluation approaches could be used; here are some examples:

1) Measuring knowledge: written or multiple choice exams with questions to determine if the learner is familiar with the various aspects of AO;
2) Measuring attitudes and values (people skills): asking the learner the extent to which he or she believes different aspects of AO are important;
3) Measuring behaviours (skills or know-how): observing the learner as he or she applies the concept in a real situation or a simulation, or asking the learner to do a self-evaluation of his or her behaviours.

Our team was particularly interested in measuring AO behaviours, that is, the actions that actually demonstrate AO. We also wanted to identify the determinants[5] of AO; in other words, the characteristics that influence the propensity of a person to act in this way. For example, one could think that a person who has a strong Francophone identity is highly aware of accessibility issues, and may demonstrate more AO behaviours. We hoped to confirm which of the probable determinants have a decisive impact on observable AO behaviours. Better knowledge of AO determinants and their impact will give us valuable insight into potential action, by highlighting the underlying aspects of AO that could be influenced by educational programs and would be important to support so that service providers would be more likely to act in this manner.

Objective of the Research Program

At the time we began these studies, our consultations and literature review had not uncovered any measurement tools to evaluate AO behaviours and determinants. Thus we had to design, produce, and validate measurement tools. We created three tools: the first addresses the way service providers perceive their own AO behaviours (see A of Figure 1); the second addresses the way service providers perceive the actions of their own organization to support AO (see B of Figure 1); and the third addresses factors that possibly determine the practice of AO, such as the ethnolinguistic vitality of the community, identity and acculturation, level of self-determination, and cultural competency (see C of Figure 1). The ultimate objective was to examine the extent to which the probable determinants (C) predict the AO of French-language services (A) by service providers who speak French, and the extent to which organizational support (B) influences these links.

Figure 1. Active Offer Behaviours

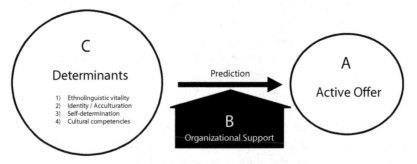

This chapter describes our research process and results. We began by identifying indicators of AO behaviour and transforming these indicators into questions in order to create Questionnaires A and B. We continued by studying the measurement properties[6] of these two questionnaires, simultaneously finding ways to measure variables we considered probable determinants of AO, so as to explore their association with AO behaviours and to refine the measurement of these variables (Questionnaire C).

Designing Tools to Measure the Active Offer Behaviours (A) and Organizational Support for Active Offer (B)

A preliminary step in designing tools to measure AO consisted of outlining a clear description of AO and its measurable characteristics and behaviours. This step was divided into two parts: first, an exhaustive review of the literature; then, second consultation with experts in the AO field.[7] This study is described in detail elsewhere (Savard, Casimiro, Bouchard, Benoit, Drolet, & Dubouloz, 2015). We will summarize the main points here, focusing on the reasons that justify the recommended actions.

A structured review of published studies provided a list of 25 organizational actions that facilitate AO. Very few articles addressed elements related to the individual behaviour of service providers (in other words, the behaviours that our educational programs on AO were trying to influence). However, we were able to transpose some organizational actions into individual behaviours to expand the list of behaviours we believed we would observe among individuals actively offering services.

Two guides (Francophone Affairs Secretariat of Manitoba, 2011; Gouvernement de l'Île-du-Prince-Édouard, 2012) specified the individual AO behaviours expected of their staff who worked in points of service that were designated bilingual. Among the behaviours are the following: staff members should wear a pin that shows they can offer services in both languages or make sure that their French-language service sign is visible; they should always greet users in both languages and continue the conversation in the official language chosen by the user; they should reply to correspondence (letter, email, etc.) in the language in which it was written. In addition, it is recommended that staff members who do not speak French immediately refer the user to a bilingual co-worker and indicate the user's choice of language. These basic directions have since been incorporated into other documents on AO (for example, Government of New Brunswick, 2015).

In the majority of documents we consulted, the order of languages used in greetings is not important. However, Manitoba's document instructs people to "Generally, use English first and French second. (In completely bilingual service centres, use French first and English second)" (Section II. p. 5). In their study of the use of French-language services in Nova Scotia, Deveau and his colleagues (2009) observed that Francophones are rarely inclined to speak French when they notice the staff member they are addressing has difficulty speaking French. They also suggest posting in French first in regions where there is a high concentration of Acadians, in order to make the use of French more prominent.

Most of the literature on organizational actions deals with the importance of producing official communications from the organization in both languages (Consortium pour la promotion des communautés en santé, 2011; Francophone Affairs Secretariat of Manitoba, 2011; Gouvernement de l'Ile-du-Prince-Édouard, 2012) and the importance of providing bilingual or French-language tools to support bilingual staff members (Bouchard, Desmeules, & Gagnon-Arpin, 2010; Consortium pour la promotion des communautés en santé, 2011). Some documents mention having Francophones represented among the organization's decision-makers (Consortium pour la promotion des communautés en santé, 2011) and having continuing education or in-service activities for staff on the importance of French-language services and the concept of AO (Deveau *et al.*, 2009; Lortie and Lalonde, 2012).

The first compiled list of AO behaviours was submitted to a group of nine experts, who suggested several relevant aspects that were either missing or not sufficiently emphasized in the literature. In their opinion, it is preferable in a Francophone minority community for the service provider—in order to make it more obvious that she or he is willing and able to speak French—to speak in French *first* when asking users whether they prefer communications to be in French or in English. A pleasant, enthusiastic, and clear "Bonjour" seems to be the best way to demonstrate this willingness. It is also important for the service provider to show she or he is ready to communicate in one language or the other, and to adapt her or his vocabulary to the cultural context of the users so that the latter feel comfortable using their "everyday French."

Regarding informational, educational, and assessment tools when the resource is available in the language of the minority, the user should systematically be offered to access the information in both official languages. For the expert group, a culturally sensitive service provider should show leadership, for instance, by undertaking to find and obtain educational material in French (information sheets, pamphlets, exercise programs, etc.) when resources are not available in the facility. Moreover, the service provider should, whenever possible, use documents that feature the French and English versions in the same document so users do not have to choose. This is because, in a minority setting, the choice may be a difficult one to make if people are not comfortable with the French vocabulary used in the social service or health field, or if they want to share the information with a caregiver or family member who is more comfortable in English.

Furthermore, service providers should ensure their French-language assessment tools are at a language level appropriate for their clients. When using standardized measures, service providers should verify whether the reliability and validity of the French versions have been examined in French and whether these measurement studies included Francophones in minority communities, and interpret the results accordingly. The experts added that if a service provider supervises interns and the client population includes a strong percentage of Francophones, she or he should ask to have interns who can speak French. The service provider should specify the language used by the client on transfer forms to facilitate the continuity of services in French when the client is referred to another organization. To demonstrate leadership, each service provider should look for every opportunity to promote French-language services, and take steps to remedy the situation when they become aware of language gaps in their organization. Service providers should also seek out opportunities for continuing education in French.

Following the suggestions of Beaulieu (2010), the experts pointed out how important it was for individuals working in an Anglo-dominant setting to feel supported by their employer if they are to put their willingness to actively offer French-language services into action. It seems imperative that indicators of organizational support for AO be measured at the same time as individual AO behaviours.

From this work, we constructed two questionnaires, one surveying 20 types of individual AO behaviour, divided into three sectors of activity, and another on their perception of 34 organizational actions that could support AO, divided into six sectors of activity. The content validity of the tools was examined through a Canada-wide Delphi survey. Relevant suggestions from the survey were incorporated and this process resulted in the creation of an experimental version of each of the two questionnaires.

The experimental version of the two questionnaires was submitted to 60 graduates of health and social service programs from the universities of Ottawa and Moncton for an initial study of its measurement properties. The measurement study has been described in more detail elsewhere (Savard, Casimiro, Benoît, & Bouchard, 2014). Results led to changes in both questionnaires to improve the quality of their measurement properties, changes that are reflected in the first official versions of the two questionnaires to measure AO. These are appended at the end of this chapter.

In the questionnaire about individual behaviours, respondents rated the frequency of their own AO behaviours by responding to a series of 23 statements, grouped according to three domains or subscales. In the questionnaire about organizational support, respondents rated their perception of the prevalence of organizational support for AO in their workplace by responding to 42 statements, grouped according to six domains or subscales. Responses to each statement assessed the frequency of the behaviour on a scale of 1 (never) to 4 (always). The experimental trial proved the questionnaires had certain measurement properties: good internal consistency,[8] acceptable temporal stability,[9] and construct validity[10] consistent with our expectations.

In their current state of development, the measures can be used as self-assessment tools for people who want to compare their own AO behaviour to an entire range of behaviours. This self-assessment can help service providers develop an initial awareness of AO principles, and help them improve their own behaviour or work with their organization to introduce practices that facilitate AO. The questionnaires also provide a means to measure AO in order to examine its determinants.

Designing a Tool to Measure the Determinants of Active Offer

Kahn's personal engagement theory (1990, 1992) served as a starting point to identify possible determinants of AO as it encompasses several concepts related to engagement at work that might foster engagement towards AO. According to Kahn, four different components define people's engagement in the workplace: the cognitive dimension, mainly concerned with the individual's identity; the emotional connection to the role performed in the workplace; the physical characteristics of their workplace, such as the location and working environment; and their existential position in relation to the meaning they give their role.

From the literature we were able to identify a series of concepts related to each of the four dimensions in this framework; we then researched existing questionnaires measuring these concepts. Since questions on the workplace environment were already included on the questionnaire on organizational support for AO, our subsequent research focused mainly on the three other dimensions (Figure 2).

Figure 2. Components of Personal Engagement

A – COGNITIVE	C – PHYSICAL
Ethnolinguistic Identity **Language Proficiency** **Language Behaviours** (Landry *et al.*, 2008) **Cultural Competency** (Campinha-Bacote, 2002)	**Subjective Vitality** (Landry *et al.*, 2008) **Workplace AtmosphereÉnvironment** (Bouchard & Vézina, 2009)
B – EMOTIONAL	D – EXISTENTIAL
Desire for integration (Landry *et al.*, 2008)	**Self-Determination** (Deci & Ryan, 1985; Guertin *et al.*, 2015; Radel *et al.*, 2013; Ryan & Deci, 2000) **Linguistic Motivation** (Landry *et al.*, 2008)

Among the work we reviewed on the linguistic minority context, we found the *Modèle intergroupe de la revitalisation ethnolinguistique* (intergroup model of ethnolinguistic revitalisation) of Landry, Allard, and Deveau (2008) well aligned with Khan's theory. After conducting various empirical studies, these authors showed the language behaviour of Francophones is closely connected to the ethnolinguistic vitality of their community. The weaker the ethnolinguistic vitality of the Francophone community is, the more closely the language behaviour of Francophones resembles that of Anglophones. The relationship the authors observed is so strong that it is described as the result of "social determinism" (ibid., p. 59). Thus, factors that originate in the psycholinguistic development of an individual (for example, the desire to belong in the minority or majority community, ethnolinguistic identity, language proficiency, and language behaviours) could have an influence on the likelihood of the person to introduce himself or herself openly as a Francophone and to make efforts to actively offer services in French. Our questionnaire about determinants of AO was informed mainly by components related to psycholinguistic development (see A, B, and C of Figure 2) and by a questionnaire designed to measure the identity construction of young Francophones who attended French-language secondary schools in minority communities (Landry, Allard, & Deveau, 2010).

As Landry and his colleagues note (2008; 2010), social determinism is potentially counter-balanced by individual self-determination (see D of Figure 2). Self-determination is the capacity of individuals to make their own choices and stems from their having three basic needs met: autonomy, competence, and relatedness (Deci & Ryan, 1985; Ryan & Deci, 2000). To this end, we included the *Échelle de motivation générale* (general motivation scale, ÉMG-18: Luc Pelletier, personal communication, October 16, 2012) in our questionnaire. The scale, based on the self-determination continuum described by Ryan and Deci (2000), includes 18 statements, three for each of the following constructs: intrinsic motivation, integration, identification, introjection, external regulation, and amotivation. The scale allows for the calculation of an index of self-determination (Radel, Pelletier, & Sarrazin, 2013). The scale of language motivation in the questionnaire developed by Landry *et al.* (2010) is also based on these concepts, but applied to the learning and use of French and English.

Last, questions on the cultural competency were added, based on the model developed by Campinha-Bacote (2002) (see A of Figure 2) that views cultural competency as a process labelled "ASKED," comprising five components: awareness, skills, knowledge, encounters, and desire. Twelve instruments to measure cultural competency were identified (Guitard, Dubouloz, Benoit, Brosseau, & Kubina, 2013) and inspired four questions on general cultural competency and 12 questions about knowledge of the needs of FMCs.

In total, the experimental version of the questionnaire on AO determinants included 202 questions (Table 1). The questionnaire provided an opportunity for us to undertake three explorations of links between the AO behaviours of service providers (A of Figure 1); certain socio-demographic variables of the service providers and their workplace; the organizational support for AO (B of Figure 1); and potential determinants arising from personal characteristics (C of Figure 1).

Table 1. Linguistic Characteristics of Sample

Variables	Dimension	Number of questions		Used in analyses*	
				Exploration 2	Exploratio n 3
Mother tongue/First official language still understood	Cognitive	2		1 (Francophone identity)	2
Linguistic identity (Francophone, Anglophone, bilingual, or other)	Cognitive	4			4
Sociolinguistic identity (for example, Francophone from minority or majority language group)	Cognitive	7			*Note 3
Language of education	Cognitive / Physical	3		Total of 3	1 (Overall Score)
Education on subjects related to AO	Cognitive	8		Total of 7	7
Self-assessment of cultural competencies • general • knowledge of Francophone minority communities	Cognitive	4 5		Total of 9	4 5
Language behaviours: Extent to which French or English is used with friends, at work, etc. Higher score indicates greater use of French	Physical	15		Total of 15	*Note 4
Linguistic insecurity in French	Emotional	6		Total of 6	6
Speak and advocate for French	Emotional	6		Total of 6	6
General motivation	Existential	18		1 Overall Rating, *Note 1	18
Sub-Total:		**78**			
Questions asked about each of the languages or linguistic communities:		French	English		
Ethnolinguistic vitality of your region	Physical	8	8	2 x total of 8	16
Pride/Protection of linguistic community	Emotional	3	3	2 x total of 3	6
Sense of competency in language	Cognitive / Emotional	5	5	2 x total of 5	10
Sense of autonomy when using language (linguistic motivation)	Emotional	5	5	2 x total of 5	10
Sense of comfort in relationships with both language groups	Emotional	5	5	2 x total of 5	10
Linguistic motivation	Existential	26	26	*Note 2	*Note 5
Language proficiency in specific tasks	Cognitive	10	10	2 x total of 10	20
Sub-Total:		**62**	**62**		**125**
Total		**202**			

*Note 1: Overall rating of self-motivation, calculate by using the following formula: Self-motivation = [3(intrinsic) + 2(integrated) +(identified) - (introjected) - 2(external) - 3(amotivation)] (Radel et al., 2013).

*Note 2: The data did not allow calculation of an overall rating of self-motivation; not used in this exploration.

*Note 3: Redundant questions with the variable "linguistic identity;" not included in factorial analysis presented below.

*Note 4: Redundant questions with the variable "Speak and advocate for French;" not included in factor analysis presented below.

*Note 5: Redundant questions with the variable "Feeling of autonomy;" not included in factor analysis presented later on.

Exploration of Determinants of Active Offer

This section will begin by describing each of the three exploratory studies, and then will present the results to outline what we have learned so far about possible determinants of AO.

First Exploration

The first study, aimed at calculating the measurement properties of the two questionnaires on AO, also allowed us to collect data on potential AO determinants. The study was conducted among graduates of health and social services programs at the University of Ottawa and the Université de Moncton. Participants were either working or had worked previously in a health care or social service position, in a province other than Quebec. Of the 1771 people invited to participate, 160 (9%) responded. Respondents were excluded if they did not have work experience outside Quebec or if they left more than 50% of the questions on Questionnaires A and B unanswered. The final sample for this study was composed of 60 people.

Data collection included a questionnaire on socio-demographic data, the two questionnaires (Questionnaire A—Individual Behaviours and Questionnaire B—Organizational Support) from the *Mesure de l'offre active de services en français en contexte minoritaire* (the Active Offer of French-language services in Minority Context Measure), and the questionnaire on possible determinants of AO (Questionnaire C). The questionnaires were published online using the FluidSurveys software.

The socio-demographic information gathered included the province or territory in which the person worked, as well as her or his area of studies and primary role at work. The data on the workplace included the working language of the facility, the proportion of clients to whom French-language services are offered, and the type of facility. A majority of respondents spoke French as their mother tongue (Table 2) and worked in Ontario, primarily in the Ottawa area (75%), or in New Brunswick (16.7%) (Table 3). In this sample, there was little variation in the psycholinguistic development of the respondents. For example, 70% of respondents had completed most of their studies in French. All of them considered themselves either Francophone or bilingual; no one selected Anglophone as the primary identity. The fact that the sample was relatively homogenous in language limited the opportunities for some analysis. This led to a second exploration with a more hetero-geneous sample.

Second Exploration

The second study explored personal factors related to AO behaviours during a clinical placement for Anglophone, Bilingual, and Francophone students in medicine from the University of Ottawa, the Northern Ontario School of Medicine (NOSM), and the *Centre de formation médicale du Nouveau-Brunswick* (CFMNB). Data collection proceeded in a similar fashion to the first exploration: socio-demographic questionnaire, Questionnaires A, B, and C online via FluidSurveys. The only differences were in the socio-demographic characteristics examined: this time they included gender, age group, program of study, mother tongue, and ability to communicate with a service user in French.

Of the 508 students in the three medical programs invited to an information session, 98 were interested in participating in the study and received the link to the questionnaires. Forty-three students completed the questionnaires, which corresponds to a response rate of 8.5% for eligible students and 44% for those who had expressed an interest in the study. A majority of respondents were from the University of Ottawa (58.1%) and from NOSM (37.2%). Only one student (2.3%) was from CFMNB.

This time, the respondents had varied linguistic profiles (Table 2). Indeed, even though they were almost all bilingual, a little less than half of the sample identified more closely with the Anglophone community, approximately a quarter with the Francophone community, and another third had a strongly bilingual identity and showed no preference for either official language community. The responses of the three unilingual Anglophones were excluded from the analysis, since their experiences differed too greatly from the reality of bilingual participants. This time, it was the small sample size that limited the types of analysis that could be applied.

Third Exploration

In order to pursue our analyses of AO determinants, the databases of the first two explorations were combined. Only the data of participants for whom less than 30% of the data were missing were retained for the last exploration. This provided a sample of 80 people.

Table 2. Linguistic Characteristics of Sample

Variables	Numbers*		
	Exploration 1	Exploration 2	Exploration 3
Mother tongue / First official language still understood			
• French	41 (68.3%)	17 (39.5%)	51 (63.8%)
• English	4 (6.7%)	22 (51.2%)	21 (26.3%)
• Other	4 (6.7%)	4 (9.3%)	7 (8.8%)
Educated in French			
• 0-66%	6 (10.0%)	20 (46.5%)	15 (20.5%)
• 67-89%	8 (13.3%)	9 (20.9%)	19 (26.1%)
• 90% and over	34 (56.6%)	14 (32.5%)	39 (53.4%)
Strongest linguistic identity			
• Francophone / bilingual Francophone	21 (35.0%)	11 (25.6%)	44 (55.0%)
• Bilingual. no preference for either	29 (48.3%)	13 (30.2%)	21 (26.3%)
• Anglophone / bilingual Anglophone	0 (0.0%)	19 (44.2%)	15 (18.8%)
Ability to speak French with a user			
• Yes, I can provide all services in French		28 (65.1%)	70 (87.5%)
• Yes, I can provide certain services in French	60 (100%)	12 (27.9%)	10 (12.5%)
• No, I cannot speak French with a user		3 (7.0%)	

* The percentages do not add up to 100% due to missing data.

Table 3. Socio-demographic Characteristics, Workplace or Internship Setting

Variables	Numbers and percentage*		
	Exploration 1	Exploration 2	Exploration 3
Province of work or clinical placement			
• New Brunswick	10 (16.7%)	1 (2.3%)	10 (12.5%)
• Ontario	49 (81.7%)	42 (97.7%)	69 (86.3%)
• British Columbia	1 (1.7%)		
Type of setting			
• Health or social service facility (hospital, rehabilitation centre, community health centre, private office, home health care organization, long-term residence or home and child protection centre, women's centre)	36 (60.0%)	43 (100%)	67 (83.7%)
• Educational institution (college, university, elementary or secondary school)	12 (20.0%)		7 (8.7%)
• Other workplace (public service, not-for-profit organization).	11 (18.3%)		6 (7.5%)
Discipline of degree			
• Medicine	10 (16.7%)	43 (100%)	44 (55.0%)
• Nursing	10 (16.7%)		8 (10.0%)
• Rehabilitation: audiology, occupational therapy, speech-language pathology, physiotherapy	12 (20.0%)		11 (13.7%)
• Other: kinesiology, nutrition, psychology, social services	25 (41.7%)		15 (18.7%)
Primary role in workplace			
• Clinical work: service provider, student	37 (61.7%)	43 (100%)	66 (82.5%)
• Non-clinical work: administration, research, teaching	23 (38.3%)		13 (16.2%)
Working language in primary workplace or internship			
• French	13 (21.7%)	14 (32.6%)	21 (26.3%)
• Bilingual	31 (51.7%)	8 (18.6%)	31 (38.8%)
• English	14 (23.3%)	21 (48.8%)	27 (33.8%)

* The percentages do not add up to 100% due to missing data

Table 3. Socio-demographic Characteristics, Workplace or Internship Setting (*continued*)

Variables	Numbers and percentage*		
	Exploration 1	Exploration 2	Exploration 3
Of the users you meet, what proportion are offered services in French?			
• 0-39%	18 (30.0%)	23 (53.5%)	32 (40.0%)
• 40-79%	24 (40.0%)	15 (34.9%)	32 (40.0%)
• 80-100%	18 (30.0%)	5 (11.6%)	16 (20.0%)
STRATEGY most often used to serve Francophone clients			
• The majority of service providers speak French in all departments and units	25 (41.7%)	19 (44.2%)	36 (45.0%)
• At least one service provider in each department or unit speaks French	15 (25.0%)	7 (16.3%)	19 (23.8%)
• Professional interpreters are available, or staff from other departments or units or family members are asked to translate	8 (13.3%)	14 (32.5%)	20 (25.0%)
• Services are provided in English only	1 (1.7%)	2 (4.7%)	

* The percentages do not add up to 100% due to missing data.

Analyses

The results are first presented using descriptive statistics (average and standard deviation). An analysis of the influence of different characteristics on individual AO behaviours ensued. Data from the first exploration were primarily used to examine how individual AO behaviours (Questionnaire A) were linked with characteristics of the workplace and organizational support (Questionnaire B). The second and third explorations were used to study the link between individual AO behaviours (Questionnaire A) and individual characteristics (Questionnaire C), while taking into account organizational support (Questionnaire B).

Testing for statistically significant differences between various groups of respondents was done using Student (dichotomous variables) and ANOVA (3-group category variables) tests. The influence of continuous variables was studied first in a univariate linear regression analysis. Multivariate linear regression analyses were also conducted to test for the simultaneous influence of different variables on AO individual behaviours.

During the third exploration, a factorial analysis was used to empirically group items on the determinants questionnaire into a certain number of factors. Factors explaining more than 2% of the variance were examined for conceptual adequacy. The internal consistency of the selected factors was calculated using Cronbach α coefficient. The influence of these factors on individual AO behaviours was examined in univariate and multivariate linear regression analyses. A factorial analysis permits grouping of items shown to be highly correlated within the same factors. Using this method (instead of the original grouping of items, Table 1) allowed us to enter a greater number of potential predictors into the regression analyses, while avoiding multicollinearity.[11]

Results

First Exploration: Links between the Characteristics of the Workplace, Organizational Support, and Individual Active Offer Behaviours

The results in Table 4 show statistically significant differences between the individual AO behaviours and perceived organizational support of service providers in Ontario and New Brunswick. We observed similar differences according to the proportion of Francophone clients in the workplace, a higher proportion being associated to more AO behaviours and greater organizational support.

Table 5 shows more AO behaviours were observed in facilities where there is a plan to have at least one service provider who speaks French in each department, compared to those relying on the services of interpreters. The difference between facilities where one service provider speaks French per department and those in which the majority of service providers speak French is not statistically

Table 4. Differences between Workplace Characteristics and AO (Dichotomous Variables)

	Measurement of AO							
	Individual behaviours					Perceived organizational support		
	n	Average total weighted score[1]	t Test			n	Average total weighted score[1,2]	t Test	
			t	p				t	p
Province of work 1. Ontario 2. New Brunswick	54	66.2 76.1	-2.72	0.012*		49	97.2 110.0	-2.38	0.028*
Proportion of Francophone clients in setting 1. 0 to 39% 2. 40% or more	55	57.7 71.5	-2.75	0.011*		50	87.2 103.0	-2.35	0.028*

1 On the questionnaire about AO behaviours and the questionnaire about organizational support, we use the weighted total according to the number of questions answered by each individual.

2 The "barriers" subscale under organizational support was converted to a single item, in which "4" means absence of barriers and "1" means existence of 5 barriers or more. This conversion was necessary because, during the first exploration, the question asked was whether or not there were barriers. The questionnaire on organizational support used for these analysis included 37 items instead of 42.

* p<0.05

Table 5. Differences between Workplace Characteristics and AO (3-Group Category Variables)

Variable	Individual AO Behaviours (n=47)					Perceived Organizational Support (n=46)				
	Average total weighted score[1]	ANOVA		Tukey Test[2]		Average total weighted score[2]	ANOVA		Tukey Test[2]	
		F	p	pair	p		F	p	pair	p
Strategy used in workplace to serve Francophone clientele										
1. The majority of service providers speak French in all departments and units	73.4	6.229	0.004*	1 vs 2	NS	109.5	18.068	0.000*	1 vs 2	0.003*
2. At least one service provider in each department or unit speaks French	68.5			2 vs 3	NS	90.9			2 vs 3	0.024*
3. Professional interpreters are available	54.8			1 vs 3	0.003*	70.7			1 vs 3	0.000*

1 Averages are calculated as for Table 5.
2 When ANOVA revealed statistically significant differences, Tukey's Tests were used post hoc to identify the groups between which differences are found
* $p<0.05$; NS = not significant, i.e., $p> 0.05$.

significant. The perceived level of organizational support is also better in workplaces where there are Francophone service providers in departments and units than it is in those which rely on interpreters.

Univariate linear regression analyses illustrate the association between AO behaviours and organizational support. The total organizational support rating is a predictor for individual AO behaviours and accounts for 36.5% of the variance observed (Table 6). When taken individually, the following subscales are also predictors of AO behaviours: "Reception and Intake," "Management and Governance," and "Support and Referrals." In particular, the "Reception and Intake" subscale explains the largest proportion of the observed variance, 40.2%, followed by "Management and Governance," explaining 24.1%.

Table 6. Relation between Individual AO Behaviours and Various Components of Organizational Support

Component of Organizational Support	Coefficient B	Standardized Beta Coefficient	CI 95% for B	p	R^2
Reception and Intake (n=51)	1.169	0.634	(0.760; 1.578)	< 0.001*	0.402
Intervention (n=49)	0.843	0.279	(-0.007; 1.693)	0.052	0.078
Support and Referrals (n=50)	1.245	0.307	(0.126; 2.364)	0.030*	0.094
Continuous Professional Development in French (n=42)	0.693	0.305	(0.001; 1.386)	0.050	0.093
Management and Governance (n=51)	1.318	0.491	(0.647; 1.989)	< 0.001*	0.241
Obstacles (n=47)	5.520	0.220	(-1.824; 12.864)	0.137	0.048
Total Organizational support (n=49)	0.403	0.605	(0.247; 0.559)	< 0.001*	0.365

* $p<0.05$

Second Exploration: Links between Determinants, Perceived Organizational Support, and Individual Active Offer Behaviours

Table 7 presents the descriptive statistics of each of the subscales in Questionnaire C (determinants of AO), and the extent to which each is associated with AO behaviours. In this sample, which includes a slightly higher number of Anglophones than Francophones, we observed that participants reported a higher competency in English than in French. In addition, they seemed more likely to defend the interests of the Francophone community than those of the Anglophone community, possibly because protecting the rights of Francophones seems more necessary. The majority of respondents (72.1%) consider their education prepared them well for the challenges of offering services in French, although their responses did not seem to demonstrate that the AO content covered in their courses was complete.

Table 7. Averages and Standard Deviations for Perceived Organizational Support and Various Determinants Examined, and Their Association with Individual AO Behaviours

			Descriptive statistics			Association with AO behaviours		
		n	Average score	Standard deviation	P of t test	Beta Coefficient	p	R²
	Perceived organizational support (/148)	39	98.0	22.4	n/a	0.790	<0.001*	0.624
	Francophone identity (/5)	39	3.49	1.43	n/a	0.560	<0.001*	0.314
	Education in French (/100)	40	73.5	22.9	n/a	0.793	<0.001*	0.629
Cultural competencies	Education on 7 subjects related to AO (/100)	40	60.1	25.2	n/a	-0.044	0.789	-
	Self-assessment of cultural competencies (/100)	40	73.3	13.4		-0.101	0.534	-
Linguistic competencies	Sense of competency in language (/100) • in French • in English	40 / 40	82.5 / 88.8	17.0 / 14.3	0.017*	0.497 / -0.332	0.001* / 0.036*	0.247 / 0.111
	Language proficiency in specific tasks (/100) • in French • in English	38 / 38	85.2 / 95.3	16.6 / 8.1	0.001*	0.599 / -0.500	<0.001* / 0.001*	0.359 / 0.250
	Linguistic insecurity in French (/100)	39	37.4	17.1	n/a	-0.361	0.024*	0.131
Affirmation of identity	Pride/Protection of linguistic community (/100) • francophone • anglophone	40 / 40	76.7 / 59.8	19.1 / 22.3	0.001*	0.700 / 0.158	<0.001* / 0.331	0.490 / -
	Speak and advocate for French	39	43.6	22.3	n/a	0.672	<0.001*	0.452
Language behaviours	Extent to which French is used with friends, at work, etc (/100)	38	43.2	20.6	n/a	0.661	<0.001*	0.437
Linguistic motivation	Sense of autonomy when using language (/100) • in French • in English	40 / 40	69.9 / 83.8	10.1 / 15.2	<0.001*	0.411 / -0.181	0.008* / 0.264	0.169 / -
Feeling of comfort	Sense of comfort in relationships (/100) • with Francophones • with Anglophones	40 / 40	78.8 / 80.4	17.7 / 12.8	0.409	0.529 / 0.019	<0.001* / 0.910	0.280 / -
Ethnolinguistic vitality	Ethnolinguistic vitality of the community (/100) • Francophone community • Anglophone community	40 / 40	64.9 / 87.1	12.6 / 12.0	<0.001*	0.260 / -0.083	0.106§ / 0.610	-0.067 / -
General motivation	Self-motivation index	38	35.7	16.1	n/a	0.214	0.198§	0.046

1 In order to simplify this table, scores for the subscales on Questionnaire C were converted to a 100-point scale, with the exception of the self-motivation rating, which was calculated using the formula in Radel *et al.*, 2013.

*p< 0,05; § p< 0,25

Univariate regression analyses demonstrate that several variables are associated with AO behaviours.

To measure the relative contribution of each AO determinant, multivariate analyses are indicated.

Various sociolinguistic characteristics are strongly correlated with each other. For example, of the 28 correlations between different variables related to the knowledge of French, its use, and Francophone identity, 13 are higher than 0.600. Correlations between different variables related to the knowledge of English, its use, and Anglophone identity are less obvious; only 4 of the 21 correlations are higher than 0.600.

In order to avoid problems with multicollinearity, multiple regression analyses were performed on organizational support and one sociolinguistic variable at a time. Just as we found with graduates in our first study, the organizational support perceived by service providers is closely correlated to individual AO behaviours ($r=0,790$, $p<0,001$) in this group of medical students. It explains 62.4% of the variance in these behaviours. Six sociolinguistic characteristics linked to the sense of competency, comfort, or affirmation in French show a statistically significant association with AO behaviours, and explain an additional proportion of variance (between 3% and 13%) beyond the variance explained by organizational support (Table 8).

Table 8. Multiple Regression Analyses using Individual AO Behaviours with Perceived Organizational Support and Sociolinguistic Variables

	Models	n	Beta Coefficient	p	Variance Explained
I	Organizational support	39	0.790	<0.001	0.624
II	Organizational support	39	0.443	0.001	0.745
	Language of education		0.491	<0.001	
III	Organizational support	39	0.704	<0.001	0.673
	Sense of competency in French		0.237	0.026	
IV	Organizational support	39	0.692	<0.001	0.669
	Francophone identity		0.238	0.032	
V	Organizational support	39	0.606	<0.001	0.744
	Pride/protection of Francophone community		0.392	<0.001	
Vi	Organizational support		0.604	<0.001	0.654
	Speak and advocate for French		0.277	0.038	
VII	Organizational support	39	0.675	<0.001	0.689
	Sense of comfort inrelationships with Francophones		0.280	0.009	

Note: Multivariate linear regression analyses, using the stepwise method, with variables associated individually with AO at $p<0.25$. Results shown are for variables remaining statistically significant ($p<0.05$) in multivariate analyses.

Third Exploration: Links between Determinants, Organizational Support, and Individual AO Behaviours

Using the grouped data from the first and second explorations, a factor analysis was conducted on 125 questions described in Table 1. The results revealed 12 factors, 11 of which included 117 questions that could have a conceptual meaning. These factors do differ from the theoretical dimensions in the model presented by Landry *et al.* (2008), although this does not represent a pronounced difference. Often, elements from two or three dimensions in the model are connected to the same factor. Five of these factors seemed associated with AO behaviours in univariate regression analyses, and four of these associations (sense of competency in French and Francophone identity; cultural knowledge; language affirmation; sense of competency in English) remain significant when the simultaneous influence of these factors and organizational support on AO behaviours is examined (Table 9).

Table 9. Univariate and Multivariate Regression Analyses (n = 80)

Factor	Number of questions	Univariate Analyses			Multivariate Analysis[1]		
		Beta Coefficient	p	R^2	Beta Coefficient	p	R^2
Perceived organizational support	37	0.698	<0.001	0.487	0.472	<0.001	
French proficiency and Francophone identity	24	0.449	<0.001	0.202	0.244	0.003	
Cultural knowledge	11	0.210	0.062	0.044	0.178	0.013	0.642
Affirmation of French language[2]	11	0.383	<0.001	0.147	0.253	0.001	
Sense of competency in English	10	-0.316	0.004	0.100	-0.217	0.003	
Linguistic competency in English	10	-0.169	0.134	-			
Ethnolinguistic vitality of the Anglophone community in the region	8	0.005	0.962	-			
General motivation: non-self-determined[3]	10	-0.034	0.765	-			
Sense of comfort with both language groups	8	0.040	0.723	-			
Ethnolinguistic vitality of the Francophone community in the region	8	0.034	0.763	-			
General motivation self-determined[2] and autonomy in use of French	11	0.062	0.585	-			
Weak sense of autonomy in the use of French and English and elements of linguistic insecurity	6	-0.049	0.667	-			

1 Multivariate linear regression, using the stepwise method, and considering only the variables individually associated with AO at p<0,25. A factor was retained when its association with AO remained statistically significant (p<0.05) in multivariate analyses.

2 Includes: Mother tongue is French, Speak and advocate for French, Pride/protection of francophone community, and one item from Sense of comfort in relationships with francophone.

3 Self-determined motivation includes intrinsic, integrated, and identified motivations. Non-self-determined motivation includes introjected motivations, external regulations, and amotivation.

The four factors associated with individual AO behaviours beyond organizational support include 56 questions. After eliminating those that reduced the internal consistency of their subscale, 48 questions remained. Table 10 presents the components of this questionnaire on determinants of AO and the internal consistency of each of its 4 subscales. The other measurement properties of this questionnaire have not yet been evaluated.

Table 10. Components of New Questionnaire on Personal Determinants of AO

Factors[1]	After reduction		Correspondence with initial questionnaire (Table 3)	
	Number of questions	Coefficient α	Variable	Number of items
Proficiency in French and Francophone identity	18	0.967	Francophone linguistic identity	1
			Sense of comfort in relationships with Francophones (listened to, trust/trusted)	2
			Language proficiency in specific tasks	10
			Sense of autonomy when using French	5
Cultural knowledge	11	0.918	Education on French minority communities	7
			Self-assessment of cultural competencies regarding Francophone communities	3
			Self-assessment in general cultural competencies	1
Affirmation of language	10	0.839	Pride / protection of Francophone community	3
			Speak and advocate for French	6
			Sense of comfort in relationships with Francophones (feeling supported)	1
Sense of competency in English and bilingual identity	9	0.88	First official language still understood is English	1
			Bilingual linguistic identity	1
			Sense of competency in English	4
			Sense of autonomy when using English	3

1 Factors resulting from factor analysis of main components with Varimax rotation.

Discussion

Our studies aimed to identify behaviours that demonstrate the AO of social services and health care in French in linguistic minority communities, to measure them, and to identify the determinants of these behaviours. Given the lack of questionnaires available to measure these concepts, we developed three questionnaires, two of which measure AO (A—Individual Behaviours and B—Organizational Support), and a third investigating possible determinants of AO (Questionnaire C). The first study allowed us to begin the quantitative validation of the two questionnaires on AO measurement, which increases our confidence in the results obtained from these questionnaires compared to non-validated in-house tools. The third study allowed us to identify some determinants of AO with a reduced questionnaire of 48 questions. Having shorter and validated questionnaires available will be useful for future research on the subject, providing a better response rate. This research supports the ultimate goal of better preparing educators and decision-makers interested in improving access to services in French by helping them make evidence-based decisions.

As far as AO determinants are concerned, the results demonstrate a strong link between organizational actions that support AO and individual AO behaviours. The organizational support they perceived explained 36.5% and 62.4% of the individual AO behaviours of health sciences graduates and medical students, respectively. These results are similar to those obtained in a qualitative study by Bouchard and Vézina (2009), which found that organizational support is seen by service providers as being a key facilitator. They are also consistent with studies suggesting that organizational identity (the values and actions of the organization) can guide an employee's behaviour (Edwards, 2009). A strong organizational identity gives meaning to the actions of employees in the workplace, and motivates them to transmit its corporate values (Ashforth & Mael, 1996). Although it seems logical that organizational support influences AO behaviours, our study is the first to demonstrate this with quantitative data.

Specifically, the first exploration suggests two categories of organizational support—"Reception and Intake" and "Management and Governance"—have the most significant influence on individual AO behaviour. In the first case, questions focused on the visibility of service provision in French in the workplace. Greater visibility may inform users and thereby raise the awareness of service providers. In the second case, there were questions on the presence of Francophones in management and decision-making bodies. These Francophone representatives may show leadership and, in so doing, guide the organization to promote AO behaviours.

The first exploration suggests the legislative environment and the characteristics of the workplace can explain certain differences in perceived organizational support. For example, service providers in New Brunswick perceive greater organizational support than those in Ontario. The legislative framework in the two provinces is clearly different. New Brunswick's *Official Languages Act* supports bilingualism in all government services offered in the province, including social services and health care (Government of New Brunswick, 2015). In Ontario, the *French Language Services Act* specifies that government services must be offered in French where numbers warrant, and that parapublic services must be offered in French in designated facilities. Obtaining this designation is voluntary for most organizations offering social services and health care (Office of Francophone Affairs, 2014).

Facilities working to ensure there are Francophone service providers in each department, rather than relying on the services of interpreters, seem to be more favourable to AO. This finding supports the recommendation of Ferguson and Candib (2002) to avoid using interpreters, as service providers of diverse culture, race, and language are preferable for many reasons. It is also a concern when, as observed, there is only one Francophone service provider in an Anglo-dominant organization. In this case, the service provider may choose not to self-identify as being Francophone or bilingual in order to avoid the inevitable increase in workload that results from being asked to interpret in other departments or units (Bouchard & Vézina, 2009; Drolet *et al.*, 2014).

Although the difference is not statistically significant, one of our observations was very surprising. We found a tendency in facilities with a majority of Francophone employees to provide less active offer than those with only one Francophone employee in each department or service. It is possible that in facilities where most staff members are Francophones, they apply fewer of the AO strategies that make French services visible. These people may rely on their capacity to speak French to those who ask (passive offer), thus bypassing the principle of AO.

The link between organizational support and individual AO behaviours during a clinical placement for students in medicine was found to be even stronger than that of graduates. This could be explained by the fact that in a learning environment, people may feel more vulnerable and find it more difficult to show leadership in their AO behaviours. Moreover, the sample of students in medicine, as compared to the graduates, included a lower proportion of people for whom French was the first language and a higher proportion of Anglophones who could speak French. Organizational support may have more of an impact on this group. Furthermore, certain psycholinguistic factors have an impact on AO, beyond those related to perceived organizational support. Although these factors are expressed slightly differently in the second and third explorations, they are similar. Affirmation of identity and competency in French were found to be significant in both studies. Cultural knowledge did not appear to be a determinant of AO behaviour among medical students, while it is for the combined sample (Exploration 3). Since the concept of AO is relatively new, it is likely that current students have received more education on the subject than the graduates, which may have increased the variance in the sample and made it possible to detect a link.

Last, a greater sense of competency in English among bilingual service providers is associated with less frequent AO behaviours. It is possible that this result is linked to a phenomenon observed among people of Francophone origin called "Francogène," whereby members of a linguistic group have the impression that their spoken French is not good enough to express themselves clearly, thus preferentially reverting to English. Forgues and Landry (2014) have noted a similar situation among users. In their study on access to French-language services, users' competency in English and identification with an Anglophone community were negatively associated with receiving services in French.

Strengths and Limitations of Our Exploratory Studies

The strength of these explorations lies in the use of validated questionnaires and the application of a recognized conceptual framework to identify probable determinants of AO. In this perspective we chose to use, in whole or in part, pre-existing questionnaires (psycholinguistic development and motivation) to measure the determinants. However, the length of the questionnaire we compiled may have limited participation. As a result, the greatest limitation of the first two explorations is the low response rate. The small number of invited people who participated affects representativity of the data (Streiner & Norman, 2008). It is probable that the participants were those most interested in the study subject, and that people who were not sufficiently aware of the importance of AO did not feel motivated to respond. Moreover, participants who did not answer several questions were kept in the studies in order to avoid reducing the sample even further. The results on different scales were converted to percentages, allowing an account for missing responses; hence, the results are approximations of the actual data would have been obtained if all questionnaires had been completed in their entirety. Samples were also limited to Ontario and New Brunswick, with a higher participation rate from Ontario. Better representation from Francophone minority communities in the remainder of Canada would be necessary in order to confirm that the results from these studies can generalized to the rest of Canada or to obtain complementary perspectives. Combining data from two studies allowed us to establish a larger sample, study individuals with fewer missing responses, and represent a more varied linguistic reality. On the other hand, the reality of students may differ from those of graduates in several ways, and these differences were amalgamated. In addition, the sample size remained rather small for factor analyses.

Ideas for Further Research

The development of measurement tools presents certain challenges and must proceed through a number of steps (Bradburn, 2004; Streiner & Norman, 2008). Recently, a Rasch modelization of the two questionnaires included in the *Mesure de l'offre active de services en français en contexte minoritaire* (the Active Offer of French Language Services in Minority Context Measure) allowed examination of other aspects of their measurement properties and will permit further refinement of these tools (Grondin, Dionne, Savard, & Casimiro, 2017). As far as the questionnaire on determinants is concerned, other studies are necessary to confirm its measurement properties. Notwithstanding this fact, we will continue refining the questionnaire, using only the factors associated with AO, in order to create a tool that will help direct learners to targeted educational or awareness-building activities tailored to their particular profile. Future studies could also examine if the frequency of AO behaviours and the determinants of these behaviours differ according to respondent group—for example, service providers from different professions, various settings (hospitals, community centres, long-term care facilities, private practice), other Canadian provinces, or from regions where there is a high density versus low density of Francophones. The realities of other OLMCs, such as Anglophone communities in Quebec or Welsh-speaking people in Wales, are potentially different from FMCs. Hence the results of these studies cannot be directly applied to these communities. However, the same procedure for identifying observable AO behaviours and for developing tools to measure these behaviours and identify their determinants could be repeated with these groups.

Conclusion

Despite their limitations, these three explorations represent, to our knowledge, the first attempts to conduct a quantitative study of AO behaviours and their determinants in a group of health care and social service providers. These explorations point to several recommendations on how AO behaviours can be optimized.

First, ensuring organizational support for AO seems to be a key factor encouraging individual AO behaviours. Therefore, it would be important to raise the awareness of senior managers (managers, directors, etc.) regarding AO. Making leaders accountable is necessary so they may establish clear guidelines for French-language services and provide staff members with the tools they need to put them into practice. Unfortunately, in some circumstances bilingual service providers are hired for their professional and linguistic skills, but senior managers do not use their expertise to its full advantage (Bouchard *et al.*, in Chapter 2; Savard *et al.*, in Chapter 9). A Canada-wide collaboration could promote strategy sharing in order to better support these employees. Our results also provide some leads as to the OA education of service providers. Besides activities designed to build the cultural knowledge of service providers, we should consider the possibility of organizing activities to foster their Francophone identity and develop their proficiency in French, or cultural events that increase their sense of belonging within the Francophone community. These activities would also be useful for improving retention rates of bilingual staff in Anglo-dominant settings (Savard *et al.*, in Chapter 9).

Finally, it appears important to continue encouraging Francophones in official language minority communities to pursue their elementary and secondary education in French schools as these programs add to their sense of competency as well as their proficiency in French. Francophone schooling is also correlated to the affirmation of Francophone identity (Association canadienne d'éducation de langue française—[ACELIF, 2006).

To summarize, although the concept of AO is a recent one, several service providers have adopted some AO behaviours. Whether or not they integrate these behaviours into their practice appears to depend on several personal and environmental factors. Personal factors are influenced by the psycholinguistic development of an individual and by his or her educational background, while environmental factors may be tied to the legal or organizational context of their workplace. Knowing these factors makes it possible to propose strategies to build awareness and create educational activities designed to meet the needs of diverse audiences (legislators, leaders, service providers) and, ultimately, to improve the quality and safety of the services provided to users in OLMCs. This three-part study allowed us to move one step closer to better understanding these concepts.

Notes

1. These studies were made possible by the financial support of the *Consortium national de formation en santé* (CNFS), *Volet Université d'Ottawa* and *Secrétariat National*, which are funded by Health Canada as part of the Roadmap for Canada's Official Languages 2013–2018. The authors would like to thank the *Réseau des services de santé en français de l'Est de l'Ontario*, and in particular Isabelle Morin for her expertise in active offer throughout the first study, as well as all those who participated in the expert group on active offer in order to substantiate the individual behaviours and organizational actions which support active offer (see note 7). As well they wish to thank the people who took part in the second study: Danièle Barbeau-Rodrigue and Lisa Graves (Northern Ontario School of Medicine), Lyne Pitre (Faculty of Medicine at the University of Ottawa), and Jacinthe Beauchamp (*Centre de formation médicale du Nouveau-Brunswick*). Finally, the authors thank all the students and research assistants who helped with the data analysis: Nicole Atchessi, Stéphanie Brûlé, Christiane Guibord, Émilie Guitard, Krista Langevin, Ziad Nsarellah, Marie-France Sauvé, Josée Venne, and all the participants who took the time to complete the online questionnaires.

2. In the remainder of this chapter, "services" will be used as a general term encompassing all types of social services and health care services.

3. The term "user" refers here to the person who receives services in different settings. This word can be considered a synonym of patient, recipient, client, etc.

4. The term "service provider" designates a person who provides services or is studying in order to provide them in the future. It can be considered a synonym of health professional, physician, social worker, personal support worker, home support worker, aid, or student in one of these professional professions.

5. According to the *Oxford Dictionary*, a determinant is defined as a "factor which decisively affects the nature or outcome of something." See https://en.oxforddictionaries.com/definition/determinant

6. Measurement properties describe the qualities of a measurement, which may include: (1) its validity—that is, its ability to accurately reflect what we want to measure and to distinguish individuals or situations in which the value of this concept may differ; (2) its reproducibility or reliability—that is, its ability to give stable results when one measurement is compared with another in a characteristic or situation which has not changed; and (3) its reference values for a group or standards to which results obtained for an individual can be compared.

7. The group of active offer experts included: Sylvain Vézina (Université de Moncton), Mai Savoie (*Consortium national de formation en santé, Volet Université de Moncton*), Gilles Vienneau (*Société Santé et Mieux-être en français du Nouveau-Brunswick*), Jacinthe Beauchamp (*Centre de formation médicale du Nouveau-Brunswick*), Florence Flower (*Collège communautaire du Nouveau-Brunswick*), Lise Lortie (*Sentiers du leadership inc.*, Ontario), Isabelle Morin and Ginette LeBlanc (*Réseau des services de santé en français de l'Est de l'Ontario*), and Jacynthe Carrière-Lalonde (*Consortium national de formation en santé, Volet Université d'Ottawa*).

8. Internal consistency, measured by Cronbach alpha, is based on the correlations between responses to different items or statements on the same test. Our results are within the desirable values of 0.70 and 0.90 for all subscales on the two questionnaires, with the exception of the optional subscale on specific interventions ($\alpha= 0.597$).

9. Test-retest reliability or reproducibility refers to how consistent the results of a test are across time, and is calculated as the correlation between the results when the evaluation test is administered on two different occasions and no change has occurred in an individual respondent between the two occasions. Our results indicate an acceptable level of test-retest reliability of the weighted scores, as the interclass correlation coefficients were higher than the minimal threshold (> 0,60) for 8 of the 10 subscales.

10. Construct validity is aimed at confirming the theoretical framework underpinning the measurement and testing hypotheses about the links between selected indicators and the phenomenon being measured. In this study, construct validity was demonstrated by moderate correlations between the scores on each subscale and the score on the questionnaire as a whole ($r > 0.70$, with the exception of one subscale). It is also demonstrated by the links between subscales on the individual behaviour questionnaire with correspondent subscales on the perceived organizational support questionnaire ($r = 0.416$ to 0.605), which means that the two questionnaires measured related, although distinct, concepts.

11. Multicollinearity is a problem that arises when certain predictor variables in the model are highly correlated with other variables already included in the model.

References

Ashforth, B. E., & Mael, F. A. (1996). Organizational identity and strategy as a context for the individual. *Advances in Strategic Management, 13,* 19–64.

Association canadienne d'éducation de langue française (ACELF). (2006). *Cadre d'orientation en construction identitaire.* Québec, QC: Patrimoine canadien/Heritage Canada..

Beaulieu, M. (2010). *Formation linguistique, adaptation culturelle et services de santé en français: Sommaire.* Ottawa: Consortium national de formation en santé et Société Santé en français.

Bouchard, L., Beaulieu, M., & Desmeules, M. (2012). L'offre active de services de santé en français en Ontario: Une mesure d'équité. *Reflets: Revue d'intervention sociale et communautaire, 18*(2), 38–65. doi:10.7202/1013173ar.

Bouchard, L., & Desmeules, M. (2011). *Minorités de langue officielle du Canada: Égales devant la santé?* Québec, QC: Presses de l'Université du Québec.

Bouchard, L., Desmeules, M., & Gagnon-Arpin, I. (2010). *Rapport national de cartographie conceptuelle: Les représentations de l'avenir des services de santé en français en francophonie minoritaire.* Ottawa, ON: University of Ottawa. Retrieved from http://www.rrasfo.ca/images/docs/publica-tions/2012/Finding%20the%20number%20of%20concepts%20for%20 mapping%20French%20Canadian%20health%20networks.pdf. Retrieved February 11, 2011.

Bouchard, P., & Vézina, S. (2009). *L'outillage des étudiants et des nouveaux professionnels: Une condition essentielle à l'amélioration des services de santé en français.* Ottawa, ON: Consortium national de formation en santé (CNFS).

Bouchard, P., Vézina, S., & Savoie, M. (2010). *Rapport du Dialogue sur l'engagement des étudiants et des futurs professionnels pour de meilleurs services de santé en français dans un contexte minoritaire: Formation et outillage, Recrutement et Rétention.* Ottawa, ON: Consortium national de formation en santé (CNFS).

Bradburn, N., Sudman, S., & Wansink, B. (2004). *Asking questions: The definitive guide to questionnaire design.* San Francisco, CA: Jossey-Bass.

Campinha-Bacote, J. (2002). "The process of cultural competence in the delivery of healthcare services: A model of care." *Journal of Transcultural Nursing, 13*(3), 181–184. doi:10.1177/10459602013003003

Consortium pour la promotion des communautés en santé (2011). *Collaborer avec les francophones en Ontario: De la compréhension du contexte à l'application des pratiques prometteuses.* Toronto, ON: Nexus Santé.

Deci, E. L., & Ryan, R. M. (Eds.). (1985). *Intrinsic motivation and self-determination in human behavior.* New York, NY: Springer.

de Moissac, D., de Rocquigny, J., Giasson, F. Tremblay, C.-L., Aubin, N., Charron, M, & Allaire, G. (2012). Défis associés à l'offre de services de santé et de services sociaux en français au Manitoba: Perceptions des professionnels. *Reflets: Revue d'intervention sociale et communautaire, 18*(2), 66–100. doi:10.7202/1013174ar.

Desabrais, T. (2010). L'influence de l'insécurité linguistique sur le parcours doctoral d'une jeune femme acadienne: Une expérience teintée de la double minorisation. *Reflets, 16*(2), 57–89.

Deveau, K., Landry, R., & Allard, R. (2009). *Utilisation des services gouvernementaux de langue française: Une étude auprès des Acadiens et francophones de la Nouvelle-Écosse sur les facteurs associés à l'utilisation des services gouvernementaux en français.* Moncton, NB: Institut canadien de recherche sur les minorités linguistiques.

Drolet, M., Savard, J., Benoit, J., Arcand, I., Savard, S., Lagacé, J., Lauzon, S., & Dubouloz, C.J. (2014). Health services for linguistic minorities in a bilingual setting: challenges for bilingual professionals. *Qualitative Health Research, 24*(3), 295–305.

Edwards, M. R. (2009). An integrative review of employer branding and OB theory. *Personnel Review, 39*(1), 5–23. doi:10.1108/00483481011012809.

Ferguson, W. J., & Candib, L. M. (2002). Culture, language, and the doctor-patient relationship. *Family Medicine, 34*(5), 353–361.

Forgues, É., Bahi, B., & Michaud, J. (2011). *L'offre de services de santé en français en contexte francophone minoritaire.* Moncton, NB: Institut canadien de recherche sur les minorités linguistiques (ICRML).

Forgues, É., & Landry, R. (2014). *L'accès aux services de santé en français et leur utilisation en contexte francophone minoritaire.* Moncton, NB: Institut canadien de recherche sur les minorités linguistiques (ICRML).

Francophone Affairs Secretariat of Manitoba (2011). *Guideline 1 –The Active Offer Concept.* Now integrated into: Francophone Affairs Secretariat of Manitoba (2017). *Guidelines Manual for the Implementation of French Language Services Based on Government of Manitoba Policy.* Available at: http://www.gov.mb.ca/fls-slf/part2_partie2_082017.pdf

Gouvernement de l'Île-du-Prince-Édouard—Secrétariat aux affaires acadiennes (2012). *Offre active de services en français—Active offer of French Services.* Wellington, PE: Author.

Government of New Brunswick—Human Resources. (2015). *Official Languages—Language of Service Policy and Guidelines.* http://www2.gnb. ca/content/gnb/en/departments/treasury_board/human_resources/content/about_us/policies_and_guidelines/language_service.html. Accessed March 2, 2017.

Grondin, J., Dionne, E., Savard, J., & Casimiro, L. (2017). Mise à l'épreuve d'une méthodologie mettant à profit les modèles de Rasch: L'exemple d'une échelle de la mesure de l'offre active de services en français. In E. Dionne & I. Raîche (Eds.). *Regards actuels et prospectifs sur l'évaluation des apprentissages complexes en éducation dans le domaine de la santé.* Presses de l'Université du Québec.

Guitard, P., Dubouloz, C-J., Benoît, J., Brosseau, L., & Kubina, L-A. (2013). *Recension exhaustive des écrits 2010–2012: Approches pédagogiques et contenus de formation significatifs pour faciliter la préparation des futurs professionnels des services sociaux et de la santé à œuvrer en contexte francophone minoritaire.* Ottawa, ON: University of Ottawa.

Kahn, W. A. (1990). Psychological conditions of personal engagement and disengagement at work. *The Academy of Management Journal, 33*(4), 692-724. doi:10.2307/256287.

Kahn, W. A. (1992). To be fully there: Psychological presence at work. *Human Relations, 45*(4), 321–349. doi:10.1177/001872679204500402.

Landry, R., Allard, R., & Deveau, K. (2008). Un modèle macroscopique du développement psycholangagier en contexte intergroupe minoritaire. *Diversité urbaine* [Special issue], 45–68. doi:10.7202/019561ar.

Landry, R., Allard, R., & Deveau, K. (2010). *École et autonomie culturelle: Enquête pancanadienne en milieu scolaire francophone minoritaire.* Ottawa, ON: Patrimoine canadien, Institut canadien de recherche sur les minorités linguistiques.

Lortie, L., & Lalonde, A. J., with the collaboration of Pier Bouchard (2012). *Cadre de référence pour la formation à l'offre active des services de santé en français.* Ottawa, ON: Consortium national de formation en santé.

Office of Francophone Affairs (2014). *French Language Services Act: Designated agencies.* Retrieved from https://www.ontario.ca/page/government-services-french. Accessed November 23, 2014.

Radel, R., Pelletier, L., & Sarrazin, P. (2013). Restoration processes after need thwarting: When autonomy depends on competence. *Motivation and Emotion, 37*(2), 234–244. doi:10.1007/s11031-012-9308-3.

Ryan, R. M., and Deci, E. L. (2000). Self-determination theory and the facilitation of intrinsic motivation, social development, and well-being. *American Psychologist, 55*(1), 68–78. doi:10.1037/0003-066x.55.1.68.

Savard, J., Casimiro, L., Benoît, J., & Bouchard, P. (2014). Évaluation métrologique de la Mesure de l'offre active de services sociaux et de santé en français en contexte minoritaire. *Reflets: Revue d'intervention sociale et communautaire, 20*(2), 83–122. doi:10.7202/1027587ar.

Savard, J., Casimiro, L., Bouchard, P., Benoît, J., Drolet, M., & Dubouloz, C. (2015). «Conception d'outils de mesure de l'offre active de services sociaux et de santé en français en contexte minoritaire.» *Minorités linguistiques et sociétés, 6*, 131–156.

Société Santé en français. (2007). *Santé en français, communautés en santé: Une offre active de services en santé pour une meilleure santé des francophones en situation minoritaire—Résumé du plan directeur 2008–2013.* Ottawa, ON: Author. Société Santé et Mieux-être en français du Nouveau-Brunswick – Réseau-action formation et recherche (n.d.). *L'offre de services dans les deux langues officielles dans le domaine de la santé: à nous *d'y voir.* Retrieved from http://www.ssmefnb.ca/images/docs/Guide%20 offre%20active%20en%20ofrancais.pdf. Accessed May 13, 2011.

Streiner, D. L., & Norman, G. R. (2008). *Health measurement scales: A practical guide to their development and use* (4th edition), Oxford, UK: Oxford University Press.

Tajfel, H. (1978). *The social psychology of minorities.* Sacramento, CA: Minority Rights Group.

Tajfel, H., & Turner, J. C. (1986). The social identity theory of intergroup behavior. In Austin, W. G., and Worchel, S. (eds.), *Psychology of intergroup relations* (pp. 7–24). Chicago, IL: Nelson-Hall.

ACTIVE OFFER OF SOCIAL AND HEALTH SERVICES IN FRENCH, Version 1.0

Answer the questions as honestly as possible

Not all of the behaviours listed in this questionnaire are carried out in normal practice. Please answer the questions as honestly as possible to reflect your current practice. The questionnaire is not meant to judge any practice or workplace.

Active Offer Behaviors	Never	Rarely	Often	Always
Welcome and Intake				
What actions do I personally take to indicate that I can offer services in French?				
1. In my workplace, I wear a form of identification to indicate that I can provide services in French (a lapel tag, for example).				
2. I ask my patients/clients whether they prefer that I communicate with them in French or English.				
3. When I don't know a patient's/client's preferred language, I say hello in French first, then in English.				
4. There are visual signs that indicate that I can offer services in French or in both official languages (for example, sign on door or desk, label on agenda).				
5. If the organization where I work fails to do so, I remind them of the importance of promoting the French-language services they offer (for example, signage, advertising, website).				
6. When I answer the telephone, I answer in French first, followed by English, as necessary.				
7. My voice mail begins with a greeting in French, followed by the English, as necessary.				
8. My email signature appears in French first.				
9. I make sure that common areas (for example, waiting rooms) are supplied with documents and materials in French (for example, brochures, magazines, newspapers, radio, television, and games).				
10. I use expressions and vocabulary familiar to the patients/clients to make them feel comfortable about speaking French with me.				

	Never	Rarely	Often	Always
Intervention When I interact with Francophone patients/clients in French . . .				
1. I take steps to obtain information or education tools for patients/clients in French, or in both official languages, even when they are not available at the organization where I work.				
2. I use education or information tools (for example, information brochures, exercise programs) that have been adapted to the French used by my patients/clients (for example, cultural, ethnic, or regulatory context).				
3. During the intake interview, I use guides or questionnaires adapted to the regional French used by my patients/clients.				
4. I help patients/clients understand statements written in French when they find the language difficult to understand.				
Specific Interventions				
1. When I use a standardized measurement tool (for example, questionnaires, scales, inventories), I make sure that the instrument has been validated in French (that is, reliability and validity of the French version has been measured). ☐ I don't use standardized measurement instruments in my workplace.				
2. I check that the validation studies of the standardized measurement tool (that is, questionnaires, scales, or inventories) included Francophone minority community members in order to better interpret the findings. ☐ I don't use standardized measurement instruments in my workplace.				
3. When a group activity is only offered in English, I find a way to offer an equivalent activity in French. ☐ I don't have group activities in my workplace.				
4. When I prepare education or information tools (for example, written documents and presentations) for patients/clients, I prepare them in French or in both official languages. ☐ I don't prepare informational and educational resources in my workplace.				
5. When I supervise clinical placements, I ask for students who can speak both official languages. ☐ I don't supervise clinical placements.				
Support and Referrals I sometimes refer Francophone patients/clients to another care provider (consultation request, institutional transfer, etc.). If yes, fill in this section. If not, skip this section.				
1. I refer to a list of employees and organizations capable of delivering services in French.				

	Never	Rarely	Often	Always
Support and Referrals (continued)				
2. I offer patients/clients the option of being referred to a Francophone care provider or organization.				
3. I specify the patient's/client's language preference in the transfer documentation.				
4. I inform the referred care provider of the patient's/client's language preference.				

Organizational Support

Reception and Intake
In my workplace, it is common practice to . . .

	Never	Rarely	Often	Always
1. Post signs in French or in Canada's two official languages.				
2. Provide lapel pins or labels indicating that services are available in Canada's two official languages.				
3. Post clear and visible signs indicating the availability of services in French.				
4. Provide information in French or in Canada's two official languages on the institution's website.				
5. Have magazines, booklets, and media in Canada's two official languages available for patients/clients.				
6. Disseminate information through French-language newspapers and radio.				
7. Recruit physicians and staff capable of delivering services in French at every service level.				
8. Hold meetings in French or in Canada's two official languages.				
9. Foster the use of French among Francophone employees or physicians.				
10. Inform patients/clients about the institution's commitment to provide services of equal quality in both of Canada's official languages.				
11. Speak French when among Francophone employees.				
12. Print organizational letterhead and business cards in French or in Canada's two official languages.				

Intervention
In my workplace, it is common practice to . . .

	Never	Rarely	Often	Always
1. Provide work tools that facilitate service delivery in French or in Canada's two official languages (for example, calendars, spelling/grammar checkers, dictionaries, and forms).				

	Never	Rarely	Often	Always
Intervention (continued)				
2. Provide a glossary of health and social services terminology in French.				
3. Offer helplines or distance specialized services in French (for example, call centres, Internet, videoconferences, and telemedicine).				
4. Check that French-language education and information tools are adapted to the patients/clients (that is, cultural, ethnic, or regulatory context).				
5. Develop education and information tools that include the French and English versions in the same document.				
6. Complete documentation, (files, reports, insurance forms, etc.), in the patient's/client's preferred language.				
Support and Referrals In my workplace, it is common practice to . . .				
1. Document the patient's/client's language preferences on the forms used for transfers.				
2. Keep an up-to-date list of professionals and organizations in the region or city who can provide services in French.				
3. Encourage staff to inform patients/clients that it is possible to be referred to French-language services in the region or elsewhere.				
Continuous Professional Development In my workplace, employees are offered training . . .				
1. To develop their French-language proficiency.				
2. On French terminology specific to their work.				
3. On the active offer of health and social services in French.				
4. On cultural and linguistic competency.				
5. On resources that foster the delivery of services in French.				
6. On the issues and challenges facing French-language minority communities.				
7. On language rights.				
8. Through professional development activities offered in French.				
Management and Governance In my workplace . . .				
1. Some management personnel are able to speak French.				
2. At least one seat on the Board of Directors is reserved for a Francophone community representative.				

	Never	Rarely	Often	Always
Management and Governance (continued)				
3. Care providers are made aware of the acts, regulations, and provincial policies related to French-language services.				
4. It is standard practice to verify the quality of services offered in French.				
5. It is standard practice to value the delivery of services in French.				
6. The official name of the organization is displayed in French or in Canada's two official languages.				
7. There is a written policy on the delivery of services in French or in Canada's two official languages.				
Obstacles In my workplace, the following factors prevent me from providing services in French as often as I would like:				
1. Union attitudes.				
2. Heavy work load.				
3. Lack of organizational leadership.				
4. Community pressure and prejudices against French-language services.				
5. Peer pressure and prejudices against the provision of French-language services.				
6. A work environment that does not facilitate the use of French.				

CHAPTER 13

The Necessity for Normalized Tests for Speech, Language, and Hearing Assessment of Young Francophone Children Living in Linguistic Minority Settings: Myth or Reality?[1]

Josée Lagacé, *University of Ottawa,* and
Pascal Lefebvre, *Laurentian University*

Abstract

Most Francophone children who are part of linguistic minority communities in Canada are bilingual. The audiologists and speech-language pathologists performing assessments to determine if children have communication disorders have called for specific tests to be developed for this particular group. However, there are more effective means of assessing communication disorders in bilingual children. This chapter reviews data from the scientific literature and highlights the gap observed between best practices and current practices regarding the use of normalized speech, language, and hearing tests with bilingual children. In order to improve the services offered to these children, recommendations are provided for university programs, professional development programs, employers, and parents.

Key Words: normalized tests, bilingualism, audiology, hearing, speech, language, speech-language pathology, best practices.

Introduction

Ensuring access to safe, quality health and social services in French to Francophone minority communities (FMCs) requires not only training more Francophone professionals who will be working there, but also preparing professionals to better meet the particular needs of FMCs. This chapter offers an example of the specific knowledge audiologists and speech-language pathologists should acquire to work more effectively with FMCs.

The lack of quality French-language assessment tools is one of the challenges reported by audiologists and speech-language pathologists working with Canada's Francophone population (Garcia & Desrochers, 1997; Garcia, Paradis, Sénécal, & Laroche, 2006; Gaul Bouchard, Fitzpatrick, & Olds, 2009). This chapter reviews the use of normalized tests to assess communication disorders in Canadian children from Francophone minority communities. First, statistics are showing that Francophones in minority language contexts are nearly all bilingual. Next, practices to assess communication disorders in bilingual children are discussed. These practices contrast with the needs expressed by speech-language pathologists and audiologists. The dichotomy observed between best practices and current practices in the use of normalized tests is then discussed and, as a last step, recommendations are made.

Linguistic Realities of Canadian Francophones Living in Minority Settings

In the fall of 2011, an interdisciplinary research team from the School of Social Work, the School of Rehabilitation Sciences, and the Faculty of Education of the University of Ottawa conducted eight focus groups with people working in a number of health and social service professions in Eastern Ontario, including speech-language pathology and audiology. The discussions focused on various aspects of health and social services offered in French in this minority linguistic community. A detailed description of the findings from the focus groups were published in Drolet et al. (2014). When the reports of comments by the speech-language pathologists and audiologists who were interviewed (see the examples in the Appendix) were analyzed, one point stood out: the lack of appropriate normalized French-language assessment tools appears to represent a major obstacle in the assessment of language and hearing abilities of Francophones in minority language settings. Responses also indicate the high rate of bilingualism of individuals does not seem to be the primary concern of speech-language pathologists and audiologists who work with them.

According to the data collected in the Canadian Census in 2012 (Statistics Canada, 2012), 4.8% of Ontarians (http://ofa.gov.on.ca/fr/franco.html) and 33.2% of New Brunswickers are Francophone; they represent three-quarters of the 4.0% of Canadians living outside Quebec who listed French as the first official language they learned. Having French as their first language, however, does not necessarily imply French is the language these Canadians use at home or in public. According to the data from the 2006 Canadian Census (Corbeil & Lafrenière, 2010), only slightly more than half of Franco-Ontarians reported that French was the language they used most often at home; approximately 10% speak English and French equally often and the rest communicate mainly in English. In public, the proportion of Franco-Ontarians who use mainly French falls to approximately 35% with friends, to 25% in their social network, and to 20% at work. The others either use both languages equally often or predominantly use English. As for Francophones in New Brunswick (Lepage, Bouchard-Coulombe, & Chavez, 2011), approximately 85% speak mostly French at home, 5% speak English and French equally often, and the rest speaks mostly English. In public, 80% of Francophones in this province nearly always speak French with their friends, 75% in their social networks, and 60% at work. Here, again, the others either use the two languages equally often or use mainly English. To summarize, English is undeniably the language of daily life especially in the case of Franco-Ontarians, but also in that of many Francophones in New Brunswick. It is not surprising that the rate of bilingualism among Francophones living outside Quebec is 87%, according to the last census (Lepage, Bouchard-Coulombe, & Chavez, 2011). Among Franco-Ontarians, the rate is 88% and among Francophones in New Brunswick, it is 72% (Corbeil & Lafrenière, 2010; Lepage, Bouchard-Coulombe, & Chavez, 2011).

However, bilingualism should not be seen as a uniform entity (Grosjean, 1989; Valdés & Figueroa, 1994; von Hapsburg & Peña, 2002), but rather as a continuum. Indeed, each French-English bilingual individual is located on a continuum between unilingual

Francophones and Anglophones. The balanced bilinguals are at the centre of this continuum, and are generally exposed to both languages from birth. This is observed in several exogamous families in which one parent speaks French, and the other English, at home. French-dominant and English-dominant bilinguals are found on either side of balanced bilinguals on the continuum. In their case, only one of the languages is generally used at home, and the second language is generally learned later (sequential bilingualism) with speakers outside the family. According to the census data (Corbeil & Lafrenière, 2010; Lepage, Bouchard-Coulombe, & Chavez, 2011), Francophones who live in minority settings are generally French-dominant bilinguals or balanced bilinguals; a minority of them are unilingual Francophones or English-dominant bilinguals.

The data so far include all age groups. However, when looking more closely at the data for youth (18 years of age and under) who have at least one Francophone parent, only a third of those living in Ontario are from families in which both parents are Francophones. Approximately 60% are from French-English exogamous families (Corbeil & Lafrenière, 2010). In New Brunswick, two thirds of them are from families in which both parents are Francophones; approximately 30% are from exogamous French-English couples (Lepage, Bouchard-Coulombe, & Chavez, 2011). The same data (Corbeil & Lafrenière, 2010; Lepage, Bouchard-Coulombe, & Chavez, 2011) show that families in which both parents are Francophone are most likely to transmit French as the mother tongue. In exogamous families, only a quarter of children in Ontario and a third in New Brunswick speak French as their first language; the others report either English or both official languages as their first language. Thus, in a minority language context, bilingualism is an undeniable reality.

The linguistic reality of the Francophone population outside Quebec has an important impact on the health and social services offered to them, particularly in terms of speech-language pathology and audiology because the expertise in these two fields relates to the disorders and the typical development of communication. For speech-language pathologists and audiologists, language does not simply represent the means of communication with their clients, it is also the focus of the services they offer. Speech-language pathologists and audiologists offering services to Francophones living in minority linguistic contexts must consider the high rate of bilingualism among their clients and be familiar with the issues this raises, particularly for younger clients. It is important to remember the typical development of communication skills among bilingual children is different from unilingual individuals (Bedore & Peña, 2008; Westman, Korkamn, & Byring, 2008).

Scientific Evidence and Best Practices in Speech-Language Pathology and Audiology Services for Bilingual Individuals

Since the 1980s, various associations and professional colleges in audiology and speech-language pathology in Canada and around the world have published position papers and practice guidelines for professionals working with bilingual clients (American Speech-Language-Hearing Association [ASHA], 1985, 2007, 2011; College of Audiologists and Speech-Language Pathologists of Ontario, 2000; Crago & Westernoff for the Canadian Association of Speech-Language Pathologists and Audiologists, 1997; Multilingual Affairs Committee of the International Association of Logopedics and Phoniatrics, 2006; Royal College of Speech & Language Therapists, 2007; Speech Pathology Australia, 2009). In these documents, bilingualism is discussed but often broader terms are used, such as minority languages, multilingualism and multiculturalism, diverse language, and cultural or ethnic communities. Furthermore, these documents emphasize the language competencies and cultural awareness of the speech-language pathologist and audiologist delivering services to bilingual individuals. The procedures used during assessments, such as the use of normalized tests, are almost unmentioned.

The next two subsections deal with more specific recommendations around best practices regarding the assessment of bilingual individuals. The first discusses recommendations specific to speech and language assessments, and the second discusses those specific to hearing assessments.

Best Practices in Speech-Language Pathology

Before directly assessing the language abilities of any child, a speech-language pathologist should document the child's perinatal, developmental, communicative, medical, and educational history. This information be obtained by reading the child's records, by interviewing significant adults such as parents and teachers, and/or by observing the child in different contexts. In the case of

Francophone children in linguistic minority communities, it is particularly important for the speech-language pathologist to gather data on the child's previous language experiences. More precisely, it is crucial for the speech-language pathologist to know how long the child has been exposed to each of the languages, and in which circumstances (for example, characteristics of the speakers, contexts, proportion of exposure, beginning of exposure). It is important to consider the language and type of educational programs the child has attended (for example, a day care centre, kindergarten, or an elementary school), and how frequently the child is or has been in this setting. By taking into account the sociolinguistic context (for instance, the majority or minority status of each of the languages), these data make it possible to determine if the child is a French-dominant, balanced, or English-dominant bilingual, and to formulate more accurate hypotheses about the typical pattern of communicative development that can be expected from him or her. The models proposed by Gathercole (2007) and MacLeod (2015) provide a mean to predict the language development of bilingual children in each of the languages they speak, in comparison with unilingual children, and take into consideration factors related to the age of exposure, the quantity of exposure, and the sociolinguistic context. Protocols such as the Alberta Language Environment Questionnaire ([ALEQ]: Paradis, 2011) or the Questionnaire for Bilingual Children (MacLeod, in progress) allow more systematic data collection on this subject. Data are usually obtained from the family and educational professionals and may be collected in person, by telephone, or through written questionnaires. Actively offering the opportunity to answer questions in French or in English must be a priority. If the professional asking the questions does not fluently speak the language of the parent who is present, or if the parents speak another language, the assistance of interpreters becomes essential.

According to Langdon (2008), a direct evaluation of the child's language skills is necessary if the family reports delays in the dominant language, especially compared to the development of her or his siblings. If there is no concern with development in the dominant language, it is important to enrich the child's linguistic experiences in the second language, and to document changes over time (over a period of approximately four to six weeks). If little progress is noted, despite increased stimulation, a direct assessment of the child's language skills is recommended.

The direct assessment of the child's language skills by a speech-language pathologist generally includes the collection and analysis of a spontaneous language sample and the delivery of standardized tests that are often normalized (Langdon, 2008). For bilingual children, including Francophones in minority settings, these two evaluations should be conducted in English as well as in French. According to Kohnert (2010), even if a dominant language can be identified in many bilingual children, this does not mean that some or all of their language skills are automatically stronger in their dominant language than in their second language. Differences in strengths stem from the fact that children often develop their skills by interacting with a variety of people, in different contexts, to reach varied communication goals. For example, a young Franco-Ontarian may use a more literary or formal French vocabulary at school while developing useful English expressions to socialize with neighbourhood friends, who may be mostly Anglophones. This can result in scores on normalized tests delivered in French that do not reflect the real abilities of the child, because many tests have been developed using the norms of a unilingual French population. To account for a bilingual child's uneven distribution of language skills between the two languages, a speech-language pathologist should obtain and review the data in both languages spoken by the child, and produce an overall profile of the child's language skills and knowledge encompassing abilities in both languages.

The results of the spontaneous language sample and normalized tests in both languages cannot be analyzed solely in comparison with norms based on unilingual children. In fact, some bilingual children who are developing normally present results similar to unilingual children with a language disorder in one of their languages. Additionally, bilingual children often make associations between the two languages during their language development (Kohnert, 2010). These associations may be positive—that is, they may allow children to transfer acquired knowledge from one language to another—or they may be negative and produce interference between the languages. Since French and English share several similar lexical, phonetic/phonemic, syntactic, and alphabetical characteristics, numerous positive transfers are possible, but the omnipresence of English can also result in anglicized sentence structure or words when the child speaks French (Döpke, 2000). Also, comparisons with unilingual norms on normalized tests do not make it possible to determine whether a bilingual child's language development is normal or not.

Developing norms for bilingual children would seem to be the ideal solution. However, as Kohnert explains (2013, p. 146), there are no normative databases incorporating both languages and the diversity of linguistic experiences and influences in any group of bilinguals. Indeed, even within a homogenous sociolinguistic group, there is a wide inter-individual variability in the language development of bilingual children. This variability may be due to different socioeconomic situations, parents' education, different family literacy practices, and intrinsic individual differences in children's aptitudes and communication styles (Kohnert, 2010). This makes the development of normative data for bilingual children much more complicated, even when languages, age, and the context of language experiences are accounted for. For example, studies by Mayer-Crittenden (2013) and Mayer-Crittenden, Thordardottir, Robillard, Minor-Corriveau, and Bélanger (2014) showed that within a group of Franco-Ontarian children in the Greater Sudbury Area, results on language evaluations vary depending on whether the children are unilingual, French-dominant bilingual, or English-dominant bilingual. Furthermore, the performance of these children on language assessments is lower than that of Francophone children in a majority setting in Quebec. One study that used the same assessment tools was conducted in the Ottawa region, with unilingual and French-dominant children; the results were almost identical to those of Francophone children in Quebec (Lefebvre *et al.*, in progress at time of printing). It seems clear, then, that developing normalized language tests for Francophones living in minority settings would not be valid given the overly wide linguistic variability of this population.

In short, normalized tests used in a bilingual context lose their efficiency and validity because they must be administered in both of the children's languages and the norms established are inappropriate. Without norms, clinicians might be tempted to compare the results between the two languages of the child in order to determine if she or he has stronger abilities in one of the languages. However, this method is not valid either, since the measurements obtained depend on the characteristics of each language. For example, measurements of the mean length of utterances cannot be compared, because the French language requires longer sentences than English (Thordardottir, 2005).

Standardized and normalized tests are usually designed to evaluate two types of abilities: first, the skills and knowledge specific to a language such as speech sounds, vocabulary, morpho-syntax, and discourse; and second, the underlying language processing abilities such as lexical retrieval and phonological memory. The latter group of skills is dependent on working memory, attention, and perception. These abilities are believed to be less influenced by linguistic experiences in each of the languages and to be important indicators of language disorders (Langdon, 2008). However, research on the topic suggests that even if these abilities are less subject to the biases introduced by linguistic experiences, measures of language processing abilities are not accurate indicators of language difficulties in a bilingual setting, since the performance of bilingual people on these tasks are not necessarily identical to those of unilinguals (De Lamo White & Jin, 2011).

It is, therefore, recommended that normalized tests be used in a non-standardized way (Crago & Westernoff 1997); that is, by modifying the administration procedures and by collecting more informal data. For example, practice items or additional time may be given. It is also recommended that one language be assessed at a time and on different days in order to decrease linguistic interference, except in the case of children who have very weak abilities in one of the languages. Testing should begin in the language with which the child is more familiar, and the child should be encouraged to answer in the language being evaluated. The use of unilingual norms can be useful, not to determine if a bilingual child has a language disorder but rather to have a better idea of the child's development in each of the languages as compared to unilingual children. By using predictive models of the language development of bilingual children as Gathercole (2007) and MacLeod (2015) propose, analyzing the performance of a bilingual child on tests normalized against unilingual children's results can determine if his or her language development follows the model of bilingual development according to the factors of age of exposure, quantity of exposure, and sociolinguistic context. In other words, it is not the gap against the norms established with unilingual children that indicates if concerns should be raised about the language development of a particular bilingual child, but rather the language portrait in both of the languages the child speaks according to the expected development of a typical bilingual child.

It is important to highlight that a different type of standardized tool exists to evaluate the language development of bilingual children, not through direct assessment conducted by a speech-language pathologist, but by means of questionnaires filled out by adults close to the child. Tools such as the Alberta Language Development Questionnaire ([ALDeQ]: Paradis, Emmerzael, & Sorenson Duncan, 2010) or the Intelligibility in Context Scale ([ICS]: McLeod, Harrison, & McCormack, 2012) enable a speech-language pathologist to obtain systematic developmental data on a child's language even if the professional does not master the language. The data are then translated into scores that makes it possible to determine if the child's development is adequate in that language or not.

It must be taken into account that interactions between the languages a child speaks are influenced by the child's age, developmental stage, exposure to each of the languages, and the requests of tasks to be accomplished (Conboy & Thal, 2006; Gildersleeve-Neumann et al., 2008; Yip & Matthews, 2000). The dynamic nature of normal language development in bilingual children means that static measurements taken at a single moment in time by normalized tests make it difficult to detect language disorders. Thus, it is imperative to measure the rate and the direction of change in the language performance of a child over time. Two assessment methods can be used by the speech-language pathologist to do this: limited training and dynamic assessment (De Lamo White & Jin, 2011; Langdon, 2008). The limited training method consists of the modelling and imitation of unfamiliar speech sounds, words, and syntactical structures (authentic or not) in a structured context. A baseline measurement allows the lack of language knowledge or skills to be confirmed, while measurements taken following the intervention evaluate the child's efficiency in learning. The dynamic assessment method consists in offering the child mediation—in the form of scaffolding—in order to identify the potential for change in the child's language skills when different levels of support are offered. The nature and level of support required to modify the learner's language skills are determined through this procedure, which also involves baseline and measurements after the intervention. It is recommended that these procedures be carried out with at least two other children the same age and with comparable linguistic experiences, and who are not suspected of having language disorders or difficulties (Langdon, 2008). This precaution will give an idea of the typical bilingual language development in a context specific to the social environment of the child.

The best practice presented up to this point in the chapter has consisted of methods for assessing bilingual children in each of their languages on separate occasions. However, these children are growing up in an environment in which adults offer models of language involving code-switching (Poplack, 1980). Code-switching is defined as using both languages within a single sentence, or juxtaposing sentences in the two languages (Cook, 2001). Contrary to popular belief, code-switching is not a demonstration of lack of familiarity with one or both languages; it is used to express specific communication goals such as the affirmation of identify among bilinguals (Kramsch & Whiteside, 2007) or to nuance the meaning of an idea (Zentella, 1997). Alternating between languages is not a random act; it is governed by its own rules (Poplack, 1980). Constantly exposed to these linguistic models, young children also adopt code-switching (Comeau, Genesee, & Lapaquette, 2003). Thus, it is a typical language behaviour and not an indication of language problems (Paradis & Nicoladis, 2007). The approach of translanguaging—that is, a bilingual person's free, flexible, and permeable use of linguistic repertories (García, 2009)—favours the idea that code-switching is an asset for bilingual children. According to proponents of this approach, the linguistic competencies of bilingual individuals are seen as being more valuable in contexts where code-switching is accepted and even encouraged (Otheguy, García, & Reid, 2015). Nonetheless, current research on the impact of translanguaging during speech-language pathologists' assessments of the language competence of bilingual children is in its infancy. More studies must be conducted before there is sufficient evidence to recommend this practice.

Thus, speech and language assessments of bilingual individuals are very different from assessments of unilingual individuals. The role of normalized tests in these assessments of the two populations is also different, and professionals need to consider relevant research on their use. The diagnosis of language disorders relies on a sociocultural approach that enables the clinician to interpret the child's language performance while taking into consideration data on her or his linguistic and cultural exposures (De Lamo White & Jin, 2011).

Best Practices in Audiology

Difficulty understanding speech in noise is the main reason for consultations in audiology (Wilson & McArdle, 2005). Not only do people with peripheral hearing loss have difficulties recognizing speech in noise, but certain people with normal hearing thresholds do as well. For instance, children and adults identified with school-based learning problems have lower speech recognition in noise performance when compared to control groups with the same hearing sensitivity (Bradlow, Kraus, & Hayes, 2003; Warrier *et al.*, 2004), as do children with auditory processing disorder (Muchnik *et al.*, 2004; Sanches & Carvallo, 2006) and children with dyslexia (Ahissar, Lubin, Putter-Katz, & Banai, 2006; Chandrasekaran *et al.*, 2009).

Bilingual adults and children are not exempt from these hearing problems, either. Indeed, several studies report a weaker performance in recognizing speech in noise among bilingual individuals as compared to their unilingual peers, especially when the task involves listening to speech in their second language (Cooke, Garcia Lecumberri, & Barker, 2008; Garcia Lecumberri & Cooke, 2006; Shi, 2011; von Hapsburg, Champlin, & Shetty, 2004).

An audiologist must be able to identify the underlying deficit of the hearing difficulties in noise. For some people, a weak performance on speech recognition in noise may be attributed to a dysfunction in auditory processing, while for others it may be related to a cognitive impairment such as an attention deficit or problems with language skills. Identifying the origin of the speech perception problems in noise is essential to develop an effective treatment plan.

When a bilingual person has difficulty understanding speech in noise, the assessment process is not simple. Problems understanding speech are intrinsic to language skills. Hence, an audiologist cannot proceed in the same manner as with a unilingual population by using tests that include verbal stimuli corresponding to the language of the client. For example, it is not always obvious to identify the language a client has learned first, or the language the client is more comfortable speaking. Even in cases in which the best known language is identified, there is no consensus on the effect of bilingualism on the ability to understand speech in noise in that language.

The age at which the second language is learned is a decisive factor of the bilingual person's speech recognition in noise ability

(Shi, 2014). Weiss and Dempsey (2008) show that participants who learned their second language before the age of seven have a better ability to recognize sentences in this language when there is noise in the environment than those who learned the language after eleven years of age. On the other hand, results obtained from tests administered in the first language learned show that speech recognition in noise changes with the number of years the bilingual person have been using the second language. The findings show that abilities to recognize speech in noise in the first language learned seem to deteriorate as the skills in the second language improve. Similar findings were reported by von Hapsburg and Bahng (2009). The administration of tests composed of verbal stimuli in the first language a bilingual person has learned to speak does not, therefore, allow an audiologist to draw an accurate portrait of the hearing ability in noise.

Where children are concerned, the audiologist must evaluate, in addition to the effects of bilingualism on the ability to perceive speech in noise, the effect of development on this ability (Fallon, Trehub, & Schneider, 2000). Indeed, children generally experience more difficulty than adults in perceiving speech in noise (Johnson, 2000; Lagacé, 2010; Picard & Bradley, 2001); this is true of unilingual children, as well. Given the dynamic nature inherent in the development of their hearing ability and the level of bilingualism of individual children, the speech recognition in noise abilities of bilingual children are variable in both languages. Evaluating the child's speech recognition in noise ability in both languages is an option to consider (Shi, 2014).

Data on the speech recognition in noise abilities of bilingual children are rare. As for adults, most studies have examined the effects of bilingualism on the speech perception in noise in the second language and the results show the same trends. For example, Crandell and Smaldino (1996) compared the performance of bilingual children to those of unilingual children on a sentence-in-noise recognition test. The test stimuli were in the second language of the bilingual participants. Bilingual children had lower sentence recognition scores in noise than unilingual participants. Bovo and Callegari (2009) also reported a difference, although it was not statistically significant, between bilingual children (with Italian as their second language) and unilingual (Italian) children on a words-in-noise task. The competing noise level had to be lower for bilingual children than for unilingual children to reach the same performance.

Few studies have examined the effects of bilingualism on speech recognition in noise abilities in the first language learned. A study aimed at developing normative data for a word in noise test, called the Test de Mots dans le Bruit ([TMB]; Lagacé, 2010), revealed that correct recognition scores of Francophone children speaking more than one language at home were lower than those speaking French only (Lagacé *et al.*, 2013). On the other end, Filippi *et al.* (2015) reported that bilingual children who learned their second language (English) at birth or during their first year of life had a higher correct sentence keyword recognition score than unilingual Anglophone children. The sentences were presented with a competing noise composed of a continuous foreign language speech. Authors suggested that exposure to a second language at birth may foster the development of auditory processing abilities. The lack of consensus in the findings of these studies suggests that the use of normalized tests when assessing speech in noise abilities of bilingual children may be of little value.

In order to draw an accurate portrait of bilingual children's ability to hear speech in noise, Shi (2014) suggests administering tests in each of the languages spoken by the child. Among other information, the audiologists may be able to determine the specific needs in each language. Although several speech-in-noise tests are available in English, few clinical tools are available and adapted for the Francophone population in Canada. Three tests have been identified: first, the French adaptation of the Synthetic Sentences Identification with Ipsilateral Competitive Message (SSI-ICM) test (Speaks & Jerger, 1965) developed by Lynch and Normandin (1983); second, a word-in-noise test called the Test de Mots dans le Bruit ([TMB]; Lagacé, 2010; Lagacé *et al.*, 2013); and third, the Canadian French adaptation of the Hearing In Noise Test ([HINT]; Nilsson, Soli, & Sullivan, 1994) developed by Vaillancourt *et al.*, 2008 (children's version) and Vaillancourt *et al.*, 2005 (adults' version).

Following Shi's recommendations (2014), audiologists should consider speech-in-noise tests that are available in the languages spoken by the bilingual child. The HINT test, for example, is available in Canadian French and in English. By comparing the speech in noise threshold obtained for the same test condition of the HINT in both languages, for example, it is possible to evaluate speech-in-noise abilities in both languages. However, the audiologist must keep in mind that the level of difficulty of each version of the test may not be equivalent. For example, while verifying the effect of bilingualism on the results obtained on two versions of the HINT test on bilingual participants, Stuart, Zhang, and Swink (2010) reported that in the continuous noise condition, the unilingual Anglophone participants had lower (better) thresholds than bilingual participants on the English version of the test. While comparing the speech in noise thresholds with the version of the HINT in the first language learned by bilingual participants (in this case, in Mandarin), bilingual participants showed better thresholds in the continuous noise condition than the Anglophone participants on the English version of the test (Stuart, Zhang, & Swink, 2010). The authors suggested the acoustical characteristics of Mandarin may be, in part, the cause of these results. Mandarin is a tonal language while English is a stress language. Since perception of tone in Mandarin would not be influenced by the presence of competing noise (Kong & Zeng, 2006), the recognition of speech in noise in this language would be easier than in English. Although the difference between the syntactic and acoustic characteristics of French and English are not as great as the one between Mandarin and English, the audiologist should be cautious about interpreting the differences in thresholds observed on the two versions of the test.

Since there is a limited number of adequate clinical tests, no one should believe it would be appropriate to develop a treatment plan based on the premise that bilingual people have difficulty hearing speech in noise. This would be contrary to best practices. Given the predictive potential of language variables such as the age of acquisition, the length of exposure to the language, the contexts of use, and other data, on speech perception in noise, Shi (2014) suggests using questionnaires to collect data on these aspects. The answers to the questionnaire, which can be provided by either the child or the parent, have been shown to be useful in helping professionals understand the results on clinical tests. One questionnaire that deals specifically with the language abilities of bilingual individuals, the Language Experience and Proficiency Questionnaire ([LEAP-Q]; Marian, Blumenfeld, & Kaushanskaya, 2007), includes items on the major variables of language, notably the age of acquisition and reading abilities, as well as items on cultural and educational background, which are also known to influence language abilities in bilingual people. The LEAP-Q is available and has been validated in several languages, including English and French.

Another way of assessing speech recognition abilities of bilingual individuals, according to the current recommendations of the American Speech-Language-Hearing Association (2015), is the use of questionnaires on auditory behaviour. According to its guidelines, particular attention must be paid to using questionnaires created in the first language of the individual being tested. If no questionnaire is available in that language, a translated version could also be considered if the adaptation has been scientifically validated. Although some English-language questionnaires can be used to evaluate hearing difficulties in children (e.g., Anderson, 1989; Barry & Moore, 2014; Fisher, 1976; Meister *et al.*, 2004; Smoski *et al.*, 1992; etc.), only home-made adaptations of these tools are available in French.

In conclusion, available data suggest that the performance of bilingual individuals on speech-in-noise tests is not comparable to that of unilingual people. Furthermore, this hearing ability is not static; it varies with the number of years of bilingualism and the degree of exposure to each language. The importance of normalized tests for the assessment of speech in noise with bilingual Francophones, then, differs from what it really should be. Results obtained with these tests must be interpreted cautiously. One effective way to assess speech recognition in noise of bilingual children consists of administering tests in the languages spoken by the child, while ensuring that the results are interpreted carefully and that language variables are taken into consideration. The use of questionnaires assessing auditory behaviour also shows promise as a method for assessing speech perception in noise.

Current State of Assessment Practices in Speech-Language Pathology and Audiology When Working with Bilingual Individuals

Jordaan (2008), who conducted an international survey of speech-language pathologists working with bilingual clients, states that the current practice does not yet reflect evidence-based best practices. In the United States and Australia, numerous studies have investigated assessment methods specifically for bilingual children (Caesar & Kohler, 2007; Guiberson & Atkins, 2012; Hammer, Detwiler, Detwiler, Blood, & Qualls, 2004; Kritikos, 2003; Roseberry-McKibbin, Brice, & O'Hanlon, 2005; Verdon, McLeod, & McDonald, 2014;

Williams & McLoed, 2012). Research essentially shows speech-language pathologists generally use English standardized and normalized tests for the evaluation of bilingual children, but they support the development of standardized and normalized assessment tools specific to a bilingual population. Moreover, their sense of self-efficacy when assessing bilingual children has been found to be related to their ability to speak their clients' languages. It should be emphasized that these studies were carried out in a context of bilingualism different from that of Canadian Francophones living and working in minority contexts. In these studies, the mother tongue of the clients is not an official language and it is rarely possible to receive schooling in this language. Thus, it may be dangerous to transpose these results to speech-language pathologists who work with Francophone children in official language minority communities.

A survey similar to those conducted in the United States and in Australia was done in Canada by D'Souza, Kay-Raining Bird, and Deacon (2012). Findings showed that bilingual and multilingual speech-language pathologists assess more clients who speak diverse languages than unilingual ones. The five methods they use the most for the evaluation of these clients are: natural observations, language samples, dynamic assessment, standardized tests in English, and standardized tests adapted for a specific client. The barriers most frequently reported by speech-language pathologists in their evaluations are: the lack of reliable assessment tools in the client's language; lack of access to a speech-language pathologist who speaks the client's language; inability to speak the client's language; the lack of knowledge of developmental norms in the client's language; and the lack of knowledge of the client's culture.

Finally, a study carried out in Ireland by O'Toole and Hickey (2012) on practices in the assessment of language disorders in children took place in a very similar context to that of Francophones in minority communities; that is, with Irish-English bilingual clients in a country with an Anglophone majority but where Irish is an official language and education in Irish is available. Participants in this study reported, among other things, that they use standardized tests, but most often also favour informal procedures. However, the interpretation of these data is difficult because of the lack of developmental norms for children living in a bilingual context.

To summarize, whether they work in Canada or in another country, speech-language pathologists continue to use normalized tests in language of the majority, and sometimes in the minority language with their bilingual clients. Most of the time they assess their clients in only one language, the same one they speak themselves. The lack of normalized tools is the most frequently reported obstacle to effective assessment of multilingual clients. Speech-language pathologists, however, use complementary procedures such as informal evaluation, spontaneous language samples, and collection of cultural and linguistic data from the family, but the lack of normative data makes the interpretation of data difficult.

The situation is not different in audiology. Even though audiologists know there is a need for tests that are sensitive to their clients' linguistic characteristics, many prefer vocal tests available in their own language because they are more comfortable using them (Ramkissoon & Khan, 2003). Since Francophones living in a linguistic minority context do not always have access to French-speaking audiologists, they are not always being evaluated with linguistically appropriate tests. As in the case of speech-language pathology, audiologists continue to use normalized tests of majority language and, occasionally, in the minority language with bilingual clients when these tests are available. It is often assumed that the performance measured speech-in-noise tests will not be influenced by a person's bilingualism if his or her language skills are considered good.

As illustrated by comments made by speech-language pathologists and audiologists working with Francophone clients in minority language contexts (see Appendix), it seems the effect of bilingualism on the development of language and hearing skills is not their major preoccupation, despite the high rate of bilingualism in this population. According to studies on the topic (Guiberson & Atkins, 2012; Roseberry-McKibbin, Brice, & O'Hallon, 2005), the initial university training received by speech-language pathologists and audiologists contributes to this situation. Even in cases where the initial training is adequate, the problem of accessing essential resources, such as clinical tests adapted to bilingual clients, prevents the clinicians from adopting the best practices that are recommended. Furthermore, the time needed to assess bilingual children is much longer than that required to assess unilingual children, especially if the recommendation to do a normalized test in each of the spoken languages is considered. Unfortunately, pressure on these professionals (in the public and private sectors, in education and health care) to offer more services in less time (Lubinski & Hudson, 2013; Ontario Speech-Language Pathologists and Audiologists [OSLA], 2015) does not create ideal conditions for this type of assessment.

Conclusion and Recommendations

Contrary to speech-language pathologists, and audiologists, claims about the priority for the development of normalized assessment tools to better serve Canadian Francophones living in minority language settings, best practices indicate that other methods requiring different resources should be considered. Moreover, it is impossible to develop normalized tests given the heterogeneity of the bilingual population. Narrowing the gap between current practice and best practices in the assessment of bilingual individuals in the areas of speech-language pathology and audiology calls for different solutions. Here are some that can be considered:

- Modifying university training programs, in order to integrate knowledge- and skill-building related to assessments in multilingual contexts into most courses and work placements; this requires training professors, instructors, and clinical supervisors in the same content;
- Fostering linguistic and cultural diversity among potential students in speech-language pathology and audiology programs, by setting quotas based on the linguistic representation of the population;
- Establishing mandatory professional development programs on these topics for speech-language pathologists and audiologists already in the workforce;
- Making the necessary resources available so that best practices can be adopted: additional time for assessments in both languages, access to professionals who speak the language of the clientele or interpreters,and more data about the linguistic and developmental characteristics of other languages;
- Developing awareness programs for Francophone parents living in a linguistic minority context to highlight the importance of assessment in both languages and their cooperation in assessing their children.

Although the assessment of Francophone children in minority language settings should be understood and conducted in the context of their bilingualism, audiologists and speech-language pathologists call for the development of normalized tests to better serve this population. It appears, however, that the real problem lies in the lack of knowledge both of the reality of Francophones in minority settings and of best practices in the assessment of communication in this bilingual context. This chapter is intended to be an educational tool that establishes a factual foundation for assessing the speech, language, and hearing of young Francophones outside Quebec. This foundation can then be used to re-frame the discourse, focusing on bilingual assessment rather than on the need for normalized tests.

Notes

1. This reflection on best practices in speech-language pathology and audiology began during interviews carried out as part of a project funded by the *Consortium national de formation en santé*. The project was aimed at better understanding the reality of health and social service professionals who work with Francophones in minority language settings.

References

Ahissar, M., Lubin, Y., Putter-Katz, H., & Banai, K. (2006). Dyslexia and the failure to form a perceptual anchor. *Nature Neuroscience, 9,* 1558–1564.

American Speech-Language-Hearing Association (ASHA). (2004). *Knowledge and skills needed by speech language pathologists and audiologists to provide culturally and linguistically appropriate services.* Retrieved from http://www.asha.org/policy/KS2004-00215/. Accessed June 18, 2015.

American Speech-Language-Hearing Association (ASHA). (2005). *(Central) Auditory processing disorders [Technical report].* Retrieved from http://www.asha.org/members/deskref-journals/deskref/default. Accessed June 18, 2015.

American Speech-Language-Hearing Association (2009). *Summary counts by ethnicity and race.* Retrieved from http://www.asha.org/uploadedFiles/2009MemberCounts.pdf. Accessed June 18, 2015.

American Speech-Language and Hearing Association (ASHA). (2011). *Cultural competence in professional service delivery [Position statement].* Retrieved from http://www.asha.org/policy/PS2011-00325.htm. Accessed June 18, 2015.

American Speech-Language-Hearing Association (ASHA. (2015). *Bilingual service delivery*. Retrieved from http://www.asha.org/Practice-Portal/Professional-Issues/Bilingual-Service-Delivery. Accessed June 18, 2014.

Anderson, K. (1989). *SIFTER: Screening instrument for targeting educational risk in children identified by hearing screening or who have known hearing loss*. Tampa, FL: The Educational Audiology Association.

Barry, J. G., & Moore, D. R. (2014). *Evaluation of children's listening and processing skills (ECLiPS)*. London, UK: MRC-T.

Bedore, L. M. & Peña, E. D. (2008). "Assessment of bilingual children for identification of language impairment: Current findings and implications for practice." *International Journal of Bilingual Education and Bilingualism*, 11(1), 1–29. doi:10.2167/beb392.0.

Bovo, R. & Callegari, E. (2009). Effects of classroom noise on the speech perception of bilingual children learning in their second language: Preliminary results. *Audiological Medicine*, 7(4), 226–232. doi: 10.3109/16513860903189499.

Bradlow, A. R., Kraus, N., & Hayes, E. (2003). Speaking clearly for children with learning disabilities. Sentence perception in noise. *Journal of Speech, Language, and Hearing Research*, 46(1), 80–97. doi:10.1044/1092-4388(2003/007).

Caesar, L. G., & Kohler, P. D. (2007). The state of school-based bilingual assessment: Actual practice versus recommended guidelines. *Language, Speech, and Hearing Services in Schools*, 38(3), 190–200. doi:10.1044/0161-1461(2007/020).

Chandrasekaran, B., Hornickel, J. M., Skoe, E., Nicol, T., & Kraus, N. (2009). Context-dependent encoding in the human auditory brainstem relates to hearing speech in noise: Implications for developmental dyslexia. *Neuron*, 64(3), 311–319. doi:10.1016/j.neuron.2009.10.006.

College of Audiologists and Speech-Language Pathologists of Ontario. (2000). *Service delivery to culturally and linguistically diverse population [Position statement]*. Retrieved from http://www.caslpo.com/sites/default/uploads/files/PS_EN_Service_Delivery_to_Culturally_and_Linguistically_Diverse_Populations.pdf. Accessed June 18, 2015.

Comeau, L., Genesee, F., & Lapaquette, L. (2003). The modeling hypothesis and child bilingual codemixing. *International Journal of Bilingualism*, 7(2), 113–126. doi: 10.1177/13670069030070020101.

Conboy, B. T., & Thal, D. J. (2006). "Ties between the lexicon and grammar: Cross-sectional and longitudinal studies of bilingual toddlers." *Child Development*, 77(3), 712–735. doi: 10.1111/j.1467-8624.2006.00899.x.

Cook, V. (2001). Using the first language in the classroom. *Canadian Modern Language Review*, 57(3), 402–423. doi: http://dx.doi.org/10.3138/cmlr.57.3.402.

Cooke, M., Garcia Lecumberri, M. L., & Barker, J. (2008). The foreign language cocktail party problem: Energetic and informational masking effects in non-native speech perception. *Journal of the Acoustical Society of America, 123*(1), 414–427. doi: 10.1121/1.2804952.

Corbeil, J., & Lafrenière, S. (2010). *Portrait des minorités de langue officielle au Canada : Les francophones de l'Ontario (Produit no. 89-642-X).* Ottawa, ON: Retrieved from http://www.statcan.gc.ca/pub/89-642-x/89-642-x2010001-fra.pdf Accessed June 18, 2015.

Crago, M., & Westernoff, F. (1997). Exposé de position de l'ACOA sur l'orthophonie et l'audiologie dans un contexte multiculturel et multilingue. *Revue d'orthophonie et d'audiologie, 21*(3), 225–226. Retrieved from http://cjslpa.ca/files/1997_JSLPA_Vol_21 /No_03_145228/Crago_ Westernoff_JSLPA_1997.pdf. Accessed June 18, 2015.

Crandell, C. C. & Smaldino, J. J. (1996). Speech perception in noise by children for whom English is a second language. *American Journal of Audiology, 5*(3), 47–51. doi:10.1044/1059-0889.0503.47.

De Lamo White, C., & Jin, L. (2011). Evaluation of speech and language assessment approaches with bilingual children. *International Journal of Language & Communication Disorders, 46*(6), 613–27. doi: 10.1111/ j.1460-6984.2011.00049.x.

Döpke, S. (2000). Generation of and retraction from cross-linguistically motivated structures in bilingual first language acquisition. *Bilingualism: Language and Cognition, 3*(03), 209–226. Retrieved from http://journals.cambridge.org/abstract_S1366728900000341. Accessed June 18, 2015.

Drolet, M., Savard, J., Benoît J., Arcand I., Savard, S., Lagacé, J., Lauzon S., & Dubouloz, C.-J. (2014). Health services for linguistic minorities in a bilingual setting: Challenges for bilingual professionals. *Qualitative Health Research. 24*(3), 295–305. doi: 10.1177/1049732314523503.

D'Souza, C., Kay-Raining Bird, E. K., & Deacon, H. (2012). Survey of Canadian speech-language pathology service delivery to linguistically diverse clients. *Canadian Journal of Speech-Language Pathology and Audiology, 36*(1), 18–39. Retrieved from http://cjslpa.ca/files/2012_ CJSLPA _Vol_36/No_01_1-87/D_Souza_KayRaining_Bird_Deacon_ CJSLPA_2012.pdf. Accessed June 18, 2015.

Fallon, M., Trehub, S. E., & Schneider, B. A. (2000). Children's perception of speech in multitalker babble. *Journal of the Acoustical Society of America, 108*(6), 3023–3029. doi: 10.1121/1.1323233.

Filippi, R., R., Morris, J., Richardson, F. M., Bright, P., Thomas, M. S. C., Karmiloff-Smith, A., & Marian, V. (2015). Bilingual children show an advantage in controlling verbal interference during spoken language comprehension. *Bilingualism: Language and Cognition, 18*(3), 490–501. doi: 10.1017/S1366728914000686.

Fisher, L. (1976). *Fisher's Auditory Problems Checklist*. Bemidji, MN: Life Products.

Garcia, L., Paradis, J., Sénéchal, I., & Laroche, C. (2006). Utilisation et satis-faction à l'égard des outils* en français évaluant les troubles de la communication. *Revue d'orthophonie et d'audiologie, 30*(4), 239–249. Retrieved from http://cjslpa.ca/detail.php?ID=937&lang=francais. Accessed June 18, 2015.

Garcia, L. J., & Desrochers, A. (1997). L'évaluation des troubles du langage et de la parole chez l'adulte francophone. *Revue d'orthophonie et d'audiologie, 21*(4), 271–293. Retrieved from http://cjslpa.ca/files/1997_JSLPA_Vol_21/No_04_229312/Garcia_Desrochers_JSLPA_1997.pdf. Accessed June 18, 2015.

García, O. (2009). *Bilingual Education in the 21st Century: A Global Perspective*. Malden, MA: Wiley-Blackwell.

Garcia Lecumberri, M. L., & Cooke, M. (2006). Effect of masker type on native and non-native consonant perception in noise. *Journal of the Acoustical Society of America, 119*(4), 2445–2554. doi: 10.1121/1.2180210.

Gathercole, V. C. M. (2007). Miami and North Wales, so far and yet so near: Constructivist account of morpho-syntactic development in bilin-gual children. *The International Journal of Bilingual Education and Bilingualism, 10*(3), 224–247. doi: 10.2167/beb442.0.

Gaul Bouchard, M.-E., Fitzpatrick, E. M., & Olds, J. (2009). Analyse psycho-métrique d'outils d'évaluation utilisés auprès des enfants franco-phones. *Revue d'orthophonie et d'audiologie, 33*(3), 129–139. Retrieved from http://cjslpa.ca/files/2009_CJSLPA_Vol_33/No_03_113-160/Bouchard_Fitzpatrick_Olds_CJSLPA_2009.pdf. Accessed June 18, 2015.

Gildersleeve-Neumann, C. E., Kester, E. S., Davis, B. L., & Peña, E. D. (2008). English speech sound development in preschool-aged children from bilingual English-Spanish environments. *Language, Speech, and Hearing Services in Schools, 39*(3), 314–28. doi: 10.1044/0161-1461(2008/030).

Grosjean, F. (1989). Neurolinguists, beware! The bilingual is not two mono-linguals in one person. *Brain and Language, 36*(1), 3–15. doi: 10.1016/0093-934X(89)90048-5.

Guiberson, M., & Atkins, J. (2012). Speech-language pathologists' prepara-tion, practices, and perspectives on serving culturally and linguisti-cally diverse children. *Communication Disorders Quarterly, 33*(3), 169–180. doi: 10.1177/1525740110384132.

Hammer, C. S., Detwiler, J. S., Detwiler, J., Blood, G. W., & Qualls, C. D. (2004). Speech-language pathologists' training and confidence in serv-ing Spanish-English bilingual children. *Journal of Communication Disorders, 37*(2), 91–108. doi: 10.1016/j.jcomdis.2003.07.002.

Johnson, C. (2000). Children's phoneme identification in reverberation and noise."*Journal of Speech, Language and Hearing Research, 43*(1), 144–156. doi: 10.1044/jslhr.4301.144.

Jordaan, H. (2008). Clinical intervention for bilingual children: An international survey. *Folia Phoniatrica et Logopaedica, 60,* 97–105.

Kohnert, K. (2010). Bilingual children with primary language impairment: Issues, evidence and implications for clinical actions. *Journal of Communication Disorders, 43*(6), 456–473. doi: 10.1016/j.jcomdis.2010.02.002.

Kohnert, K. (2013). *Language disorders in bilingual children and adults.* San Diego, CA: Plural Publishing.

Kong, Y.Y., & Zeng, F.G. (2006). Temporal and spectral cues in Mandarin tone recognition. *Journal of Acoustical Society of America, 120*(5), 2830–2840. doi: 10.1121/1.2346009.

Kramsch, C., & Whiteside, A. (2007). Three fundamental concepts in SLA and their relevance in multilingual contexts. *Modern Language Journal, 91*(s1), 905-920. doi:10.1111/j.1540-4781.2007.00677.x.

Kritikos, E. P. (2003). Speech-language pathologists' beliefs about language assessment of bilingual/bicultural individuals. *American Journal of Speech-Language Pathology, 12*(1), 73–91. http://doi.10.1044/1058-0360(2003/054)

Lagacé, J. (2010) Développement du Test de Mots dans le Bruit: Mesure de l'équivalence des listes et données préliminaires sur l'effet d'âge. *Acoustique canadienne, 38*(2), 19–30. Retrieved from http://jcaa.caa-aca.ca/index.php/jcaa/article/view/2219/1966. Accessed June 15, 2015.

Lagacé, J., LeBlanc, L., Boisvert, V., Arseneau, M. J., & Breau-Godwin, S. (2013). Mise à jour sur le développement du Test de Mots dans le Bruit. *Acoustique Canadienne, 41*(2), 65–72. Retrieved from http://jcaa.caa-aca.ca/index.php/jcaa/article/view/2620/2350. Accessed June 15, 2015.

Lagacé, J., Leblanc, L., Noël, A., Boudreau, M., & Bourdages Gauvin, E. (2015). *Development of normative data for a Canadian French words-in-noise test and the effect of bilingualism on the performance.* 12th Congress of The European Federation of Audiology Societies, Istanbul, May 27 to 30, 2015.

Langdon, H. W. (2008). *Assessment & intervention for communication disorders in culturally & linguistically diverse populations.* Clifton, NY: Thomson Delmar Learning.

Lefebvre, P., Desmeules, P., Boucher, M.-L., McKennedy, G., Leblanc, M., St-Laurent, G., Pollabauer, E., & Roy, S. (in progress at time of printing). Performance des enfants franco-ontariens de la région d'Ottawa à des épreuves d'évaluation du langage.

Lepage, J.-F., Bouchard-Coulombe, C., & Chavez, B. (2011). *Portrait des minorités de langue officielle au Canada: Les francophones du Nouveau-Brunswick (Produit no. 89-642-X).* Ottawa. Retrieved from http://www.statcan.gc.ca/pub/89-642-x/89-642-x2011005-fra.pdf. Accessed June 18, 2015.

Lubinski, R. & Hudson, M.W. (2013). *Professional issues in speech-language pathology and audiology* (4th edition). Clifton, NY: Delmar Cengage Learning.

Lynch, A., & Normandin, N. (1983). *Adaptation en français du test Synthetic Sentence Identification*. Unpublished paper. Montréal, QC: Université de Montréal.

McLeod, A. A. N. (in progress at time of printing). *Questionnaire pour les enfants bilingues*.

MacLeod, A. A. N. (2015). *La pratique orthophonique avec les enfants bilingues (Supporting documentation)*. Formation continue de l'Ordre des orthophonistes et audiologistes du Québec, Montréal, QC.

Marian, V., Blumenfeld, H.K., & Kaushanskaya, M. (2007). The Language Experience and Proficiency Questionnaire (LEAP-Q): Assessing profiles in bilingual and multilinguals. *Journal of Speech, Language, and Hearing* Research, *50*(4), 940–967. doi:10.1044/1092-4388(2007/067). (Different versions of the questionnaire are available at: http://www.bilingualism.northwestern.edu/leapq/co).

Mayer-Crittenden, C. E. (2013, July 30). *Compétences linguistiques et cognitives des enfants bilingues en situation linguistique minoritaire* (Unpublished doctoral dissertation). Sudbury, ON: Laurentian University/Université Laurentienne. Retrieved from https://zone.biblio.laurentian.ca/dspace/handle/10219/2015. Accessed June 18, 2015.

Mayer-Crittenden, C., Thordardottir, E., Robillard, M., Minor-Corriveau, M., & Bélanger, R. (2014). Données langagières franco-ontariennes: effets du contexte minoritaire et du bilinguisme Franco-Ontarian speech data: the effects of a minority context and bilingualism. *Revue canadienne d'orthophonie et d'audiologie, 38*(3). Retrieved from http://cjslpa.ca/files/2014_CJSLPA_Vol_38/No_03/CJSLPA_Fall_2014_Vol_38_No_3_Paper_3_Mayer-Crittenden_et_al.pdf

McLeod, S., Harrison, L. J., & McCormack, J. (2012). The intelligibility in context scale: Validity and reliability of a subjective rating measure. *Journal of Speech, Language, and Hearing Research, 55*(2), 648–656. doi:10.1044/1092-4388(2011/10-0130).

Meister, H., von Wedel, H., & Walger, M. (2004). Psychometric evaluation of children with suspected auditory processing disorders (APDs) using a parent-answered survey. *International Journal of Audiology, 43*(8), 431–437. doi:10.1080/14992020400050054.

Muchnik, C., Roth, D. A.-E., Othman-Jebara, R., Putter-Katz, H., Shabtai, E. L., & Hildesheimer, M. (2004). Reduced medial olivocochlear bundle system function in children with auditory processing disorders. *Audiology & Neurotology, 9*(2), 107–114. doi:10.1159/000076001).

Multilingual Affairs Committee of the International Association of Logopedics and Phoniatrics. (2006). Recommendations for working with bilingual children. *Folia Phoniatrica et Logopaedica, 58*(6), 458–464. doi: 10.1159/000096570.

Nilsson, M., Soli, S. D., & Sullivan, J. A. (1994). Development of the Hearing in Noise Test for the measurement of speech reception thresholds in quiet and in noise. *Journal of the Acoustical Society of America, 95*(2), 1085–1099. doi:10.1121/1.408469.

Ontario Speech-Language Pathologists and Audiologists (OSLA). (2015). *Maximizing Speech-Language Pathologists' Capacity in Ontario's Health Care System.* Toronto, ON. Retrieved from https://www.osla.on.ca/uploads/SLP%20Scope%20of%20Practice%20Submission20June%20 2015.pdf. Accessed January 9, 2017.

Orthophonie et Audiologie Canada. (2015a). *Fiche de renseignements: La profession d'audiologie.* Retrieved from http://oac-sac.ca/sites/default/files/resources/Audiologists_ FRENCH_Who we are info sheet.pdf. Accessed June 18, 2015.

Orthophonie et Audiologie Canada. (2015b). *Fiche de renseignements: La profession d'orthophonie.* Retrieved from http://oac-sac.ca/sites/default/files/resources /SLPs_FRENCH_Who we are info sheet.pdf. Accessed June 18, 2015.

Otheguy, R., García, O., & Reid, W. (2015). Clarifying translanguaging and deconstructing named languages: A perspective from linguistics. *Applied Linguistics Review, 6*(3), 281–307. doi:10.1515/applirev-2015-0014.

O'Toole, C. & Hickey, T. M. (2012). Diagnosing language impairment in bilinguals: Professional experience and perception. *Child Language Teaching and Therapy, 29*(1), 91–109. doi:10.1177/0265659012459859.

Paradis, J. (2011). Individual differences in child English second language acquisition: Comparing child-internal and child-external factors. *Linguistic Approaches to Bilingualism, 1*(3), 213–237. doi:10.1075/lab .1.3.01par.

Paradis, J., Emmerzael, K., & Sorenson Duncan, T. (2010). Assessment of English language learners: Using parent report on first language development. *Journal of Communication Disorders, 43*(6), 474–497. doi:10.1016/j.jcomdis.2010.01.002.

Paradis, J., & Nicoladis, E. (2007). The influence of dominance and sociolinguistic context on bilingual preschoolers' language choice. *International Journal of Bilingual Education and Bilingualism, 10*(3), 277–297. doi:10.2167/beb444.0.

Picard, M., & Bradley, J.S. (2001). Revisiting speech interference in classrooms. *Audiology, 40*(5), 221–244. doi:10.3109/00206090109073117.

Poplack, S. (1980). Sometimes I'll start a sentence in Spanish y termino en espanol: Toward a typology of code-switching. *Linguistics, 18*(7–8), 581–618.

Ramkissoon, I., & Khan, F. (2003). Serving multilingual clients with hearing loss: How linguistic diversity affects audiologic management. *The ASHA Leader, 8*(3), 1–27. doi:10.1044/leader.FTR1.08032003.1.

Roseberry-McKibbin, C., Brice, A., & O' Hanlon, L. (2005). Serving English language learners in public school settings: A national survey. *Language, Speech & Hearing Services in Schools, 36*(1), 48–61. doi:10.1044/0161-1461(2005/005).

Royal College of Speech & Language Therapists. (2007). *Good practice for speech and language therapists working with clients from linguistic minority communities.* London, UK. Retrieved from http://www.rcslt.org/members/publications/publications2/linguistic_minorities. Accessed June 18, 2015.

Sanches, S. G., & Carvallo, R. M. (2006). Contralateral suppression of transient evoked otoacoustic emissions in children with auditory processing disorder. *Audiology and Neurotology, 11*(6), 366–372. doi: 10.1159/000095898.

Shi, L.-F. (2011). How "proficient" is proficient? Subjective proficiency measure as a predictor of bilingual listeners' recognition of English words. *American Journal of* Audiology, *20*(1), 19–32. doi:10.1044/1059-0889 (2011/10-0013).

Shi, L.-F. (2014). Speech audiometry and Spanish-English bilinguals: Challenges in clinical practice. *American Journal of Audiology, 23*(3), 243–259. doi: 10.1044/2014_AJA-14-0022.

Smoski, W. J., Brunt, M. A., & Tannahill, J. C. (1992). Listening characteristics of children with central auditory processing disorders. *Language, Speech and Hearing Services in School, 23*(2), 145–152. doi:10.1044/0161-1461.2302.145.

Speaks, C., & Jerger, J. (1965). Method for measurement of speech Identification. *Journal of Speech Language and Hearing Research, 8*(2), 185. doi:10.1044/jshr.0802.185.

Speech Pathology Australia. (2009). *Working in a culturally and linguistically diverse society [Position statement].* Melbourne, Australia. Retrieved from http://www.speechpathologyaustralia.org.au/library/position_statements/Working in a Culturally and Linguistically Diverse Society.pdf. Accessed June 18, 2015.

Statistics Canada. (2012). *Le français et la francophonie au Canada (Produit no. 98-314-X2011003).* Ottawa, ON: Retrieved from http://www12.statcan.gc.ca/census-recensement/2011/as-sa/98-314-x/98-314-x2011003_1-fra.pdf. Accessed June 18, 2015.

Stuart, A., Zhang, J., & Swink, S. (2010). Reception thresholds for sentence in quiet and noise for unilingual English and bilingual Mandarin-English listeners. *Journal of the American Academy of Audiology, 21*(4), 239–248. doi:10.3766/jaaa.21.4.3.

Thordardottir, E. T. (2005). Early lexical and syntactic development in Quebec French and English: Implications for cross-linguistic and bilingual assessment. *International Journal of Language & Communication Disorders*, 40(3), 243–278. doi:10.1080/13682820410001729655.

Vaillancourt, V., Laroche, C., Giguère, C., & Soli, S.D. (2008). Establishment of age-specific normative data for the Canadian French version of the Hearing in Noise Test for Children. *Ear & Hearing, 29*, 453–466. doi:10.1080/14992020500060875.

Vaillancourt, V., Laroche, C., Mayer, C., Basque, C., Nali, M., Eriks-Brophy, A., Soli, S. D., & Giguère, C. (2005). Adaptation of the HINT (Nearing in Noise Test) for adult Canadian Francophone populations. *International Journal of Audiology, 44*(6), 358–369. doi:10.1080/14992020500060875.

Valdés, G., and Figueroa, R. A. (1994). The measurement of bilingualism. In G. Valdés & R. A. Figueroa (Eds.), *Bilingualism and testing: A special case of bias. Second language learning.* (pp. 49–69). Norwood, NJ: Ablex.

Verdon, S., McLeod, S., & McDonald, S. (2014). A geographical analysis of speech-language pathology services to support multilingual children. *International Journal of Speech-Language Pathology, 16*(3), 304–16. doi: 10.3109/17549507.2013.868036.

von Hapsburg, D., & Bahng, J. (2009). Effects of noise on bilingual listeners' first language (L1) speech perception. *Perspective on Hearing and Hearing Disorders: Research and Diagnostics, 13*(1), 31–26. doi:10.1044/hhd13.1.21.

von Hapsburg, D., Champlin, C. A., & Shetty, S. R. (2004). Reception thresholds for sentences in bilingual (Spanish/English) and unilingual (English) listeners. *Journal of the American Academy of Audiology, 15*(1), 88–98. doi:10.3766/jaaa.15.1.9.

von Hapsburg, D., & Peña, E. D. (2002). Understanding bilingualism and its impact on speech audiometry. *Journal of Speech, Language, and Hearing Research, 45*(1), 202–213. doi:10.1044/1092-4388(2002/015).

Warrier, C. M., Johnson, K. L., Hayes, E. A., Nicol, T., & Kraus, N. (2004). Learning impaired children exhibit timing deficits and training-related improvements in auditory cortical responses to speech in noise. *Experimental Brain Research, 157*(4), 431–441. doi:10.1007/s00221-004-1857-6.

Weiss, D., & Dempsey, J.J. (2008). Performance of bilingual speakers on the English and Spanish versions of the Hearing in Noise Test (HINT). *Journal of the American Academy of Audiology, 19*(1), 5–17. doi: 10.3766/jaaa.19.1.2.

Westman, M., Korkman, M., & Byring, R. (2008). Language profiles of monolingual and bilingual Finnish preschool children at risk for language impairment. *International Journal of Language and Communication Disorders, 43*(6), 699–671. doi:10.1080/13682820701839200.

Willilams, C.J., & McLeod S. (2012). Speech-language pathologists' assessment and intervention practices with multilingual children. *International Journal of Speech-Language Pathology, 14*(3), 292-305. doi:11 0.3109/17549507.2011.636071

Wilson, R.H., & McArdle, R. (2005). Speech signals used to evaluate the functional status of the auditory system. *Journal of Rehabilitative Research and Development, 42*(4), 79–94. doi:10.1682/JRRD.2005.06.0096.

Yip, V., & Matthews, S. (2000). Syntactic transfer in a Cantonese–English bilingual child. *Bilingualism: Language and Cognition, 3*(3), 193–208. doi:0.1017/S136672890000033X.

Zentella, A.C. (1997). *Growing up bilingual.* Maiden, MA: Blackwell.

Appendix

Themes	Examples of Quotations
Homemade adaptation of tools	. . . I'd say it's hell, really, we have nothing to use, and you know, we have things we translated on the fly, and. . . . . . So, there are some tools that are available and might be useful, but they are generally American. . . and that means we would do our own "homemade" translation. We don't have the money to hire translators, so we'd have to translate the tools. . . . Often it's problems with the normative data. You know, you have. . . You use a French adaptation of the tool, but the norms were developed for Anglophones. Then you think, "How can we adapt them? How can we interpret our results if the norms haven't been developed with the same?
Limited number of tools adapted into French	. . . But in French, there's almost nothing... . . . For us, at the XX hospital, we don't have tools in French, so what happens for functional assessments is that we either adapt a tool, we do a homemade translation of it, but we can't. . . the results aren't. . . [reliable]. . . . There aren't many Francophone, French tools. . . it's not that it's really a problem, but it's hard for Francophone clients to ask for Francophone, French, care and treatment, services, and it's hard for them to speak up, to say something...
Academic activities to adapt tools	. . . But there are tests that need to be done with words, like repeating a sentence, for example. . . So that, of course, is pretty lucky, because at Université XXX they can, you know, do research projects and establish the norms, that kind of thing . . . She did some adaptations of testing tools, and that was published in our scholarly journals, and we had access to those tools.
Additional time required to work on adaptations of tools	vand photocopied, and all crooked, and full of mistakes, and we. . . we never had the time to fix them up. We don't have time. . . I'm embarrassed when my students come to the clinic, really embarrassed, but I tell them: "Listen, it's been xx years that I've been trying to clean it up, now, but I'm too busy." . . . What I find hardest, myself, is that whatever we have, we have great programs in English, they're often available in French, but they require a lot of adapting, a lot of changes, a lot of work by Francophone speech-language pathologists...
Different appearance of tools adapted into French	. . . And the French-language ÉVIP is pitiful compared to the English-language version, the Peabody vocabulary test. It's the same test, but the pictures are much more attractive in the English version, they're all in colour and everything, and in French they're black and white.

CHAPTER 14

Bilingual Health Care in Quebec: Public Policy, Vitality, and Acculturation Issues[1]

Richard Y. Bourhis, *Université du Québec à Montréal*

Abstract

The first part of this chapter offers the Interactive Acculturation Model (IAM), which provides an intergroup approach to minority/majority group relations in multilingual settings. The ethnolinguistic vitality framework is the first element of the IAM as it describes the relative strength and weaknesses of linguistic communities in contact. Four language policies regulating the status of linguistic communities constitute the key second element of the IAM. Third, the acculturation orientations of minority and majority group speakers are described as they interact to yield harmonious, problematic or conflictual intergroup relations. As an application of the IAM, the second part of the chapter analyzes bilingual health care policies for official language minorities in Canada and Quebec. A detailed analysis of bilingual health care institutions serving the English-speaking communities of Quebec closes with a case study of a recent Quebec Government health care law that threatened to undermine the institutional vitality of the Anglophone minority of Quebec.

Key words: Interactive Acculturation Model (IAM), English-speaking communities of Quebec, health care policies.

Introduction

The first part of this chapter describes the Interactive Acculturation Model (IAM), which offers an intergroup approach to relations between linguistic minority and majority groups within multilingual settings such as Quebec (Bourhis, Moise, Perreault, & Senecal, 1997). In the first part of the IAM we examine the ethnolinguistic vitality of language minorities and majorities in contact situations across multicultural settings. The second part of the model provides an analysis of language policies regulating the status of minority and majority language communities in multilingual societies. The third part of the IAM examines acculturation orientations adopted by linguistic minority and majority group speakers whose intergroup relations may range from harmonious to problematic to conflictual conflicting outcomes.

Using the IAM and ethnolinguistic vitality framework as a conceptual framework, the second part of the chapter analyzes bilingual health care institutions supporting the well-being of the Anglophone minority within the Francophone setting of Quebec. The recent Quebec Ministry of Health adoption of Bill 10, centralizing the governance of the health care network, provides a case study of how the Anglophone minority had to mobilize quickly to safeguard its institutional vitality in the province. As a former elite minority within Quebec, the declining Anglophone minority must remain vigilant to maintain and develop its historical health care institutions in an intergroup setting dominated by the Francophone majority in full control of most public and private institutions of the province (Carter, 2012).

The Interactive Acculturation Model

The Interactive Acculturation Model (IAM) applies to many types of linguistic majority/minority group relations (Bourhis, 2001). Linguistic minorities may be national ones established before the creation of a country, such as indigenous communities in Australia, Canada, Mexico, and the United States. Linguistic minority communities can be regional ones present since the creation of the state, such as the Anglophones of Quebec and the Francophones of Ontario, New Brunswick, and Manitoba. Immigrant linguistic communities are born outside their country of settlement, such as the Chinese, Hispanics, and Italians in Canada and the United States. For many such linguistic communities, language and accent are cues to their category membership and remain a key dimension of their social identity for many generations (Giles & Watson, 2013).

Ethnolinguistic Vitality of Language Groups

An important feature of the Interactive Acculturation Model (IAM) is the vitality of the linguistic minorities and majorities often targeted by government integration and language policies (Figure 1). Ethnolinguistic vitality is defined as *"that which makes a group likely to behave as a distinctive and collective entity within the intergroup setting"* (Giles, Bourhis, & Taylor, 1977, p. 308). The more vitality an ethnolinguistic group has, the more likely it is that it will thrive as a strong collective entity. Conversely, ethnolinguistic groups that have little or no vitality are more vulnerable and likely to assimilate and eventually cease to exist as distinctive language groups within intergroup settings (Bourhis & Landry, 2012).

Figure 1. Interactive Acculturation Model (IAM)

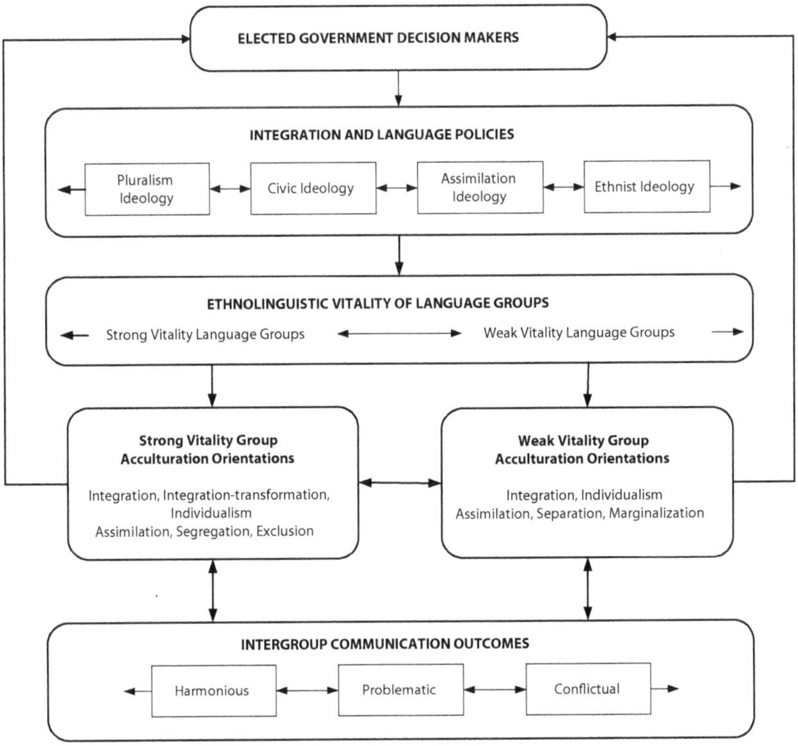

Government integration and language policies as they relate to the ethnolinguistic vitality and acculturation orientations of strong/weak vitality communities, resulting in harmonious to conflictual intergroup outcomes.

Most linguistic minority and majority communities have an enduring desire to maintain and transmit their language and culture to the next generation. As proposed in the Reversing Language Shift model ([RLS]: Fishman, 1991), this is especially the case within the proximal daily home-family-neighborhood network of minority speakers. However, maintaining this proximal network of ingroup language users is not sufficient for the survival and development of language minorities who must also seek some control of their educational, health care, commercial, and regional government institutions (Fishman, 2001). The ethnolinguistic vitality framework provides a conceptual bridge within the Interactive Acculturation Model by analyzing the full range of socio-structural variables affecting the strength of minority and majority language communities. As seen in Figure 1, three broad socio-structural dimensions influence the vitality of ethnolinguistic groups: demographic, institutional control, and status factors (Giles *et al.*, 1977; Giles & Johnson, 1987).

Demographic variables are those related to the absolute number of speakers composing the language group and their distribution throughout the urban, regional, or national territory. Number factors refer to the language community's absolute group numbers, birth rate, mortality rate, age pyramid, mixed marriages, and patterns of immigration and emigration. Distribution factors refer to the numeric concentration of speakers in various parts of the territory, their proportion relative to outgroup speakers, and whether or not the language community still occupies its ancestral territory. These demographic factors can be based on combinations of the following linguistic indicators often found in census data: mother tongue, knowledge of a first (L1) and second (L2) language, and use of L1 and/or L2 language at home. Taken together, these indicators can be used to monitor demolinguistic trends such as language maintenance in L1, language shift to L2, inter-generational transmission of the mother tongue, and language loss. Within democracies, demographic factors constitute a fundamental asset for ethnolinguistic groups, as "strength in numbers" can be used as a legitimizing tool to grant language communities the institutional support they need to develop within multilingual societies.

Institutional control is defined as the degree of power one group has over its own fate and that of outgroup language communities. The extent to which a language group has gained informal and formal control in the institutions of a city, region, or country contributes to its institutional completeness. Informal control refers to the way a language minority has organized itself as a pressure group to extend the use of its own language for local in-group activities such as advocacy, cultural production, sports, leisure, and commerce. Relatedly, the Reversing Language Shift (RLS) model proposes incremental stages in which linguistic minorities strategically build their institutional control from their family-home-neighbourhood networks to local own group language schools and health services, municipal governance, and work settings (Fishman, 1991). Following such gains, linguistic minorities can then seek more formal control for their language community in majority decision-making spheres including national education, health care, social services, the police, justice, the economy, and mass media, and within established cultural, sport, and religious institutions. The presence of quality leaders who can head the formal and informal institutions representing language minorities also contributes to the institutional control of language communities. Language groups who gained strong institutional control within state and private institutions are in a better position to safeguard and enhance their collective language and cultural capital compared to minorities who lack such institutional control. Language groups need to achieve and maintain a favourable position on the institutional control front if they wish to develop as distinctive collective entities within multilingual states.

Status variables are those related to a language community's social prestige, its socio-historical status within the state, and the prestige of its language and culture locally, nationally, and internationally. The more status a language community is ascribed to have, the more vitality it is likely to possess. Language minorities sometimes succeed in getting their regional or national governments to adopt language laws that officially recognize the status of their minority language as co-official languages for use in education, health care, judiciary, and government services. Communities whose language enjoys high status can more readily mobilize to maintain or improve their vitality position within their region than those whose language has low status. For instance, Quebec's mobilization for language laws enshrining the status of French relative to English was facilitated by the prestige of French as the national language of France and its international prestige as the language of the Francophonie network of countries (Bourhis, Montaruli, & Amiot, 2007). Conversely, lesser recognized Aboriginal languages in Francophone majority Quebec undermine the capacity of indigenous minorities to obtain the educational support they need to revive their ancestral language communities (Fettes, 1998; Taylor, Caouette, Usborne, & Wright, 2008). The experience of belonging to a high versus low-status language community is more vivid when status differentials between ethnolinguistic groups are perpetuated through language ideologies (Phillipson, 1988), linguicism (Bourhis, Montreuil, Helly, & Jantzen, 2007), and stereotypes towards "valued" and "devalued" languages, dialects and accents (Giles & Watson, 2013).

Demographic, institutional control, and status dimensions combine to affect, in one direction or the other, the overall vitality of ethnolinguistic groups. A language community may be weak on demographic variables but strengthening on institutional control thanks to language planning efforts, resulting in a medium vitality position. In contrast, a linguistic minority may be weak on demographic, institutional control, and status dimensions, resulting in low-vitality prospects. The objective vitality framework can be used as a heuristic to describe the relative position and wellness of language groups in numerous bilingual and multilingual settings in Canada and the world (Bourhis & Landry, 2012).

The public policy relevance of the ethnolinguistic vitality framework is evident in the revised Canadian *Official Languages Act*, which states in its preamble:

> Whereas the Government of Canada is committed to enhancing the *vitality* [emphasis added] and supporting the development of English and French linguistic minority communities, as an integral part of the two official language communities of Canada, and to fostering full recognition and use of English and French in Canadian society. (Canada, 2005)

The Commissioner of Official Languages, Statistics Canada, and numerous Canadian government studies also use the vitality framework to analyze the prospects of Francophone and Anglophone official minority communities across Canada (Corbeil, Grenier, & Lafrenière, 2007; Johnson & Doucet, 2006; Senate Canada Report, 2011).

Subjective Vitality Perceptions

How speakers perceive the vitality of their own language community relative to salient outgroups may be as important as objective assessments of group vitality. The subjective vitality questionnaire (SVQ) was designed to measure group members' assessments of in/outgroup vitality on items constituting the demographic, institutional control, and status dimensions of the objective vitality framework (Bourhis, Giles, & Rosenthal, 1981). A review of vitality research using the SVQ indicates that despite some perceptual biases, group members are realistic in perceiving their overall vitality position along the lines suggested by objective assessments of ethnolinguistic vitality (Abrams, Barker, & Giles, 2009; Allard & Landry, 1994; Harwood, Giles, & Bourhis, 1994; Sioufi, Bourhis, & Allard, 2016). As proposed in the cultural autonomy model (CAM), mobilisation to develop minority language vitality depends on strong collective ingroup identification which itself is nurtured by ideological legitimacy, social proximity of ingroup speaker network, and degree of institutional control (Bourhis & Landry, 2012; Landry, Allard & Deveau, 2013; Montaruli, Bourhis, & Azurmendi, 2011).

Integration and Language Policies

In multilingual settings, free market forces usually favour the ascendancy of the dominant language majority and its institutions, often to the disadvantage of weaker vitality linguistic minorities whose demographic base and institutional control is undermined by the sheer power of dominant majorities (Fishman, 1991). As a counterpoint to free market forces, linguistic minorities often need language policies to provide the institutional support they need to maintain their vitality in public settings where the dominant majority may be unaware, indifferent, or hostile towards vulnerable linguistic minorities (Fishman, 2001). Though low-vitality language minorities can be given a say in the development of such language policies in democratic states, their weaker demographic position and institutional control undermines their ability to influence government adoption of the language laws needed to sustain the use of their minority language in key public domains such as education, health care, and the workplace.

As proposed in the IAM (Figure 1), language policies can be seen as the most demanding and expensive types of state integration policies affecting linguistic minorities and majorities. Cultural pluralism policies developed to apply only in the language of the dominant language majority do not have as systemic an impact on majority institutions as do integration policies that include the addition of minority language use within public and private institutions of the majority community. From the point of view of linguistic minorities, integration policies that include cultural sensitivity can be bolstered by provisions that include the offer of stable minority language services embedded within state and private institutions. Inclusion of linguistic minority speakers using their own group language within the organizational structure of majority government services such as bilingual health care, education, and the judiciary not only provides institutional support for linguistic minorities, but also offers much needed administrative and support jobs for minority speakers in such organizations. Minority bilingual employees may then transform features of majority institutions from within making them more responsive to the needs of the linguistic minority communities they serve without undermining services offered in the language of the majority (Bourhis, 1991; 1994).

The IAM proposes that high-vitality majority groups have the demographic base and institutional control to establish the state language policies that best serve their interests relative to linguistic minorities. It remains that high- and low-vitality language communities often compete to promote the institutional vitality of their respective language groups. Through negotiation or imposition, the outcome of this competition is reflected in the language policies that are eventually adopted by ruling governments of multilingual countries (Ricento, 2009; Shohamy, 2006).

As seen in Figure 1, the IAM proposes four clusters of state ideologies that shape the language and integration policies of multilingual states (Bourhis, 2001). These language policies reflect integration ideologies that can be situated on a diversity continuum ranging from the pluralist, the civic, and the assimilationist to exclusionist ideologies. Each ideological cluster produces specific language and cultural policies concerning the maintenance or assimilation of weaker vitality language minorities within a given state. This ideological continuum also provides the public policy backdrop needed to contextualize the type of citizenship and integration strategies adopted by societies towards immigrants and linguistic minorities (Banting & Kymlicka, 2012; Bloemraad, Korteweg, & Yurdakul, 2008). The sustained implementation of these pro-diversity (pluralism) to intolerant (exclusionist) language and cultural policies can impact intergroup harmony and social cohesion. At the interpersonal level, such public policies foster a social climate that may affect the social identity of minority group speakers, their identity management strategies, and their bilingual/multilingual communication strategies (Bourhis, Sioufi, & Sachdev, 2012). The sustained impact of these language policies eventually affects the capacity of linguistic minorities to transmit their language to the next generation of speakers, thus affecting the language maintenance versus language loss prospects of linguistic minorities.

In democracies, the *pluralism ideology* implies language majorities and minorities should adopt public values, including acceptance of the democratic process, obedience to Civil and Criminal codes, and endorsement of the Constitution and/or Charters of Rights and Freedoms (this includes anti-discrimination laws protecting vulnerable ethnolinguistic minorities against prejudice, discrimination, and linguicism). Such public values may also include the responsibility of citizens to learn one or more languages adopted as official or co-official languages of the national state or in specific regions of the state. The pluralism ideology upholds that the state has no right to regulate the private values of citizens, whose individual liberties in personal domains such as the home and private relations must be respected. Private values include freedom of association in the linguistic, cultural, political, and religious spheres, as well as freedom for linguistic minorities to learn and speak the language of their choice in private settings of the home, family, and neighborhood network.

The pluralism ideology implies that in addition to implementing knowledge and use of the majority language, the state may also financially and socially support the maintenance of the linguistic, cultural, and religious distinctiveness of its minorities. Such minorities are seen as enhancing the diversity and economic adaptability of the larger society. The pluralism ideology proposes that because both high- and low-vitality language communities pay taxes, some state funds should be allocated to support minority language schooling, health care, and social services. The ideology assumes that the culture and institutions of the dominant majority may need to be transformed through "reasonable accommodation" to serve the linguistic, cultural, and religious needs of minority groups and to promote social cohesion (Kymlicka, 1995).

An example of a language policy inspired by pluralism is Canada's *Official Languages Act*, which recognizes the equality of

French and English as co-official languages in Canada, especially for the provision of federal government bilingual services to the Canadian population where numbers warrant (Jedwab & Landry, 2011). The Canadian bilingualism policy was recognized as paving the way for the adoption of the 1988 *Multiculturalism Act*, an official pluralism policy adopted for the support of immigrant cultural diversity and integration, equity treatment of minority communities, combating racism and discrimination, and fostering intercultural and interfaith understanding (Bloemraad, 2006; Gao & Wong, 2015).

As in the case of the pluralism ideology, the civic ideology assumes both majority and minority linguistic communities should adopt the public and private values of the state. Unlike the pluralism ideology, the civic ideology does not fund the activities of linguistic and cultural minorities. However, this ideology does respect the right of individual citizens to both organize as community groups and financially to maintain or promote their respective languages through after-hours schooling, weekend cultural and religious activities, and private linguistic health clinics and ethnolinguistic entrepreneurship.

In multilingual states, the civic ideology amounts to state funding of the linguistic and cultural interests of the dominant language group, often portrayed as the neutral unifying embodiment of the nation from past to present. It is in the name of a neutral state that the civic ideology legitimizes the absence of official recognition and financial support of its linguistic and cultural minorities. The survival of linguistic and cultural minorities is thus left up to free market forces, which, as the language planning literature demonstrated, usually favor in the long run the dominant language and culture of the majority (Fishman, 2001). Under the pretext of neutral non-intervention in linguistic issues, the civic ideology may, in effect, accelerate the language shift and language loss of linguistic minorities in multilingual states.

The assimilation ideology expects citizens to adopt the public values of the nation-state. It also demands that minorities should abandon their own linguistic and cultural distinctiveness for the sake of adopting the language and values of the dominant language majority. Some countries expect this linguistic and cultural assimilation to occur voluntarily and gradually over time across the generations, but other states impose assimilation through regulations repressing the linguistic and cultural distinctiveness of minority groups in public domains such as the school system, health care, municipal governance, commerce, and mass media. Usually, it is the economically and politically dominant language group that is more successful in imposing its language and culture as the unifying founding myth of the nation state. For the greater cause of national unity, assimilationist policies are designed to accelerate the language and culture loss of its linguistic minorities. Dominant language majorities endorsing assimilationist policies often portray language minorities as a threat to the authenticity, homogeneity, and indivisibility of the nation state (Barker & Giles, 2004; Crawford, 2000). State policies encouraging or enforcing linguistic assimilation resulted in the partial assimilation of not only first- to third-generation immigrants established in the United States (Ricento,1998), but also of indigenous national minorities of Canada (Taylor *et al.*, 2008) and of historical regional language minorities such as the Breton, Basque, and Provençal in France (Blanchet, 2016).

Linguistic minorities sometimes face a dilemma at the local level when a civic or a pluralist language policy is adopted, but at the state level an assimilationist policy is imposed by the language majority. Multilingual cities may adopt more pluralist policies to facilitate the linguistic and cultural integration of immigrant urban populations than is the case at the national level, where assimilationist policies may better reflect dominant majority preferences. Likewise, public and private organizations in urban centres may adopt pluralist integration policies as their organizational culture to better serve the linguistic diversity of their local employees and clients. City core health clinics and hospitals serving multilingual/multicultural patients may adopt mainly pluralist organizational cultures for linguistic minorities, whereas hospitals serving culturally homogeneous majority group patients in suburbs and regions may adopt a more assimilationist or civic organizational culture.

As in the case of the assimilationist ideology, the exclusionist ideology may force linguistic minorities to give up their own language and culture for the sake of adopting the language of the dominant majority (Skutnabb-Kangas, 2000). Unlike the assimilationist ideology, the exclusionist ideology makes it difficult for linguistic minorities to be legally or socially accepted as authentic members of the majority, no matter how much minorities assimilate linguistically and culturally to the dominant group. The exclusionist ideology usually defines "who can be" and "who should be" citizens of the state in ethnically or religiously exclusive terms (Bloemraad *et al.*, 2008). This ideology is sometimes enshrined in the notion of "blood belonging," whereby only members of selected racial groups can gain full legal access to citizenship (Kaplan, 1993). In such states, the nation is defined as being composed of a kernel ancestral ethnolinguistic group as determined by birth and kinship. Linguistic minorities and immigrants who do not share this kinship may never be fully accepted as legitimate citizens of the state.

A case in point of the exclusionist ideology was the Canadian policy of residential schools, designed to force the linguistic, cultural, and religious assimilation of 150,000 First Nations children across Indian reservations in Canada from 1880 to 1996. Aboriginal children were taken from their parents by white authorities and forced to stay in 132 boarding schools designed to assimilate them to English and the Protestant church in English Canada, and to the French language and Catholic church in Quebec. Indigenous languages and cultures were disparaged through institutional linguicism and pupils were forbidden to speak their languages in class or amongst each other. Poor quality food, unsanitary conditions, and inadequate winter clothing accounted for the deaths of over 3,000 children in residential schools. The scope and violence of this policy of forced deculturation of aboriginal children were fully documented in the Truth and Reconciliation Commission (Canada, 2016), while in 2008 an official statement of apology and plea for forgiveness was expressed in the Canadian Parliament to the First Nations, Inuit, and Métis communities for the wilful destruction of their languages and cultures.

Intergroup Tensions Over Competing Language Policies

In democracies, language policies usually reflect the prevalent ideological orientations of the dominant language majority (Figure 1). In each country, the majority of the population may endorse the assimilationist ideology, whereas the civic ideology receives moderate support, and exclusionist and pluralist ideologies are endorsed by fewer majority group members. Depending on economic, political, demographic, and military events occurring at the national and international levels, politicians elected by the majority of citizens can shift language policies from one ideological orientation to the other. Political tensions may emerge between factions of the majority holding rival ideological views on language policies. The polarization of ideological positions regarding language issues may lead to the formation of regional nationalist parties whose main platform advocate greater status and use of minority languages as was the case in the Basque Country, Catalonia, Flanders, and Quebec. Majority group backlash movements and political parties may succeed in shifting language policies from a pluralism position to an assimilationist or exclusionist ideology (for example, the English Only movement in the United States, the Vlaams Belang in Flanders and the Front National in France). However, mobilized ethnolinguistic minorities with efficient leadership may succeed in convincing majorities and their governments to change existing assimilationist language policies to more tolerant approaches, such as the civic and pluralist language policies.

Once language policies are adopted by the state at the local or national level, the government apparatus applying such language laws in effect stabilize and legitimize the inclusion or exclusion of minority languages, not only in public domains of language use but eventually in private everyday discourse. The long-term application of assimilationist and exclusionist language policies by dominant majorities can succeed in eroding the inter-generational capacity of language minorities to maintain and develop their heritage language and culture. Thus, both top-down and bottom-up pressures can shift language policies from one pole of the ideological continuum to the other over time and in different cities or regions of a state. Taken together, language and integration policies applied at the local and national level can have a substantial impact on multilingual communication, on language assimilation, language revival, and on the acculturation orientations of linguistic minorities as well as members of the dominant language majority.

Acculturation Orientations of Strong/Weak Vitality Communities

Acculturation is the process of bidirectional change that occurs when two ethnolinguistic groups come in sustained contact with one another (Berry, 2006). Psychological acculturation refers to changes experienced by individuals whose ethnolinguistic group is collectively experiencing acculturation (Berry, 1997). Acculturation processes involve changes in the cultural and linguistic repertoire of individual speakers whose own language group is in sustained contact with high- or low-vitality outgroups (Bourhis et al., 1997). Individuals experiencing extensive cross-cultural contact with linguistic outgroups may shift from being unilingual in their mother tongue (L1) to being bilingual or trilingual in L2 and L3, while their progeny may become unilingual in the dominant language of the majority (Giles, Bonilla, & Sperr, 2012).

The struggle of linguistic minorities to maintain their own language and culture may not only depend on their objective/subjective vitality positions and state language policies, but also on acculturation orientation endorsed by individual members of minority and majority ethnolinguistic communities. A premise of the IAM model is that not all members of a majority group hold the same opinions about how minorities and majorities should relate with each other. By virtue of their strong vitality position, dominant language majorities play a major role in shaping the acculturation orientations of linguistic minorities by telling them how they should integrate culturally and linguistically. The IAM proposes that dominant language groups can endorse three welcoming and three unwelcoming acculturation orientations toward linguistic minorities.

The welcoming orientations adopted by dominant majorities are integration, integration-transformation, and individualism. Integrationists accept and value that minorities maintain aspects of their own heritage cultures and languages. They also wish minorities to learn and adopt their majority language and culture. Dominant majorities adopting integration-transformation accept and value the maintenance of minority languages and cultures. Such majority members are also willing to adapt and transform aspects of their own majority culture and institutions for the sake of facilitating the incorporation of minorities within the majority setting. Individualists majority members define themselves and minorities as individuals rather than as members of us-them categories. Because personal qualities count most, individualists interact with minorities regardless of their race, language, culture, or creed.

The three unwelcoming orientations are assimilation, segregation, and exclusion. The assimilationist orientation corresponds to the traditional concept of absorption, whereby dominant majority members expect linguistic minorities to relinquish their heritage language and culture for the sake of adopting the language and culture of the majority society. Dominant majority members endorsing the segregationist orientation accept that minorities maintain their heritage language and culture as long as such minorities stay separate from majority group members. Segregationists disfavour cross-cultural contacts with minorities as such relations could dilute the authenticity of the majority culture and undermine the status and use of the majority language. Members of the dominant majority who endorse the exclusionist orientation are not only intolerant of the maintenance of minority group languages and cultures but also fear that such minorities may contaminate the authenticity of the majority if they adopt their dominant language and culture. Basically, exclusionists believe minorities can never be incorporated as rightful members of the majority society and would prefer such minorities to leave.

These dominant majority acculturation orientations can be assessed using the host community acculturation scale (HCAS) and research has documented these acculturation orientations in Canada, the United States, and Europe (Arends-Toth & van de Vijver, 2004; Bourhis, Barrette, El-Geledi, & Schmidt, 2009; Bourhis, Barrette, & Moriconi, 2008; Navas, Fernandez, Rojas, & Garcia, 2007; Rohmann, Florack, & Piontkowski, 2006; Zagefka & Brown, 2002).

As proposed in Figure 1, it is the elected members of the dominant majority that are most likely to influence government language policies towards linguistic minorities. For example, elected language majority members whose acculturation orientation is integrationist and integration-transformation are likely to favor the pluralism ideology of providing publicly funded institutional support for the maintenance of minority languages in health care and schools. In contrast, elected language majority members endorsing the assimilationist orientation are likely to endorse language policies along the civic to assimilationist segments of the ideological continuum. Assimilationists are unlikely to support any state funding for minority language services while supporting government measures eroding the transmission and use of minority languages. Exclusionist majority members are likely to prefer assimilationists or ethnic language policies repressing the use and transmission of minority languages.

As seen in Figure 1, the IAM proposes linguistic minorities may adopt one of five acculturation orientations, depending on their desire to maintain their heritage language and culture and their wish to adopt the language and culture of the dominant majority (Bourhis, 2001). The integrationism orientation reflects a desire to maintain key features of the linguistic and cultural minority identity while adopting aspects of the majority culture including its dominant language. Linguistic minorities who adopt the assimilationism strategy essentially relinquish their own linguistic and cultural identity for the sake of adopting the language and culture of the dominant majority. Those who adopt the separatism strategy have a desire to maintain their heritage language and culture while rejecting key aspects of the dominant culture and sometimes its language. The marginalization orientation characterizes minority individuals who feel estranged from both their own heritage language community and that of the dominant language majority. Alternatively, linguistic minority members who dissociate themselves from both their ethnolinguistic origin and the dominant majority may do so not because they feel marginalized but simply because they prefer to identify themselves as individuals rather than as members of either a minority or majority. Such individualists reject group ascriptions per se and prefer to treat others as individual persons with their qualities and achievements rather than as all the same as members of contrasting language groups.

These five acculturation orientations can be more or less adopted by members of a particular linguistic minority. A majority of individuals from a linguistic minority may endorse an integrationist orientation, whereas only a few individuals from that minority group may endorse assimilation or separation. While most individuals from one language minority may adopt the assimilationist orientation, speakers from another background may prefer the separatist orientation following systemic linguistic discrimination from the majority. Research on acculturation orientations endorsed by minorities interacting with dominant majority communities is ongoing (Barrette, Bourhis, Personnaz & Personnaz, 2004; Berry, Phinney, Sam, & Vedder, 2006; Bourhis, *et al.*, 2009; Nguyen & Benet-Martínez, 2013).

Intergroup Relations Outcomes

It is by combining the five acculturation orientations of linguistic minorities with the six acculturation orientations of high-vitality majorities that we see the interactive nature of the IAM framework. The model proposes that during intergroup contact the interaction of majority and minority group acculturation orientations can either be concordant or discordant, and can produce relational outcomes ranging from harmonious to problematic to conflictual (Bourhis *et al.*, 1997). The most harmonious relational outcomes occur when both high-vitality majority group speakers and linguistic minority speakers are concordant in sharing the integrationist or individualist acculturation orientations. It is under such circumstances that the IAM predicts harmonious outcomes including effective cross-cultural and bilingual communications, mutually positive interethnic attitudes and stereotypes, low intergroup tension, low acculturative stress, and absence of linguicism between dominant majority and linguistic minority groups (Montreuil & Bourhis, 2004).

Problematic outcomes emerge when members of the dominant majority and the linguistic minority experience some discordance in their acculturation orientations, with some agreement and some disagreement with regard to their preferred profile of acculturation orientations (Zagefka & Brown, 2002). Problematic outcomes may emerge when dominant majority speakers insist minorities assimilate linguistically to mainstream society, while minorities prefer integration strategies that maintain their heritage language while allowing them to acquire competence in the majority language.

Dominant majority speakers endorsing the segregationism or exclusionism orientations are likely to experience conflictual outcomes regardless of the acculturation orientations endorsed by immigrant and linguistic minorities (Rohmann *et al.*, 2006). In addition to miscommunicating with linguistic minorities, exclusionists and segregationists are likely to be prejudiced towards such minorities and to discriminate against them in employment and housing while opposing institutional support in health care and education for linguistic minorities. Exclusionists are more likely to organize as right-wing political parties to disparage the language of minorities seen as diluting or contaminating mainstream culture and values. Under such circumstances, linguistic minorities who have low vitality are likely to be more vulnerable and suffer more acculturative stress and assimilation pressures compared to medium vitality linguistic minorities whose "strength in numbers" and institutional control can better shield them collectively against abuses from segregationist and exclusionist language majorities. Of linguistic minorities targeted by exclusionists, those with a separatist orientation and medium vitality are most likely to resist majority group intolerance. In de-facto multilingual countries, devalued linguistic and immigrant minorities may adopt the separatist acculturation orientation bolstering the intensity of their linguistic network within their own-group urban or territorial enclaves as of way of minimizing their contact with antagonistic dominant majority members (Barrette *et al.*, 2004;

Bourhis *et al.*, 2009). As implied in Figure 1, the IAM proposes that conflictual relational outcomes may be attenuated by state language policies that are situated at the pluralistic and civic pole of the continuum. Conversely, conflictual relational outcomes may be accentuated by language policies that are situated at the assimilation, and especially exclusionist pole of the ideological continuum.

Bilingual Health Care in Canada and Quebec

Vitality and Language Policies in Canada

Canada can be situated at the pluralist side of the ideological continuum of language policies proposed in the IAM. With French and English as its two official languages, Canada has one federal linguistic policy and separate linguistic policies within each of its ten provinces and three territories. Canada's *Official Languages Act* of 1969 provided bilingual federal services in both languages where numbers warranted across Canada, thus providing many jobs to bilingual Francophone and Anglophone public servants thus promoting national cohesion especially during the threat of Quebec separation (Jedwab & Landry, 2011). The Act included the establishment of the Office of the Commissioner of Official Languages, which reports annually on the progress of French and English language services in the Federal administration and its agencies. The act was enhanced in 1988 to bolster provisions concerning federal services in French and English to the public, enhanced use of French and English as the language of work in the Federal administration. It committed the federal government to enhance the vitality of English and French official minorities in cooperation with provincial and municipal governments (Jedwab & Landry, 2011). The 1982 Canadian Charter of Rights and Freedoms enshrined English and French as the two official languages of Canada and in Article 23, it guaranteed primary and secondary schooling for French and English official language minorities across the country. The official bilingual policy recognized the right of Canadians to know the official language of their choice without having to learn the other official language.In 2005 the Canadian Government amended Part VII of the Official Language Act as follows:

> 41. The Government of Canada is committed to a) enhance the vitality of the English and French linguistic minority

communities in Canada and supporting and assisting their development, and b) fostering the full recognition and use of both English and French in Canadian society.

42. The Minister of Canadian Heritage, in consultation with other Ministers of the Crown, shall encourage and promote a coordinated approach to the implementation by federal institutions of commitments set out in section 41. (Canada, 2005)

In further support of the institutional vitality of the French and English official language communities, the federal government funded the Roadmap for Canada's official language minorities during three five-year terms from 2003 to 2018, amounting to a total investment of over \$3 billion dollars (Canadian Heritage, 2013). Overall, language planning efforts testify to the federal government commitment to a policy of pluralism designed to develop the vitality of the Francophone minorities in English majority provinces in the rest of Canada (ROC) and of the Anglophone minority within Quebec (Landry, 2014). Though national polls have shown consistent support for Canadian bilingual policies over the past few decades amongst both Francophone and Anglophone citizens (Fraser, 2006; Jedwab & Landry, 2011), some Francophone minority stakeholders in the ROC as well as Quebec Francophone nationalists have considered such Canadian language planning efforts as "too little too late" and unlikely to stem the assimilation of Francophones minorities in the ROC (Corbeil, 2007; Curzi, 2014; Gilbert, 2010).

According to the 2011 Census, 17% of the Canadian population are bilingual, meaning they have sufficient knowledge of English and French to conduct a conversation in either language. It is in Canada's 'bilingual belt' where one finds the most French-English bilinguals in the country: the proportion of Canadians who have knowledge of both official languages is highest in Quebec (43%), followed by New Brunswick (33%) and Ontario (11%). In New Brunswick and Ontario, Francophones are virtually all French/English bilinguals and remain double linguistic minorities at both the provincial and Canadian levels (Sioufi, Bourhis, & Allard, 2016). In Quebec, Francophones have dual status: they constitute the dominant language majority within the province but remain a linguistic minority nationally in Canada. Anglophones in Quebec also have dual status as they constitute a linguistic minority provincially while remaining part of the dominant linguistic majority across Canada. In Quebec 36% of majority Francophones are bilingual while as many as 70% of minority Anglophones are bilingual (Bourhis, 2012b). Though the three provinces of the bilingual belt each adopted policies that can be situated at the pluralist pole of the integration continuum, each province remains distinct in the degree of institutional support granted to official language minorities, as is evident from differing bilingual policies in their respective health care systems.

Bilingual Health Care in Canada

The Canadian healthcare system can be described as a state owner operator model characterized by universal healthcare where all citizens have access to health services regardless of their financial situation, as well as a decentralized system giving provinces responsibility for the organization and delivery of health services (Snowden & Cohen, 2011). The 1984 Canada Health Act specifies the conditions provinces must respect to receive federal transfer payments. The Act states "the primary objective of Canadian health care policy is to protect, promote, and restore the physical and mental well-being of residents of Canada and to facilitate reasonable access to health services without financial or other barriers." Provincial and territorial governments are responsible for the management, organization, and delivery of health services for their residents, including insured health services provided by hospitals and medical practitioners. The private market provides coverage for health services that are not insured by the public plan. Although most medical practitioners are in private practice, and hospitals are private non-profit organizations, remuneration for physicians and hospital services are subject to provincial government regulation.

Given that health is a provincial jurisdiction, the Federal official bilingual policies do not apply to health care delivery across Canadian provinces. Consequently, the delivery of services in the language of official minority communities is subjected to provincial laws, policies, and norms (Tremblay & Prata, 2012). Because healthcare is a provincial jurisdiction and official languages are federal responsibilities, the federal government must collaborate with provinces to improve access to health services for official language minorities. Through Health Canada the federal government contributes to improving access to health care services for the two official language minorities mainly by funding community organizations and by working with post-secondary health care teaching institutions including medical schools. The federal government committed $170 million for the 2013-2018 period to improve training, networks, and access to French and English minority language health services (Canadian Heritage, 2013). Two community organizations are funded by the federal government: one for Francophone minorities in every province except Quebec—Société Santé en Français—and one for the Anglophone minority in the majority French-speaking province of Quebec, the Community Health and Social Services Network (CHSSN). The provision of French/English bilingual health services is seen as both a quality of health issue for linguistic minority patients and as a national goal of providing Francophone and Anglophone minority communities with the institutional support they need to manage and receive quality health care in both official languages (CHSSN, 2007, 2016a; DIHI, 2015; Health Canada, 2007; FCFA, 2001). Such bilingual health services have been especially well-developed within Canada's bilingual belt of New Brunswick, Quebec and Ontario (Bourhis & Montreuil, 2017).

In Canada, as elsewhere in the world, the provision of health care in both official languages for minorities whose knowledge of the majority language is weak or absent does play a role in alleviating the language barriers to health services experienced by such minorities. Language and cultural barriers experienced by such minority patients make it difficult to establish good caregiver-patient rapport and, as a consequence, the patient may receive less attentive care and experience less satisfaction with the medical treatment than patients for whom there is no language barrier (Kirmayer, 2012; Lussier & Riel-Salvatore, 2014). In both Canada and the United States, there is growing evidence that language and income barriers can limit access to health care services, health care usage, and preventive care for vulnerable linguistic minorities (Bowen, 2001; Pocock, 2016; Yeo, 2004). Language barriers can also have an impact on follow-up appointments, the quality of health care received, satisfaction of linguistic minority patients, and the communicative effectiveness of health care encounters in hospital settings (Flores, 2006; Sarver & Baker, 2000).

Canadian studies show linguistic minority status can combine with income barriers to health resulting in wellness disparities between linguistic majorities and minorities (Bouchard & Desmeules, 2013). Canadian survey data showed the impact of income and linguistic minority status on aspects of public health such as mental health, diet, obesity and physical inactivity (Leis & Bouchard, 2013).

Empirical studies on language barriers and bilingual communication in health care settings is emerging (Meuter, Gallois, Segalowitz, Ryder, & Hocking, 2015). Studies using Communication Accommodation Theory provide a conceptual framework to explain when, how, and why people adjust their communicative behavior during bilingual encounters within health care situations (Dragojevic, Gasiorek, & Giles, 2014; Watson, Hewett & Gallois, 2012).

Before discussing specific aspects of the bilingual health care systems in Quebec it is worth addressing the cost of bilingual health care in some Canadian provinces and in comparable countries of western economies. The 2015 bilingual health care expenditures per capita adjusted in U.S. dollars (U.S. $1. = CND $0.70) were as follows: the two autonomous French and English bilingual health care systems in New Brunswick cost $4,520 per person; followed by the partial French/English bilingual system in Ontario at $4,241, and the declining bilingual system of Quebec at $4,058 (Bourhis & Montreuil, 2017). These different types of bilingual health care systems compare well with the per capita expenditures of some unilingual English health systems including British Columbia at $4,208; Alberta at $4,990; and Saskatchewan at $4,789 (CIHI, 2015). Among 29 countries of the OECD that had comparable accounting systems in 2013, expenditure per person on health care in U.S. dollars remained highest in the United States with its primarily private unilingual English system costing $9,086. The health care cost per person for Canada as a whole including some bilingual systems was $4,569, followed by the unilingual health systems of France at $4,361, Australia at $4,115 and the United Kingdom at $3,364. Taken together, these trends suggest that health care systems offering different levels of bilingual services can be cost neutral as they are not more expensive than unilingual health systems in western economies.

Vitality, Acculturation and Language Policies in Quebec

Based on mother tongue census data, Francophones remain the majority in Quebec: growing from 4,860,410 inhabitants (80.7%) in 1971 to 6,164,700 inhabitants (79%) in 2011. Allophones, who have neither French nor English as a mother tongue, grew through immigration from 6.3% of the population in 1971 (390,400) to 12.8% of the population in 2011 (1,003,500). In contrast, the Anglophone minority dropped from 13% of the population in 1971 (788,800) to 8.3% of the population (647,600) in 2011. Census data in 2011 showed that 80% of Anglophones live in the greater Montreal region. However, the other 20% of Anglophones are dispersed across different regions of the province including: 5.9% in the Outaouais region, 5.1% in the Eastern Townships, 1.7% in the Quebec City region and 1.7% across Eastern regions of the Province. It is in these regions that the demographic and institutional vitality of Anglophone minorities has declined the most in the province.

As the high-vitality majority, Francophones control all the Ministries of the Quebec Government and most Municipalities, along with much of the Quebec economy and its mass media (Bourhis, 2012b). In 1977 the separatist Parti Québécois Government adopted the Charter of the French Language (Bill 101) designed to increase the status of French relative to English in the province (Corbeil, 2007). Bill 101 promotes and protects French in Quebec as the language of work, communications, commerce, and business in public and private organizations in the province, including the francization of the linguistic landscape. With a work force of 230 employees, the Office québécois de la langue française (OQLF) oversees all aspects of Bill 101, including the granting of Francization certificates to business firms of more than 50 employees that have proven that they can work in French at all levels of the firm, including communications with clients.

Quebec language planning in favour of French may be credited amongst other factors: having 95% of the whole Quebec population maintain or gain a knowledge of French; maintaining 82% of all its citizens as French speakers at home; and, having 86% of all Quebec Allophones attend French rather than English schools. Also, the proportion of Francophones bilinguals increased from 25% in 1971 to 39% in 2011. In contrast, the proportion of Anglophones who were French-English bilinguals increased from 37% in 1971 to 69% in 2011, while Allophones who became French/English bilinguals grew from 33% in 1971 to 50% in 2011 (Bourhis 2012b; Bourhis & Sioufi, 2017).

In the Quebec labour market, studies showed that the economic returns for knowing French increased substantially since Bill 101, whereas returns for knowing English or other languages steadily decreased. Also, the growth of ownership of the Quebec economy by Francophones rose to 75%, while as many as 95% of Francophone employees used French most often at work (Vaillancourt, Lemay, & Vaillancourt. 2007). By the 2011 Canadian census, the median income of Quebec individuals by mother tongue shifted to the advantage of Francophones at $28,841/year; $25,718 for Anglophones and only $20,033 for Allophones many of whom are immigrants.

Though the Francophone majority succeeded in consolidating its demographic and institutional ascendancy over the Anglophone minority, Quebec nationalist discourse continues to nurture feelings of collective threat to French by highlighting that, although Quebec Francophones constitute 80% of the provincial population, they remain a minority of only 23% within Canada and less than 2% within North America (Curzi, 2014). Given their declining demographic and institutional vitality, Quebec Anglophones felt besieged and voted with their feet; there has been a net-outmigration of 300,000 Anglophones to the rest of Canada during the last 40 years (Stevenson, 1999). In contrast, the net out migration of majority Francophones to the ROC was only 40,000, while that of minority Allophones was 104,000. This out-migration coupled with low birth rate and Quebec laws restricting access to English schooling accounts for the 60% decrease in the English school system: from 256,251 pupils in 1971 to 105,205 pupils in 2012, the largest decline in an English school system in Canada which continues to this day (Bourhis & Foucher, 2012). Though the English language is not threatened in Quebec, it is acknowledged that the vitality of the English-speaking communities of Quebec is in decline on the demographic and institutional support fronts (Bourhis, 2014; Bourhis & Sioufi, 2017). In response, the Quebec Community Groups Network (QCGN) is a federation of 53 English-speaking associations defending and developing their community vitality across the Province (Jedwab & Maynard, 2012).

Bilingual Health Care for Anglophones in Quebec

French-language health care institutions, established in the nineteenth century, were funded mostly by the French Catholic Church until they were gradually taken over by the Quebec Government as a universal health care system in the 1970s (Lemieux, 2013). By 2015, Quebec had 60 hospitals and health centres, most of which were unilingual French serving the Quebec population. English language health care institutions, also founded in the 19th century, were run by Protestant and Catholic religious orders and supported by substantial philanthropic funding from the historical Anglophone economic elites. When the Quebec Government established its universal health care system, it granted many existing English language health care institutions with a bilingual status designed to serve the health needs of both Francophone and Anglophone patients.

The 1991 law on Health and Social Services (LHSS) specified the right of English-speaking persons to receive services in their language. The Quebec Ministry of Health and Social Services defined an English-speaking person as "someone who, in relation with an establishment providing health and social services, feels more comfortable expressing his needs in English and receiving services in this language" (Quebec, 2006). This definition of an English-speaking person is closest to the Canadian census definition of first official language spoken (FOLS) derived from three census questions: knowledge of official languages, mother tongue and home language. In the 2011 census, over one million English FOLS speakers constituted 13.5% of the Quebec population. This Anglophone population served by Quebec Health & Social Services institutions is highly diversified culturally and ethnically and is made-up of not only Quebec born English mother tongue speakers but also immigrants (34%) and visible minority groups (28%). A study by the Institut national de santé publique du Québec noted language is "a determinant of health status or as a factor acting on other determinants," while also recognizing "Income inequalities are greater in the Anglophone population of Quebec at every level when compared with Francophones" (INSPQ, 2012). Pocock (2016) summarized the health care consequences of socioeconomic status (SES) for Quebec's Anglophone population as follows:

> . . . we note that there is a prevalence of low SES among the English-speaking communities of Quebec (Canadian Heritage, 2015a). This is a health risk factor and points to a population that may be reliant on public health services not only due to a greater rate of illness but also because they cannot cover the expense of private care. After New Brunswick Francophones, Quebec's English-speaking populations display the greatest socio-economic vulnerability when aspects such as low education levels, unemployment and labour force participation and low income tendencies are analysed. Relative to the Francophone majority of Quebec, English speakers show much higher unemployment rates. This gap has grown in recent decades and is more marked among workers age 25–44 than for the older workers in the 45–64 age group (Canadian Heritage, 2015b). (cited in Pocock p. 5)

We have used the terms English-speaking and Anglophone interchangeably for the sake of convenience and in line with Quebec

Health ministry documents. In line with the LHSS law, each regional planning agency developed a plan of access to health and social services in English by identifying the institutions that offered such services to the English-speaking population in its region. The plan recognized Francophone institutions offering certain services in English, as well as designated bilingual institutions offering all services in English and French. The Ministry of Health "Cadre de référenc" regulation defined a recognised health or social service institution in the following terms:

> *Un établissement reconnu (R) est un établissement qui fournit ses services à des personnes en majorité d'une langue autre que le français et qui a obtenu de l'Office québécois de la langue française une reconnaissance en vertu de l'article 29.1 de la Charte de la langue française.*
> (Bill 101, Quebec, 2006)

To have a designated status, the Ministry selected from among the institutions recognized under section 29.1 of Bill 101 those required to make all their services accessible in English. This choice was based on the historical origins of such institutions that also included having over half their clientele being served in a language other than French. A designated bilingual health or social service institution was defined in the "Cadre de reference" regulation as:

> *Un établissement désigné est un établissement que le gouvernement désigne parmi les établissements reconnus. Il s'agit d'un établissement tenu de rendre accessible en langue anglaise aux personnes d'expression anglaise les services de santé et les services sociaux qu'il offre.*
> (Quebec, 2006)

The bilingual status of these recognized and designated health institutions is revised every 3 years based on Canadian census data on the number of non-French mother tongue population within pertinent catchment areas of the institutions concerned. The historical Anglophone institutions recognized as bilingual by section 29.1 of Bill 101 benefited from a "grandfather" clause that protected their bilingual status even if subsequently their clientele fell under the 50% non-French mother tongue cut-off. Only the board of directors of such bilingual institutions could ask for their bilingual status to be withdrawn in favour of a unilingual French status. Though Anglophone stakeholders have traditionally had an input in defining bilingual status regulations, it is the Francophone majority which controls the legal status and development of bilingual health and social services institutions across the province, a vulnerability that can vary depending on the acculturation orientation and good will of the Health Minister and/or the political party in power (Bourhis, 2014).

Finally, the LHSS law stipulated that health services to which English-speaking minorities were entitled depended on available human, financial and material resources of institutions named in the access plan. Of course, the LHSS law stipulated that all Quebec Health institutions with a majority French-speaking clientele were defined as unilingual French institutions whose governance, health professionals and unionized employees had no legal obligation to provide any services in English to their patients.

By 2010, under the LHSS law, 42 Health & Social Service institutions obtained Recognized or Designated bilingual status in Quebec of which 28 were in Montreal. These bilingual status institutions were usually hospitals and health centres created and funded by the historical Anglophone communities of Montreal and other regions of the province. Bilingual status health institutions within the McGill University Health Centre (MUHC) were the Royal Victoria Hospital, Montreal General Hospital, Montreal Children's Hospital, Montreal Neurological Institute and Montreal Chest Institute. Other important Montreal bilingual status health institutions included the Jewish General Hospital, Saint Mary's Hospital, the Queen Elizabeth Health Centre and the Lakeshore General Hospital. Bilingual status health institutions serving Anglophone and Francophone communities in other regions of the province included the Jeffery Hale / St. Brigid's hospital and home in Quebec City, the Brome-Missisquoi-Perkins Hospital in the Eastern townships, the Pontiac Community Hospital in Shawville and the Barrie Memorial Hospital in Ormstown.

All health care professionals in Quebec, from physicians to nurses to bio-medical technicians, must pass written and spoken French language tests conducted by the OQLF. Bill 101 stipulates non-Francophone health care professionals not able to pass this test are not allowed to work in either French or bilingual health institutions in the Province of Quebec. Many Francophone institutions offering services in English face numerous challenges: shortage of human resources able to provide health services in both English and French; decline of English-speaking patients in regions of the province other than Montreal where Anglophones remain concentrated; difficulty in planning bilingual services due to lack of information on the needs of minority language speakers; and, ambiguities of the Bill 101 legal framework for bilingual health care institutions (Ouimet, Trempe, Vissandjé, & Hemlin, 2013). Cost effective solutions to the lack of linguistic proficiency of health professionals exist, including access to a bank of professional interpreters for facilities with a low proportion of minority language patients.

In a survey of the linguistic skills of health professionals in Quebec, results showed the proportion of doctors with knowledge of English as a first or second language was sufficient to serve the communicative needs of Anglophone patients across most regions of the province (Trempe & Lussier, 2011). However, the study also revealed the proportion of nursing staff, social workers, psychologists and other health professionals with a knowledge of English as a first or second language was well below the proportion needed to serve the needs of Anglophone minority patients present in most regions of the province. Despite such challenges, over 7000 Francophone health professionals have received English language training in culturally sensitive health care for minority Anglophone populations residing in Montreal and other regions of the province (Riel-Salvatore, 2011).

Levels of satisfaction expressed by Quebec Anglophones regarding their access to health services in English reflect many challenges. In a 2005 survey conducted among 3,000 Quebec Anglophones, the average satisfaction rate at the provincial level toward access to services in English was consistently below 50% (Carter, 2012). The 2005 survey also revealed physicians in local private clinics were generally more likely to offer services in English than those working in public health centres and hospitals. In many regions of Quebec, less than 50% of English-speaking respondents could be served in English in primary care units. It remains that weakening the demographic vitality of the English-speaking communities of Quebec further jeopardizes Anglophones' capacity to claim health and language rights, especially in regions of the province where Anglophones constitute small, aging and isolated minorities.

In 2006, Statistics Canada conducted a large representative post-census study known as the Vitality of Official Language Minorities survey. This survey included self-report items on many demographic and institutional support features of the vitality of the Anglophone minority population of Quebec (N= 5,200 adults) and of the Francophone minority populations in each of the English majority Provinces (N= 17,500 adults). This national survey allowed an analysis of key bilingual health care issues rated by minority Anglophones in Quebec and minority Acadians in New Brunswick and Franco-Ontarians in Ontario (Gagnon-Arpin, Bouchard, Leis, & Bélanger, 2014). The declining bilingual health care system in Quebec has had some impact on Anglophone access to English-language health care. Results showed that 26% of Anglophones reported that it would be difficult or very difficult to obtain their health care in English, and of those, 74% reported that the problem was a lack of English-speaking health care providers. As many as 92% of Anglophones felt it was important to obtain their health care in English, and 77% felt at ease when requesting services in English. As many as 81% of Anglophones reported having used English with their family doctor in the last 12 months, while 26% reported being without a family doctor. Survey results also showed that access to bilingual health care services declined especially in regions of Quebec where the concentration of the Anglophones was low. The converse was true in regions where Anglophone communities were more concentrated. The more isolated Anglophone minority communities became within a given region, the more precarious their institutional support became in health care and social services, thus undermining the overall vitality of such regional Anglophone minorities.

A recent study conducted with a population of Quebec Anglophones showed that those who were unilingual English were more likely to declare poor health (Falconer & Quesnel-Vallée, 2014). Multiple logistic regression analyzes showed that the poor health of such unilingual Anglophones could not be attributed to their older age, lower income and lower education. Unilingual Anglophones also reported lower use of health services compared to Anglophones who had some knowledge of French. As is the case for Francophone minorities in New Brunswick and Ontario, when services are not actively offered in the minority language, Anglophones do not always claim these services either because they are too shy, fear increasing waiting time, or do not wish to impose an undue burden on health professionals (Bourhis & Montreuil, 2017).

In the provincial Survey on Community Vitality, English-speaking respondents results showed that while 32% reported having received public health information in English in 2005, this proportion declined to 26% in 2015 (CHSSN, 2016a, b). The 2015 survey also showed that only a minority of Anglophones (43%) reported being satisfied with the English language health and social services they received in their region. However, it was the English speakers whose health was poorest who expressed the highest levels of dissatisfaction with the amount of care they obtained in English. While, province-wide, as many as 74% of Anglophones reported being served in English in hospital emergency rooms and out-patient clinics, it was Anglophones in regions other than the Island of Montreal who were less likely to be served in English: 48% of Anglophones in the Eastern townships: 53% in the city of Laval (CHSSN, 2016a, b). Supported by the Official Languages Health Contribution Program, the CHSSN recently launched 20 collaborative action programs with the Quebec Ministry of Health to improve Anglophone access to health and social services in English. The CHSSN also launched partnerships with Anglophone communities to improve their access to English language services in Montreal and across regions of the province (Carter & Pocock, 2017; Pocock, 2016).

The health services to which English-speaking minorities are entitled must be defended or claimed in times of health structure reforms by the Quebec Ministry of Health and Social Services. As noted by Carter:

> The legislative provisions that guarantee the right to services in English, within system limits, also guide the multitude of players that comprise the health and social services system. Experience has taught community leaders that when the integrity of the legislation is maintained, progress is made. When that integrity is questioned for whatever reasons, it is not only a threat to English language services, but to the future of English-speaking communities as well. Communities must be "fire hall ready" to respond to any new political scenarios that may stimulate old debates about the legitimacy of legislative guarantees. It is also clear that sustaining progress and meeting new challenges will continue to require cooperation between the provincial and federal levels of government, with formal recognition of English-speaking communities as full partners. (Carter, 2012, pp. 243–243)

Bill 10: A Case Study of Health Care Centralisation in Quebec

The Quebec Government adopted Bill 10 in 2014, a law modifying the organization and governance of the provincial health network (Quebec, 2014). While crafting the bill, Montreal and regional Anglophone minority communities were not consulted by the Minister and its Ministry of Health and Social Services. In the name of cost saving and rationalisation, Bill 10 abolished regional planning bodies while the number of government boards for hospitals, senior homes, and other health and social service centres were reduced from 182 to only 34 mega bodies across the province, known as Regional Integrated Health and Social Services Centres ([RIHSSC]; Centre intégré de santé et de service sociaux [CISSS]). Anglophone communities across the province stood to lose 22 of their historical bilingual designated boards as a result of Bill 10, thus reducing their representation in the governance of their hospital and health/social service institutions now subsumed under Francophone majority RIHSSC mega centres. Anglophones were left with majority control of only one bilingual health care centre in the province, namely the McGill University Hospital Centre in Montreal. Bill 10 measures were seen to weaken Anglophone community links to their local health care foundations and volunteer networks established and nurtured across decades of community mobilization.

In line with earlier LHSS legislation and Bill 101, Bill 10 provided no entitlement for Anglophone patients to have their health records in English. Doctors or health professional can decide whether to write such records in French or English. Health or social services institutions can require such documents to be written only in French. In line with the Bill 101, hospital and health/social service institutions may only post signs on their premises in English if they have the status of designated bilingual institution. All others health institutions in the province may only post in French. All bilingual designated institutions must include French on their signs and posters along with English or in some cases another language. If a sign or poster is needed for public safety, it may be written in both French and another language, even if the institution is not designated. As in earlier LHSS legislation, Bill 10 agencies may enter agreements with other jurisdictions to send patients to the other regions, use technology or interpreters to provide services in English.

Dr Victor Goldbloom, the first member of Quebec's Jewish community to serve in the provincial cabinet in the 1970s, Canada's Commissioner of Official language from 1991 to 1999, and keen observer of health care issues in Quebec, voiced his concern about the impact of Bill 10 on the delivery of health and social services for the diverse Anglophone and cultural communities across the province.

> In 2014 the Quebec government brought forward legislation abolishing the agencies. I personally thought that this was an error that it would make the administration of the health care system more remote from and less responsive to the public we serve... I deeply regretted the proposal to amalgamate eight or ten institutions in each area into one, particularly since doing so would eliminate some 90 per cent of the dedicated community volunteers serving on their boards. I was concerned at the possible loss of the ethnic and religious specificity of particular community institutions. The Minister of Health gave assurances that rights to health care and social services in English would be maintained, but I am unconvinced that this commitment would provide permanent protection against a later decision by a less sympathetic government. It seemed to me that an English-speaking community of this size should not be considered to have rights only if it represented at least 51 per cent of the clientele or the staff of a given entity. (Goldbloom, 2015, p. 180–181)

As with other proposed laws, Bill 10 was submitted for public hearings by the Quebec government's Committee on Health and Social Services in the autumn of 2014: numerous briefs were submitted by Anglophone stakeholders and community groups to the government public hearings on Bill 10. Critiques of the bill were expressed in the brief submitted by the Quebec Community Groups Network (QCGN, 2015). Key concerns provided in the QCGN brief to the public hearings on Bill 10 are presented below in their original sequence of presentation. Interestingly, these concerns not only reflect a keen awareness of institutional vitality issues but also share many challenges faced by Francophone minorities when defending their institutional vitality in the ROC.

7. QCGN, its members and partners, share serious concerns expressed by other groups about Bill 10 such as the extreme rapidity of implementation, centralization of control and management of the system, and submerging of social service mandates in vast health oriented structures.

12. We believe Bill 10 would be a catastrophe for the 22 recognized and designated <u>public</u> institutions it dismantles. Only the *McGill University Health Centre* would retain this status.

14. Bill 10 would remove the right of recognized and designated institution boards to preserve the status accorded under the *Charter of the French language* (Bill 101), as these boards will no longer exist. There is no guarantee that a board of new regional institutions would preserve the bilingual status of a facility.

16. Adoption of Bill 10 as tabled would rupture a fundamental part the legacy of legislative guarantees made to the English-speaking communities over time. In our view Bill 10 must not extinguish the existence of recognized and designated institutions, and the guarantees they embody.

17. The third paragraph in the preamble of *La Charte de la Langue Française* says: "Whereas the National Assembly intends to pursue this objective (establishing the predominance of the French language) in a spirit of fairness and open-mindedness, *respectful of the institutions of the English-speaking community of Québec*, and respectful of the ethnic minorities, whose valuable contribution to the development of Quebec it readily acknowledges."

18. How does the Minister and his government respect the public health and social service institutions of the English-speaking communities when it contemplates a bill that would end their existence, save for one?

19. Recognized and designated institutions represent the legacy of the Liberal Party to English-speaking communities resulting from the reform of the Health and Social Service Act (S-4.2) carried out in 1991. That reform continued the institutions' participation in the public health and social service system, mindful

of the preamble of the Charter, adding specific provisions to S-4.2 that recognized the special character of the institutions' connection to and duties towards English-speaking communities. Adoption of Bill 10 in its current form would, we repeat, rupture this legacy.

20. Designated facilities with no corresponding governance structure would be hollow guarantees of continuity in the relationship between the English-speaking community and the institutions it considers so important.

23. If the services would continue to exist in English in the 'designated *facilities'*, one might ask why is this matter so important to our communities? Because recognized and designated *institutions* are more than just services in English. They play leadership roles in their communities. They are organizations that attract community members, citizens who want to be invited onto their boards of directors, to their foundation and fundraising activities, into their auxiliaries and volunteer services, their banks of foster families, and onto their owning corporations. If the recognized and designated institution disappears these relationships and activities would inevitably be affected and put in question, and would ultimately impact negatively on the vitality of the community. The new institution inheriting the designated facilities, and the community would both be losers in this scenario. Existence of advisory committees as proposed in article 131, which are not guaranteed to exist, would by no stretch of the imagination replace the capacities of recognized and designated institutions.

26. In regions where there are no, or very few, designated institutions, members of the English-speaking community must compete for a place in governance structures with members of the majority community. With the number of such seats drastically reduced under Bill 10, the opportunities for members of these small English-speaking communities to access a board seat would fall from few to none.

27. Under Bill 10 the selection of board members of the newly constituted institutions would be highly centralized in the hands

of the Minister, with no direct avenue for community designation to boards. This approach to the governance of health and social services institutions would have a dramatic and disproportionately negative effect on the English-speaking minority communities of the province, for whom a visible participation in the control and management, particularly of the institutions they founded and nurtured over many decades, is an important and irreplaceable part of the infrastructure of community life.

30. Recognized and designated institutions, and community participation in governance are the two subjects that cut to the heart of the relationship between the English-speaking communities and the institutions they use and contribute to the public system. Participation from the community in governance, and the mechanisms that support that participation require a new paradigm, not tinkering with the one put forward in the law (Bill 10). As other interveners have argued in a more global way, let Quebecers participate in the governance of this important network of institutions. Their participation breathes life into institutions. We are fully willing to contribute to such a reconsideration of this subject.

37. We firmly believe the Minister and his government have a legislative responsibility to treat the institutions issuing from the English-speaking community with the respect the preamble of the Charter calls for, and in keeping with the spirit of reforms made to S-4.2 to date that affect those institutions.

38. We also believe that clear mechanisms whereby members of the community can access seats on governance boards without being dependent on the approval of this minister are essential to the vitality of both the institutions and the community.

As seen above, Anglophone stakeholders and community groups submitted strong representations to the Health Minister Gaétan Barrette to amend features of Bill 10 during the 2014 public hearings. Following intense rounds of private negotiation between Anglophone stakeholders and the Health Minister, Bill 10 was amended in February 2015 to recognize the status of existing designated bilingual health care institutions across the province as they had been in the

LHSS law. In addition, each of the 34 new Regional Integrated Health and Social Services Centres (RIHSSC) were made responsible for implementing bilingual access plan for Anglophone minority communities taking account of their linguistic, ethno-cultural and demographic requirements for the recruitment and assignment of health personnel required to provide French/English bilingual services. Other amendments stipulated that each of the RIHSS must have at least one English speaker on its board and each board may have an advisory committee on cultural and language issues, where a former designated bilingual institution has become a designated bilingual "installation" of the RIHSSC. Importantly, the advisory committee could exercise a veto power over important decisions such as relinquishing the status of a designated bilingual installation. In line with the QCGN request, both the Centre de l'île de Montréal RIHSSC and the Centre ouest de l'île de Montréal RIHSSC were granted bilingual status in the amendments to Bill 10. Some special representation was guaranteed for the historical Anglophone minority using the Jeffery Hale/St Brigid's bilingual status hospital within the Francophone majority RIHSS mega-board of Quebec City.

The Montreal Gazette main editorial concerning these last-minute amendments to Bill 10 acknowledged the rapid Anglophone community mobilization to safeguard its designated bilingual institutions as follow:

> To their credit, members of Quebec's English-speaking minority-fearing the loss not only of community control over institutions, but the erosion of legal guarantees ensuring access to English services- worked doggedly behind the scenes to wring important concessions, to minimize the extent to which English-language services would be collateral damage of the reform. To his credit, Health Minister Barrette, who has not otherwise shown much flexibility, was sensitive to these concerns.

However, the editorial also highlighted some institutional losses for the Anglophone community despite efforts to amend Bill 10:

> The governing boards of the Jewish General Hospital, Batshaw Youth and Family Services, the West Island Rehabilitation Centre, Quebec City's Jeffrey Hale / St Brigid's—proudly built, nurtured and governed by their respective communities—will

effectively be extinguished. The amalgamated boards that will now run them will have fewer seats and thus fewer opportunities for the involvement of the citizens who have a stake in their operations. (Montreal Gazette, 2015a)

Overall, Anglophone stakeholders and community groups were relieved and thankful for the last-minute amendments to Bill 10 agreed by the current Minister of Health. Clifford Lincoln, a widely respected retired Liberal MNA of the Quebec National Assembly stated that English-speaking health care rights had been "affirmed in such an integrated way that it would make it much more difficult for future governments to touch them anymore" (Montreal Gazette, 2015b). On the Bill 10 amendments, Eric Maldoff, chief negotiator with the Minister of Health concluded: "We have maintained some of our legal status, maintained and enhanced some of our bilingual status, and got advisory committees to enable the community to have some meaningful engagement with the integrated centres" (QCGN, 2016). Pleading for continuing community mobilization, Maldoff warned that amendments to Bill 10 would be of no avail if members of the Anglophone minority did not actively participate as health-care administrators in their designated bilingual institutions and within the new French majority RIHSS mega boards (Montreal Gazette, 2015b).

Despite favourable Bill 10 amendments maintaining the designated status of bilingual health care institutions, the reduction of the number of regional health care boards and resulting centralisation by the Ministry of Health through the RIHSSS mega Francophone boards are problematic for minority Anglophone communities across the province. It remains that the actual provisions of bilingual health care for Anglophone minority individuals are entrusted to majority Francophone administrative board of the RIHSSS directly answerable to the current Minister of Health and its Ministry of Health public servants enforcing Bill 10. Such vulnerabilities are felt less intensively where the proportion of English-speaking population is large, long-standing and well-organized, such as the Montreal Island with its numerous bilingual status health institutions. However, most other regions of the province have declining and aging English-speaking populations who are much more vulnerable, especially when they have few existing designated bilingual health care institution and little capacity for effective Anglophone representation on the French majority RIHSSC boards and health institutions.

The Bill 10 debate served as a wake-up call for many Quebec Anglophone stakeholders. For many it was time to seriously consider the Commissioner of Official languages suggestion that Quebec needs some kind of permanent office of Anglophone affairs in Quebec. The case for such an office was detailed in a local English Montreal weekly as follows:

> Graham Fraser, a distinguished political journalist and author before he was appointed commissioner in 2006, repeated the call this fall . . . that having such an office, with a minister responsible, would be logical, especially in the context of the controversy over Bill 10 . . . In spite of a decidedly cool reaction in the French-language media and the governing Liberals, who feel Anglo views are well represented by the three MNAs from the majority English ridings, Fraser continues to believe that this idea makes good sense . . . When Bill 10 was introduced, it was concerned community leaders, including those in the QCGN that made it clear that the needs of the English community were not being taken in consideration. Fraser believes much of the controversy could have been avoided had there been a permanent government structure in place with a mandate to monitor and advise on issues affecting Anglo rights. (*The Senior Times*, 2015, p. 7)

In perhaps his political testament to the English-speaking communities of Quebec before his retirement from office, Graham Fraser is quoted in the article on lessons drawn from the Bill 10 debate:

> QCGN has expressed its satisfaction mixed with relief following some last minute amendments to Bill 10. But it was clear that Bill 10 was drawn up without taking account the needs of the English community. It took months of constant negotiating to result in the necessary amendments to the bill . . . Ontario's Office of Francophone Affairs, created in 2007, and Commissioner of French Language Services, are examples of institutions that can offer input to any proposed legislation to ensure that language rights and services are respected. Part of the reason for having a coordinating office that can act as a

> reference point for the English community is that it depoliticizes
> it so that it becomes part of the institutional reflex—less visible,
> less controversial . . . I think French-speaking Quebec as a soci-
> ety is full of strength, vitality, and energy, and is in a position
> now that it can assume its role as a responsible majority society.
> (*The Senior Times*, 2015, p. 8)

Declaring how he cared about the vitality of the English community
and their institutions in the province, the Quebec Prime Minister
appointed a Minister for relations with the English-speaking community in October 2017 (Montreal Gazette, 2017). In the same year,
the Liberal Prime Minister established a Secretariat for English-
speaking affairs with a mandate to advise present and future
Ministers of the Quebec government of the concerns and needs of
the English-speaking communities of Quebec in key public services
such as health and social services.

Conclusion

The Quebec context is distinctive within Canada in that it adopted
strong legislative measures promoting the ascendency of the French
language (Bill 101) while having to abide by a Canadian Constitution
seeking to protect the institutional vitality of the declining Quebec
Anglophone minority especially in education. Though Francophones
now constitute the dominant high-vitality majority community in
the province, government pro-French policies are often adopted as
if Quebec Francophones remain a besieged minority, while collateral
damage caused by such laws can be substantial for the vitality of the
Anglophone minority (Bourhis & Sioufi, 2017). The rapid mobilisation
of Anglophone stakeholders to negotiate amendments to Bill 10
showed that this minority, like Francophone ones in the ROC (for
example, the Montford Hospital case in Ontario), had the ideological
clarity to defend their health care institutional vitality.

Elected Francophone MNAs in the Quebec National Assembly
whose integrative orientations favour the maintenance of bilingual
health institutions understand they should do so discretely to avoid
the stigmatizing attention of Francophone assimilationists unsympa-
thetic toward the maintenance of historical English language institutions in the Province. This discretion is also pertinent for integrative
health care professionals and support staff willing to use English and

other languages with vulnerable ethnolinguistic minorities in local unilingual French health care institutions. Evidence suggests that many Francophone and Anglophone health professionals with a long history of collaboration are keen to maintain their good relations and to converge to the linguistic and cultural communicative needs of their vulnerable minority patients despite top down Health Ministry laws and regulations (Pocock, 2016). More research is needed to explore how the acculturation orientations and bilingualism of health care providers affect the quantity and quality of the care they provide to vulnerable minority group patients in unilingual and bilingual health care institutions (Schwartz & Unger, 2017).

Future research on bilingual health care systems must further explore the fundamental issue of how much linguistic minority patients improve their health outcomes when they are cared in their own language rather than only in the language of the dominant majority. The Quebec case study suggests bilingual health institutions include bilingual communications not only with patients but also between health care providers, support staff, administrators and members of governing boards. Health institutions endorsing pluralism as their organizational culture are more likely to sustain and develop bilingual health services that are integrative than institutions which implicitly or explicitly endorse the assimilationist ideology. Quebec could improve the wellness of its Anglophone and Allophone patient population by developing its support of bilingual status health and social services across all regions of the province.

As seen in the per capita cost of bilingual versus unilingual health care there is evidence that offering cost-neutral bilingual health care can contribute to public health for linguistic minorities without undermining majority group health services. It is safe to assume that maintenance of bilingual health care institutions do have beneficial health effects for both the Francophone majority and English-speaking minorities they serve, which in the long run should save public funds for all Quebec taxpayers. Beyond the classic biomedical model of health care, studies suggest that both language and cultural sensitivity in the delivery of health care services can contribute to the wellness of majority and minority patients in increasingly multicultural and multilingual health environments.

Notes

1. This chapter is dedicated to the memory of Victor C. Goldbloom (1923–2016), a steadfast defender of minority rights in Quebec. I wish to thank Jim Carter, Annie Montreuil and Joanne Pocock for their judicious comments on earlier versions of this chapter.

References

Abrams, J. Barker, V., & Giles, H. (2009). "An Examination of the validity of the subjective Vitality questionnaire." *Journal of Multilingual and Multicultural Development*, 30, 59–72

Allard, R., & Landry, R. (1994). "Subjective ethnolinguistic vitality: A comparison of two measures." *International Journal of the Sociology of Language*, 108, 117–144.

Arends-Toth, J., & van de Vijver, J.R. (2004). "Domains and dimensions in acculturation: Implicit theories of Turkish-Dutch." *International Journal of Intercultural Relations*, 28, 19–35.

Banting, K., & Kymlicka, W. (2012). "Is there a Backlash against Multiculturalism Policies? New Evidence from the Multiculturalism Index." *Gritin Working Papers Series*, 14. Universitat Pompeu Fabra. www.upf.edu/gritim

Barker, V., & Giles, H. (2004). "English-only policies: Perceived support and social limitation." *Language and Communication*, 24, 77–95.

Barrette, G., Bourhis, R.Y., Personnaz, M., & Personnaz, B. (2004). "Acculturation orientations of French and North African undergraduates in Paris." *International Journal of Intercultural Relations*, 28, 415–438.

Berry, J.W. (1997). "Immigration, acculturation and adaptation." *Applied Psychology: An International Review*, 46, 5–34.

Berry, J. W. (2006). "Context of Acculturation." D. L. Sam & J.W. Berry, (Eds.). *The Cambridge Handbook of Acculturation Psychology*. 27–42. Cambridge and New York: Cambridge University Press.

Berry, J., Phinney, J.S., Sam, D., & Vedder, P., (Eds.). (2006). *Immigrant youth in cultural transition: Acculturation, identity and adaptation across nations*. Mawah, NJ : Lawrence Erlbaum.

Blanchet, P. H. (2016). *Discrimination: Combattre la Glottophobie*. Paris: Textuel.

Bloemraad, I. (2006). *Becoming a citizen: Incorporating Immigrants and Refugees in the United-States and Canada*. Berkeley: University of California Press.

Bloemraad, I., Korteweg, A., & Yurdaku, G. (2008). "Citizenship and Immigration: Multiculturalism, Assimilation, and Challenges to the Nation-State." *Annual Review of Sociology*, 34, 153–179.

Bouchard, L., & Desmeules, M. (2013). "Linguistic Minorities in Canada and Health." *Health Care Policy*, 9, 38–47.

Bourhis, R.Y. (1991). "Organizational communication and accommodation: Towards some conceptual and empirical links." H. Giles, J. Coupland, & H. Coupland, (Eds.). *Context of Accommodation: Developments in Applied Sociolinguistics.* 270–303. Cambridge and New York: Cambridge University Press.

Bourhis, R.Y. (1994). "Official language policies and the language of work in the Canadian Federal Administration: The linguistic work environment survey." *International Journal of the Sociology of Language,* 105–106, 217–266.

Bourhis, R. Y. (2001). "Acculturation, language maintenance and language loss." J. Klatter-Falmer & P. Van Avermaet (Eds.). *Theories on Language maintenance and loss of minority languages: Towards a more integrated explanatory framework.* 5–37. New York: Waxmann Verlag.

Bourhis, R.Y. (2012a). *Decline and Prospects of the English-Speaking Communities of Quebec.* Ottawa: Canadian Heritage.

Bourhis, R.Y. (2012b). "Social Psychological Aspects of French-English Relations in Quebec: From Vitality to Linguicism." R.Y. Bourhis, (Ed.). *Decline and Prospects of the English-Speaking Communities of Quebec.* 313–378. Ottawa: Canadian Heritage.

Bourhis, R.Y. (2014). Vitality challenges facing the English-speaking communities of Quebec. Montreal, QC: *Working Papers in Health Care Access for Linguistic Minorities.* WP-HCALM, Volume 1, 1–10. https://richard bourhis minorityhealthcareaccess.com

Bourhis, R.Y., Barrette, G., El-Geledi, S., & Schmidt (2009). "Acculturation orientations and social relations between immigrant and host community members in California." *Journal of Cross-Cultural Psychology,* 40, 443–467.

Bourhis, R.Y., Barrette, G., & Moriconi, P.A. (2008). Appartenances nationales et orientations d'acculturation au Québec. *Revue Canadienne des Sciences du Comportement/Canadian Journal of Behavioural Science,* 40, 90–103.

Bourhis, R.Y., & Foucher, P. (2012). *The Decline of the English School System in Quebec.* Moncton, NB: Institut canadien de recherche sur les minorités linguistiques (ICRML). www.icrml.ca

Bourhis, R.Y., Giles, H., & Rosenthal, D. (1981). "Notes on the construction of a "Subjective vitality questionnaire" for ethnolinguistic groups." *Journal of Multilingual and Multicultural Development,* 2, 145–155.

Bourhis, R.Y., & Landry, R. (2012). "Group vitality, Cultural autonomy and the Wellness of Language Minorities." R.Y. Bourhis, (Ed.). *Decline and Prospects of the English-Speaking communities of Quebec.* 23–69. Ottawa: Canadian Heritage.

Bourhis, R. Y., Moise, L. C., Perreault, S., & Senecal, S. (1997). "Towards an interactive acculturation model: A social psychological approach." *International Journal of Psychology,* 32, 369–386.

Bourhis, R.Y., Montaruli, E., & Amiot, C. (2007). "Language planning and French-English bilingual communication: Montreal field studies from 1977 to 1997." *International Journal of the Sociology of Language*. 105, 187–224.

Bourhis, R.Y., & Montreuil, A. (2017). "Acculturation, vitality, and Bilingual Health care. S. J. Schwartz & J. Unger," (Eds.). *The Oxford Handbook of Acculturation and Health*. 49–74. New York: Oxford University Press.

Bourhis, R.Y., Montreuil, A. Helly, D., & Jantzen, L. (2007). "Discrimination et linguicisme au Québec. Enquête sur la diversité ethnique au Canada." *Canadian Ethnic Studies/Études ethniques au Canada*. 39, 31–49.

Bourhis, R.Y., & Sioufi, R. (2017). Assessing forty years of language planning on the vitality of the Francophone and Anglophone communities of Quebec. *Multilingua*, 36, 627-661.

Bourhis, R.Y., Sioufi, R., & Sachdev, I. (2012). "Ethnolinguistic interaction and multilingual communication." H. Giles, (Ed.). *The Handbook of Intergroup Communication*. 100–115. New York: Routledge/Taylor & Francis.

Bowen, S. (2001). *Language barriers in access to healthcare*. Ottawa, Ontario: Health Canada.

Canada (2005) *Official Languages Act*. Ottawa, Canada. Government of Canada. http://laws-lois.justice.gc.ca/eng/acts/)-3.01/Canada (2016). Truth and Reconciliation Commission of Canada. *Honouring the Truth, Reconciling for the future. Summary of the final report of the Truth and Reconciliation Commission of Canada*. Winnipeg: www.trc.ca

Canadian Heritage (2013). *Framework for Enhancing the Vitality of Official-Language Minority Communities* (OLMCs). https://gcgnevents.files.wordpress.com/2014/05/vitality-framework-precis-2014-15-01.pdf

Canadian Heritage (2013). *Roadmap for Canada's Official Languages 2013-2018: Education, immigration, communities*. Ottawa: Canadian Heritage.

Carter, J. (2012). What future for English-Language Health and Social Services in Quebec? In R.Y. Bourhis (Ed.). *Decline and Prospects of the English-Speaking communities of Quebec* 215–244. Ottawa: Canadian Heritage.

Carter, J. & Pocock, J. (2017). *Report on the Health and Social Services Priorities of English-speaking Communities in Quebec*. Montreal, QC: CHSSN. www.chssn.org

CHSSN (2007). Community Health and Social Services Network. *Investing in the Health and vitality of Quebec's English-Speaking Communities, A Community Action Plan 2008-2013*. Montreal: http://www.chssn.org/Document/Download/CHSSN

CHSSN (2016a). Community Health and Social Services Network and Pocock, J. Baseline Data Report 2015–2016. *English-language Health and Social Service Access in Quebec*. Based on CHSSN-CROP (2015). Survey on Community Vitality. Montreal: www.chssn.org

CHSSN (2016b). Community Health and Social Services Network and Pocock, J. Baseline Data Report 2015–2016. *CHSSN-CROP 2015 Survey on Community Vitality.* Findings on English-speaking Community Vitality Across Key Sectors. Montreal: www.chssn.org

CIHI (2015). Canadian Institute for Health Information. Health System Descriptors for Peer Countries, Canada and Provinces. https://www.cihi.ca/en/health-system-performance/ performance-reporting/ international/oecd-interactive-tool-peer-countries-can.

Corbeil, J.C. (2007). *L'Embarras des Langues. Origines, conception et évaluation de la politique linguistique Québécoise.* Montréal, Québec: Québec Amérique.

Corbeil, J.P., Grenier, C., Lafrenière, S. (2007). *Minorities Speak Up: Results of the Survey on the Vitality of the Official Language Minorities.* Ottawa: Statistics Canada. Demography Division.

Crawford, J. (2000). *At war with diversity: US language policy in an age of anxiety.* Bristol, UK: Multilingual Matters.

Curzi, P. (2014). French the common language of Quebec. In: R. Clément & P. Foucher, eds. *Fifty Years of Official Bilingualism.* 15–19. Ottawa: Invenire

Dragojevic, M., Gasiorek, J., & Giles, H. (2014). "Communication Accommodation Theory." Berger, C.P. & Roloff, H. eds. *International Encyclopedia of Interpersonal Communication.* New York: Wiley.

Falconer, J., & Quesnel-Vallée, A. (2014). Les disparités d'accès aux soins de santé parmi la minorité de langue officielle au Québec. *Recherches sociographiques, 553,* 511–529.

FCFA (2001) Fédération des communautés francophones et acadienne du Canada (2001). *Santé en français – Pour un meilleur accès à des services de santé en français.* Ottawa: Étude coordonnée pour le Comité consultatif des communautés francophones en situation minoritaire.

Fettes, M. (1998). "Life on the Edge: Canada's Aboriginal Languages under Official Bilingualism." T. Ricento & B. Burnaby, (Eds.), *Language and Politics in the United States and Canada: Myths and Realities.* 117–149. Mahwah, NJ: Lawrence Erlbaum.

Fishman, J. (1991). *Reversing Language Shift.* Bristol, UK: Multilingual Matters.

Fishman, J. A. (Ed.) (2001). "Why is it so hard to save a threatened language?" J.A. Fishman, (Ed.), *Can threatened languages be saved?* 1–22. Bristol, England: Multilingual Matters.

Flores, G. (2006) "Language barriers to health care in the United States." *New England Journal of Medicine, 355,* 229–231.

Fraser, G. (2006). *Sorry I don't Speak French: Confronting the Canadian Crisis that Won't go Away.* Toronto: McClelland & Stewart.

Gagnon-Arpin, I., Bouchard, L., Leis, A. & Bélanger, M. (2014). « Accès et utilisation des services de santé en langue minoritaire. » R. Landry, (Ed.), *La vie dans une langue officielle minoritaire au Canada.* 195–221. Québec: Presse de l'Université Laval

Gao, S., & Wong, L. (2015). *Revisiting Multiculturalism in Canada*. Rotterdam and Boston: Sense Publishers.

Gilbert, A. (2010). *Territoires Francophones: Études géographiques sur la vitalité des communautés francophones du Canada*. Québec: Septentrion.

Giles, H., Bonilla, D., & Speer, R.B. (2012). "Acculturating intergroup vitalities, accommodation and contact. In J. Jackson (Ed.), *Routledge Handbook of Intercultural Communication*. 244–259 London and New York: Routledge

Giles, H., Bourhis, R. Y., & Taylor, D. (1977). "Towards a theory of language in ethnic group relations." In H. Giles, (Ed.), *Language, ethnicity and intergroup relations*. 307–348. London: Academic Press.

Giles, H., & Johnson, P. (1987). "Ethnolinguistic identity theory: A social psychological approach to language maintenance." *International Journal of the Sociology of Language, 68,* 69–99.

Giles, H., & Watson, B. (Eds.) (2013). *The social meanings of language, dialect, and accent: International perspectives on speech styles*. New York: Peter Lang.

Goldbloom, V.C. (2015). *Building Bridges*. 180–181. Montreal: McGill-Queen's University Press.

Harwood, J., Giles, H., & Bourhis, R.Y. (1994). The genesis of vitality theory: historical patterns and discoursal dimensions. *International Journal of the Sociology of Language*, 108, 167– 206.

Health Canada (2007). *Building on the foundation. Working toward Better Health Outcomes and Improved vitality of Quebec's English-Speaking Communities.* Ottawa: Report to the Federal Minister of Health.

INSPQ (2012). Institut national de santé publique du Québec. The Socio-economic Status of Anglophones in Quebec. http://chssn.org/pdf/EN/INSPQ/SituationSocioEconoAngloQC.pdf

Jedwab, J., & Landry, R. (2011). *Life after Forty: Official Language Policies in Canada*. Montreal: McGill-Queens University Press.

Jedwab, J., & Maynard, H. (2012). "Politics of Community: The evolving Challenges of representing English-Speaking Quebecers." R. Y. Bourhis, (Ed.), *Decline and Prospects of the English-Speaking Communities of Quebec*. 277–311. Ottawa: Canadian Heritage.

Johnson, M., & Doucet, P. (2006). *A Sharper view: Evaluating the Vitality of Official Language Minority Communities*. Ottawa: Office of the Commissioner of Official Languages.

Kaplan, W. (1993). Who belongs? Changing concepts of citizenship and nationality. In W. Kaplan (Ed.), *Belonging: The meaning and future of Canadian citizenship*. Montreal: McGill-Queen's University Press.

Kirmayer, L. (2012). "Rethinking Cultural competence." *Transcultural Psychiatry*, 49, 149– 164.

Kymlicka, W. (1995). *Multicultural citizenship: A liberal theory of minority rights*. Oxford: Oxford University Press.

Landry, R. (2014) (Ed.). *La vie dans une langue officielle minoritaire au Canada.* Québec: Les Presses de l'Université Laval.

Landry, R., Allard, R., Deveau, K. (Eds.) (2013). *The vitality of the English-speaking Community of Quebec. A Sociolinguistic Profile of Secondary 4 Students in Quebec English Schools.* Ottawa : Canadian Heritage.

Leis, A., & Bouchard, L. (2013). « La santé des populations de langue officielle en situation minoritaire. » Editorial. *Canadian Journal of Public Health,* 104 (6) S3–S4.

Lemieux, V. (2013). *Le système de santé au Québec: Organisations, acteurs et enjeux.* Sainte-Foy, Québec: Presses de l'Université Laval.

Lussier, D., & Riel-Salvatore, H. (2014). Development of language tasks including the affective dimensions in a survey questionnaire defining health professional language competence. *12th International Conference on Communication in Healthcare.* Amsterdam, Netherlands.

Montaruli, E., Bourhis, R.Y., & Azurmendi, M.J. (2011). Identity, language, and ethnic relations in the Bilingual Autonomous Communities of Spain. *Journal of Sociolinguistics,* 15, 94– 121.

Montreuil, A., & Bourhis, R. (2004). "Acculturation orientations of competing host communities toward valued and devalued immigrants." *International Journal of Intercultural Relations,* 28, 507–532.

Montreal Gazette (2015a). Editorial: "Dark days for Quebec health care." February 9. http://montrealgazette.com/opinion/editorial-dark-days-for-quebec-health-care

Montreal Gazette (2015b). "Coalition of Anglophones groups satisfied with 'net gain' in Bill 10." G. Vendeville. February 9, 2015.

Montreal Gazette (2017). "Weil's appointment as anglos minister not an electoral move, Couillard insists." P. Authier. October 12, 2017.

Meuter, R., Gallois, C., Segalowitz, N., Ryder, A., & Hocking, J. (2015). "Overcoming language barriers in healthcare: a protocol for investigating safe and effective communication when patients or clinicians use a second language." *BMC Health Services Research,* 15, 371.

Navas, M.S., Fernandez, P., Rojas, A., & Garcia, M.C. (2007). "Acculturation strategies and attitudes according to the relative acculturation extended model: The perspective of Natives versus Immigrant." *International Journal of Intercultural Relations,* 31, 67–86.

Nguyen, A.D., & Benet-Martinez, V. (2013)." Biculturalism and Adjustment: A Meta-analysis". *Journal of Cross-Cultural Psychology,* 44, 122–159.

Ouimet, A.-M., Trempe, N., Vissandjée, B., & Hemlin, I. (2013). *Language adaptation in health care and health services: Issues and strategies.* Montréal: Institut national de santé publique du Québec.

Phillipson, R. (1988). "Linguicism: structures and ideologies in linguistic imperialism." T. Skutnabb-Kangas & J. Cummins (Eds.), *Minority*

Education: From shame to struggle. 339–358. Bristol, UK: Multilingual Matters

Pocock, J. & CHSSN Team (2016). Meeting the Challenge of Diversity in Health: The Networking and Partnership Approach of Quebec's English-speaking Minority. *Journal of Eastern Townships Studies,* 46.

Quebec (2006). *Cadre de référence pour l'élaboration des programmes d'accès aux services de santé et aux services sociaux en langue anglaise pour les personnes d'expression anglaise, 2002-2006.* Quebec: Santé et Services sociaux. www.msss.gouv.qc.ca

Quebec (2014). *Bill 10: An Act to modify the organization and governance of the health and social services network, in particular by abolishing the regional agencies.* Québec: 41st legislature of the National Assembly.14-010a.pdf. http://www.assnat.qc.ca

Ricento, T. (1998). National Language Policy in the United States. In T. Ricento & B. Burnaby (Eds.), *Language and Politics in the United States and Canada: Myths and Realities,*85–112. Mahwah, NJ: Lawrence Erlbaum.

Ricento, T. (2009). *An Introduction to Language Policy: Theory and Method.* New York: John Wiley.

Riel-Salvatore (2011). Le projet de formation et de maintien en poste des professionnels de la santé de l'Université McGill. *Actes du Colloque International du Plurilinguisme et Monde du Travail.* Journées des droit linguistiques. University of Teramo, Italy.

Rohmann, A., Florack, A., & Piontkowski, U. (2006). The role of discordant acculturation attitudes in perceived threat: An analysis of host and immigrant attitudes in Germany. *International Journal of Intercultural Relations,* 30, 683–702.

Sarver, J., & Baker, D.W. (2000). Effect of language barriers on follow-up appointments after and emergency department visit. *Journal of Internal Medicine,* 355, 229–231.

Schwartz, S.J. & J. B. Unger (Acculturation and Health: State of the field and recommended directiona. In S.J. Schwartz & J.B.Unger (Eds.) *The Oxford Handbook of Acculturation and Health.* 1–14. New York: Oxford University Press.

Senate Canada Report (2011). *The Vitality of Quebec's English-speaking communities: From myth to reality.* Ottawa: Report of the Standing Senate Committee on Official Languages.

Senior Times. *Quebec should create Anglo office, Fraser says.* Irwin Block, March 11, 2015, 7–8.

Shohamy, E. (2006). *Language Policy: Hidden agendas and new approaches.* London: Routledge.

Sioufi, R., Bourhis, R., & Allard, R. (2016). "Vitality and ethnolinguistic attitudes of Acadians, Franco-Ontarians and Francophone Quebecers: two or three solitudes in Canada's bilingual belt?" *Journal of Multilingual and Multicultural Development*, 37, 385–401.

Skutnabb-Kangas, T. (2000). *Linguistic genocide in education-or worldwide diversity and human rights?* Mahwah, NJ: Lawrence Erlbaum.

Snowden, A., & Cohen, J. (2011). *Strengthening Health Systems through Innovation: Lessons Learned.* Ottawa: International Centre for Health Innovation.

Stevenson, G. (1999). *Community Besieged. The Anglophone Minority and the Politics of Quebec.* Montreal: McGill-Queen's University Press.

Taylor, D.M., Caouette, J., Usborne, E., & Wright, S.C. (2008). Aboriginal Languages in Quebec: Fighting Linguicide with Bilingual Education. *Diversité Urbaine*, Autumn, 69–89.

Tremblay S., & Prata G. (2012). Study on linguistically and culturally adapted health services: a Pan-Canadian portrait. *Société Santé et Mieux-être en français du Nouveau Brunswick* (SSMEFNB).

Trempe, N., & Lussier, M.-H. (2011). *Knowledge and Use of the English Language by Healthcare and Social Services Professionals in Québec.* Montréal, Canada: Institut national de santé publique du Québec.

Vaillancourt, F., Lemay, D., & Vaillancourt, L. (2007). *Laggards No More: The Changed Socioeconomic Status of Francophones in Quebec.* Toronto: C.D. Howe Institute, No. 103. www.cdhowe.org

Watson, B.M., Hewett, D. G. & Gallois, C. (2012). Intergroup communication and Health Care. In H. Giles (Ed.), *The Handbook of Intergroup Communication.* 293–305. New York: Routledge.

Yeo, S. (2004). Language barriers and access to care. *Annual Review of Nursing Research*, 22, 59–75.

Zagefka, H., & Brown, R. (2002). The relationship between acculturation strategies and relative fit in intergroup relations: Immigrant-majority relations in Germany. *European Journal of Social Psychology*, 32, 171–188.

New Insights into Safe, Quality Services in Official Language Minority Communities

Pier Bouchard, *Université de Moncton,*
Jacinthe Savard, *University of Ottawa,*
Sébastien Savard, *University of Ottawa,*
Sylvain Vézina, *Université de Moncton,* and
Marie Drolet, *University of Ottawa*

Background

In this chapter we return to the theoretical framework underpinning this volume, the model of strategic analysis that contributes to a better understanding of the role of the actor and the system in making an active offer in the official language of the user's choice. Strategic analysis (Chapter 1) offers us new insights and knowledge based on the analyses and the various perspectives presented in these chapters. The model has proven to be valuable, especially as it can take account of the complexity of power and the rules that characterize and govern relations among the actors involved. It allows us to analyze the issues and challenges associated with the active offer of services in the official languages provided by the health and social service sector and, more broadly, with organized systems of action.

When they adopt this approach, researchers uncover the actors' objectives and strategies in order to comprehend the dynamics of their relationships and the coherence of the system of action. In our conclusion, we focus particularly on four key concepts of strategic analysis—issues, actors, systems, and strategies[1]—which connect the ideas and observations outlined in this volume. Putting the ideas into this perspective will enable us to do an in-depth analysis of our subject: the accessibility and the active offer of services in official language minority communities (see Table 1).

Table 1. Strategic Analysis and General Reference Framework

Issues of accessibility and the active offer of French-language services in linguistic minority communities	
Issues of communication, quality and safety of services, language rights, organizational issues, bilingualism, shortage of Francophone or francophile professionals, etc.	
Actors	**System**
Expectations and objectives of actors, attitudes, opinions, interests, actions, possible solutions.	Symbolic structure, political structure, policy and regulatory structure, organizational structure, and service trajectory.
Key actorsOLMC, SSF, CNFS, QCGN Health Canada, departments and ministries, educational institutions, facilities, managers, professionals and service providers, individuals and/or natural caregivers, community organizations, etc.	*Charter*, Official Languages Acts, Roadmap, public policy, responsibilities, process and practices of active offer, etc.
Dynamics and interplay of actors	
Rationality of behaviours, assets of actors, zones of uncertainty, influence, strategies and interplay of actors, dependence and interdependence, power relations, conflicts, system of action	
Strategies used by actors to foster active offer	
Policy levers and legal measures Education and engagement of future professionals to promote active offer Organizational culture that fosters active offer Leadership of social actors and the community Attraction and retention of bilingual service providers Mobilization, collaboration, and networking	

Issues

Each of the chapters in this volume discuss one or several issues related to the health and well-being of official language minority communities (OLMCs) and, in particular, Francophone minority communities (FMC). The core issue for the authors is that of access to social services and health care in the user's language. It is especially important that services be of comparable quality to those offered to the majority. Access to these services is considered essential because of the link that has been established between language and the quality and safety of services; it also enhances the vitality of OLMC communities by providing an opportunity to use and affirm an individual's language rights. According to a number of people, access to these services can only be achieved when active offer practices are developed.

The second issue dealt with in this volume is the active offer of social services and health services in the official language of the minority. What OLMCs want is a health and social service system that recognizes their language and culture, one in which all members of the public are informed from the moment they enter or contact a point of service that services can be received in the official language of their choice. This should happen without a user's having to ask for those services. For Francophones in Canada, a desire to halt the process of assimilation and to acknowledge the vulnerability of people in communities that are often isolated underlies active offer.

The issue of having the linguistic majority population recognize the needs of OLMCs was clearly described. The majority language group still tends to be unaware of the particular needs of members of the linguistic minority, since in some regions most members of OLMCs are bilingual, or will include linguistic minority communities in the overall category of minority groups or "other" cultures, towards which there is a certain awareness and cultural sensitivity.

Besides the issue of quality of services, there is another more specific issue: that of users' safety. A close link has been established between the quality of communication and safety, so the challenge is to eliminate or at least reduce the language barriers that threaten the safety of social service and health care users. These barriers affect the quality of communication and trust in the relationship between the individual and the service provider. In Francophone minority communities, literacy is a major challenge for communication (see Chapter 5). By promoting active offer, FMCs want to be able to guarantee safe, quality services (Chapter 4; Chapter 5). In Canada, communication in both official languages is an essential element of quality and safety of services.

Another issue is the lack of appropriate resources for evaluating and responding to the needs of these communities (Chapter 8). Lagacé and Lefebvre (Chapter 13) list examples of elements that should be taken into consideration in speech-language pathology and/or audiology assessments of Francophone children who live in linguistic minority contexts and have been raised in a bilingual environment.

This leads us to issues concerning the resources available in the health and social service sector and in OLMCs. In terms of access to financial and human resources, the issue of bilingual staff is a concern for many researchers in this volume. Evidently, the shortage of bilingual staff—or simply a poor use of these employees—and the fact that they often suffer from overwork and professional burnout are serious problems. Some of the chapters in this volume highlight the multiple challenges bilingual staff members must deal with and the impact the challenges have on related matters such as recruitment and retention (Chapter 8: Chapter 9). Organizational support can definitely help staff meet these challenges (Chapter 7; Chapter 12) but, as Vézina points out (Chapter 10), we should be cautious since, paradoxically, emphasis on bilingualism can negatively affect the implementation of active offer when unilingual staff members show resistance to increasing bilingual positions and services.

The last issue to raise in this category is that of the awareness and preparation of professionals in post-secondary programs and in the labour force. The objective here is to better prepare professionals to work in linguistic minority settings (Chapter 2; Chapter 11). This involves defining and proposing appropriate strategies. Actors are at the centre of a process to co-construct the concept of active offer, and especially to improve the health and social service sector, which relies on an active offer of services in the official language of the minority.

Relations Among Actors

In this section, we hope to define the role of the actors involved who, each in their own way, advocate for and protect their own particular interests within a complex system. To properly explain the system we are studying—that is, every component related to the delivery of social and health services in OLMCs—we will begin with an outline of the primary actors involved, the interests they protect, the resources and assets they have to help them reach their objectives, and the limitations and barriers they must deal with. After presenting the actors' characteristics we will try to describe the way the system of action operates, and how it has developed out of the interactions and interdependent actions of the actors.

Actors Involved

The *official language minority communities* (OLMCs) are the central player of this system. Their objectives are to receive quality, safe health care and social services when they face health or social challenges. OLMCs have a number of characteristics, resources, and assets that play in their favour and help them protect their interests. First, the use of either of Canada's official languages is protected by the *constitution of Canada*, through the *Canadian Charter of Rights and Freedoms* enshrined therein, as well as by provincial laws and policies (Chapter 3). Federal, provincial, and territorial governments cannot neglect the rights and needs of OLMCs, which are protected by important Canadian laws (Chapter 4; Chapter 7). For example, French minority communities have demonstrated their ability to rally together for important causes, and this has enabled them to dedicate energetic and visible efforts when action is necessary, as was the case in the famous 1997 Hôpital Montfort affair in Ottawa, when the community was able to have the provincial government's decision to close the only French-language hospital in the area overturned after a high-profile campaign. On the other hand, communities must also deal with substantial limitations. The first of these is their low numbers and the fact they are spread out over a very large territory. Since they are often a small minority of the population, it is harder for them to make their needs a priority, or even have them acknowledged, in the various communities where they live. The case of New Brunswick is unique in this respect because Francophones comprise one-third of the population; this gives the French-speaking population a significant power to exert influence on the system.

Users in OLMCs often suffer from what might be called a complex, stemming from their minority status. As a result, they do not always feel it is appropriate to advocate for their rights or the services to which they are entitled (Chapter 2; Chapter 6). For example, people in FMCs often accept that not being able to obtain services in their own language is a fact of life that comes with living in a province with an Anglophone majority. When they find themselves in a situation where they are highly vulnerable, such as when they are facing a health problem, a psychological crisis, or a social issue, some OLMC users are not comfortable or confident enough to ask for services in their own language out of fear that a negative reaction might be reflected in a poorer quality of services or significant delays before being treated. This behaviour, which is reasonable from the perspective of someone in the minority group, has the perverse effect of being interpreted by actors in the majority group as proof there is no real need for services in the minority language and, therefore, as justification for the status quo.

The federal government and provincial/territorial governments are responsible for funding and structuring the distribution and organization of health care and social services to the population. They have legislative and regulatory powers to determine the rules of the game, allowing them to mandate the active offer of services and to enforce the rights of official language communities. Governments are elected officials, and have the legitimate right to intervene in the lives of their citizens. On the other hand, their power is fragile, and the asset of their democratic mandate must also be viewed as a limitation: their citizens can easily vote to replace the elected officials who represent them in the next election. Because of this, governments tend to be cautious and to make decisions that will solve or attenuate the problems of the electorate and improve their living conditions. At the same time they attempt to make sure that the solutions they propose will be understood and accepted by voters. Resources they can use to fund public programs are also limited, given that increasing taxes is rather unpopular with citizens and businesses. The needs that have to be met are not limited, however; they are constantly increasing. Governments have to make choices about the use of public funding and this inevitably upsets some individuals or groups. Often the people with the least influence are the ones most affected by the decisions.

Managers of health care and social service facilities have the responsibility to offer adequate services to the population within a limited budget, legislative constraints, and complex and rigid collective agreements. When a specific group, such as an OLMC, asks for special measures to respond to a specific need, managers have to decide whether that need is enough of a priority to justify investing the necessary money, given the fact that they are accountable for the funds and this might mean cutting other expenditures or services in the organization. Depending on their position in the hierarchy, they have some leeway in their actions and have decision-making power—which may be limited but is also real—and the capacity to allocate resources and formulate policies within their organization.

In facilities designated as bilingual, or in areas where numbers warrant, managers are also obligated to provide a set minimum of services in the official languages. If they do not, they may be accused of putting patient safety at risk or exposed to legal consequences. Because of this, they want to recruit bilingual employees, yet they remain concerned about the challenges associated with bilingual-designated positions. Staffing these positions creates challenges in organizing the workload, greater mobilization of resources, and, as Vézina (Chapter 10) points out, tensions between bilingual and unilingual employees in the workplace. The multiple, inter-related levels of management add to the complexity of these relationships, because managers of different units and departments are constantly competing for resources that are limited, if not rationed. Since organizational support is essential if professionals in a facility are to be able to actively offer services (Chapter 12), there is a crucial zone of uncertainty whenever an individual tries to increase behaviours that promote active offer.

Bilingual service providers must offer services in both official languages to the population served by their facility if the province or facility in which they work officially mandates it. They at least have the advantage of speaking the minority language, which gives them some control over the zone of uncertainty. As Drolet *et al.* (Chapter 6) mention, they can create a form of alliance or complicity with their clientele and this can exert pressure on organizations to improve service delivery to OLMCs. They often want to contribute to an increase in services in the minority languages and even to be able to work in their mother tongue. When the facility is designated bilingual, they have better access to permanent positions and opportunities for promotion since they are sought after for a rare and in-demand competency (Chapter 9). Their privileged status can provoke envy and resentment on the part of unilingual employees. It can also happen that their employer refuses to let them leave to take on another position that is not designated bilingual because they are precious assets in their current position. Bilingual service providers frequently face excessive workloads because they are asked to act as interpreters for their unilingual colleagues (Chapter 2; Chapter 8), which may lead them to hide the fact they are bilingual in organizations where this competency is not valued and/or its implications are not acknowledged.

Unilingual service providers occupy the largest number of positions in the system, including management positions. Some unilingual employees are opposed to the active offer of services in both official languages. They would prefer these services not play such a large role in the organization as they are afraid their inability to respond to the demand will hamper their opportunity to advance in their careers. Some do not like the idea of active offer becoming an official organizational policy: they will react negatively, and sometimes aggressively, to any increase in the visibility of the minority language in the work place, and they have strength of numbers— the advantage of working in an environment in which operations basically take place in the language of the majority. This privilege seems completely natural to them.

Dynamics of Actors

Members of OLMCs want to receive services in their language because this access can have a significant impact on their health, well-being, and living conditions. Where there are sufficient numbers of OLMC members they can create community organizations to affirm their rights. These groups can exert pressure on leaders and decision-makers in the public sector to allocate the resources necessary to respond to their needs, since their rights are protected under the *Canadian Charter of Rights and Freedoms* and by certain provisions in provincial and territorial legislation (Chapter 3; Chapter 7).

Nonetheless, when a language community is very small, it represents a meagre percentage of the electorate and has a limited ability to exert pressure. Governments have to listen to the minority in order to have a proper understanding of their cause since members of the community can appeal to the courts to force governments to introduce policies and measures to comply with legislation—for instance, asking for an organization to be designated bilingual as in

Ontario, or, as in New Brunswick, lobbying for health authorities to be established according to specific language parameters. Still, deciding to allocate resources for services to OLMCs can prove to be contentious when it upsets a segment of the linguistic majority; they may well resent the fact that a smaller community monopolizes available resources.

In certain regions where there is a significant concentration of the minority population, OLMCs can organize to act as a pressure group. Governments are more likely to provide resources to health care and social service facilities so they will be able to put active offer and linguistically appropriate services into place. Because these facilities are constantly short of resources to fulfill their mission, they will accept and, in certain cases, advocate for and benefit from these resources.

All the same, with these resources comes the obligation to recruit bilingual employees and offer them positions that are designated bilingual. This is often a major challenge, particularly in rural and/or remote areas where the shortage of qualified service providers is a reality that even affects recruitment from the majority group (Chapter 9). Sometimes the difficulty in finding bilingual service providers will lead managers to hire unilingual employees on the condition that they learn the minority language once they are working. Results of this strategy are often disappointing because a number of employees who start learning a second language will abandon their plans and because there are few definitive measures in place to ensure compliance with this hiring condition. Managers do not want to put too much effort into controlling language standards, especially since the results are likely to confront them with realities that are hard to deal with. They may have to dismiss employees and/or hire other bilingual employees, the latter of which is hard to do when there is an inadequate pool of resources. Moreover, dismissals are apt to fuel resentment among unilingual professionals who feel that staffing bilingual positions is a concession to political pressure rather than an effort to meet a true need in the population.

Indeed, unilingual employees tend to believe there are enough colleagues who can offer services in both official languages without the organization creating more positions reserved for bilingual staff; the demand does not seem to justify it. Many believe there is no problem, because users can communicate without much difficulty in the language of the majority. They do not realize the importance of providing services in both official languages in order for users from the minority to have quality services and, in particular, to ensure their safety.

On the other hand, managers, like service providers, are responsible for maintaining quality and safety when they deliver services, and this requires effective communication. They are also obligated to behave ethically; this means, among other things, taking measures for informed consent on the part of the user and protection of the user's confidentiality. A number of testimonials reveal failures in professional ethics and situations that compromise patient safety, due to the lack of adequate services in the minority language. These failures represent a significant zone of uncertainty, which is open to the influence of decisions designed to tilt the system in favour of active offer.

System and Levers of Action

In order to describe the system of health care and social services and the levers of action actors in this system have available to them, we first turned to Champagne, Contandriopoulos, Picot-Touché, Béland, and Nguyen (2005). These authors describe the health care system as an organized system of actions in which various *structures* (physical, organizational, symbolic) define a social space where four major groups of *actors* (professionals, managers, commercial representatives, and political representatives) interact in order to accomplish collective projects that contribute to achieve the ends of the system. Moreover, following the Chronic Care Model (CCM) developed by Wagner and his colleagues in 1996, and a variation of this model known as the Expanded Chronic Care Model (ECCM) (McCurdy, MacKay, Badley, Veinot, & Cott, 2008),[2] we recognize that the person seeking services and/or the person's caregivers and the community to which they belong are active actors in the system. In addition, to ensure continuity of services in the official minority language during a person's service trajectory, we need to consider integration of services and coordination mechanisms between various service organizations (Couturier, Gagnon, Belzile, & Salles, 2013; Tremblay, Angus, & Hubert, 2012).

Inspired by these authors, we present our own model developed by the GReFoPS (Savard *et al.*, 2017) to illustrate levers of actions available to OLMCs to promote active offer of services in the official minority language. At the centre of this model, illustrated in Figure 1, is the service trajectory that consists of the encounter(s) of one or more health or social service provider(s) and the person seeking a service. This user is often supported by one or more caregiver(s) who may or may not be present during the encounter. The two primary groups of actors evolve in a social space influenced by different types of structures that we categorized as follows:

- A symbolic structure, comprising values, beliefs, and representations of society, including the image of health care and social services as well as equity, etc.
- A political and regulatory system, comprising laws, regulations, and ministerial directives governing the health and social service system in each province or territory. The numerous reforms of the health care system desired by the actors involved in it are generally accomplished through legal amendments and new regulations and directives that, in turn, shape organizational structures. Organizational structures, comprise rules that determine the distribution and organization of resources as well as the volume and type of resources in each facility that offers services.

It should be noted here that care and services are delivered within a given community. Besides formal health and social service organizations, communities may also create services structured by their own organizational rules, such as social and economic organizations, and support groups.

A more in-depth analysis of each of these structures allows us to better understand how the health care and social services system operates and where the actors within the system play their roles.

Symbolic Structure

The importance society places on health and social justice—its representations of health and its determinants, its conception of regulation, and its ideas about the responsibilities and the roles of actors (for example, the role of the government vs. individual responsibility)—are symbolic elements influencing health policies and the organization of health and social service systems. They also influence the way each of the actors in the system perceives his or her own role

Figure 1. Framework for the Analysis of Health and Social Services Access and Integration for Official Language Minority Communities

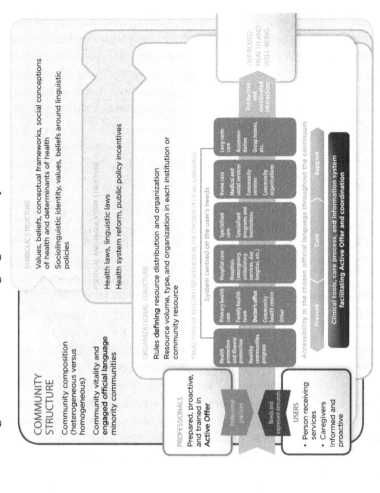

Source: Savard et al., 2017.
Inspired by: Barr et al., 2003; Champagne et al., 2005; Couturier et al., 2013; Tremblay et al., 2012

in the system. For example, as infectious and short-term illnesses decrease and chronic diseases increase, we are witnessing a shift in perception toward giving individuals greater responsibility to determine their own health outcomes and lifestyle choices. These changes in collective values bring about a transformation in the health and social service system, leading to greater cooperation between the person, her or his close caregivers, and service providers (Bodenheimer *et al.*, 2002). In the twenty-first century, person-centred or patient-centred care, user satisfaction, access to care for disadvantaged populations and vulnerable persons, and patient safety are important values in our health and social service system.[3] Moreover, various efforts are observed whereby appropriate, responsive care is adapted in a cultural perspective.

For its part, the Government of Canada recognizes linguistic duality as a basic element of Canadian identity and supports a number of initiatives to assist official language minority communities; the *Roadmap for Canada's Official Languages 2013–2018* (Canadian Heritage, 2013) is a good example. The importance placed on this value varies considerably within the Canadian population, however, and this is true for Francophones as well as Anglophones.

It would certainly be desirable for the language of the minority and the identity construction of OLMCs to have greater value and prominence. This could stimulate the OLMC's demand for services and lead to a greater awareness of the needs of these communities on the part of actors within the majority group. For service providers from the minority, a greater affirmation of their identity could encourage them to act more confidently in favour of active offer. However, wagering on the value of bilingualism and the affirmation of OLMCs would limit the zone of influence toward linguistically appropriate services, because bilingualism is sometimes a source of tension, as Vézina (Chapter 10) points out.

Political and Regulatory Structure

The political and regulatory structure comprises laws, regulations, and ministerial directives governing the health and social service system on the national level and in each of the provinces and territories. This may include laws or policies specifically addressing the provision of health care and social services such as the *Canada Health Act*, laws and policies related to health care and social services in different provinces, or laws with a larger scope that affect activities and operation in several fields (for example, Canada's *Official Languages Act* or language laws and policies in various provinces). Several authors in this volume have described ways in which the legal context has influenced the development of social services and health services in French in OLMCs. Laws and policies vary from one province to another and provide a restrictive or broad legal framework that has an impact on the planning of French language services. For instance, there may be an obligation to offer services in French, or simply an obligation to consult Francophone community groups without a stipulation to provide particular services in French. Changes in health care policies, such as those that are part of reforms designed to place the user—both the person receiving services and that person's family and/or close caregivers—also contribute to the political and regulatory structure.

Organizational Structure

Organizational structure, which deals with the quantity, volume and distribution of human, physical, and financial resources allocated to health care and social services, is influenced by the political and regulatory structure. But within the policies, regulations, and directives there is a certain amount of leeway for managers to decide how to organize resources they are asked to manage. Another element in the organizational structure is the formal links established by managers to coordinate the services offered by different resources. Resources are distributed and divided in various ways, among different geographical territories: public, private, and community services; primary, secondary, and tertiary care; and a range of client groups. When managers overlook the variable of language while making decisions about the distribution of resources, their decisions can have a negative impact on access to services in the official language of one's choice.

In several chapters (Chapter 7; Chapter 9; Chapter 10), the authors clearly demonstrate how organizational culture and leadership plays a vital role in ensuring linguistically appropriate services. Similarly, the distribution of resources among public, private, and community services may have an influence on access to services because, even in provinces that regulate the language of services, private services are rarely subject to these rules. Another example is the allocation of resources to highly specialized services, especially in the area of medical care. Decisions can result in bilingual resources being dispersed too widely among different organizations, each one with a mandate to treat a specific social or health problem. Counter-balancing this situation are organizations with broad mandates and sensitivity to the linguistic dimension that may have, overall, sufficient bilingual staff members; even these facilities might not distribute human resources evenly and appropriately, and therefore may be unable to provide and coordinate services in both official languages on a regular basis.

The lack of bilingual service providers, and in particular professionals equipped to deal with the challenges of active offer, remain a very real problem in some OLMCs. In this regard, the *Consortium national de formation en santé* (CNFS) is an important resource for educational institutions that train future professionals (Chapter 2; Chapter 11). However, increasing the number of professionals capable of expressing themselves in both official languages is an inadequate solution if these resources are not used effectively (Chapter 5; Chapter 9). For optimal human resource planning, it is absolutely essential to understand the needs and interests of these professionals, attract them to facilities offering services in the minority language, and give them recognition and support their work, so they can work effectively and efficiently and facilitate equitable access to services.

Community Resources

Improving population health is not solely the responsibility of the health system; rather, it depends on multidisciplinary and multi-sectoral actions, including healthy and positive living environments, strong community action, and public policies fostering health and well-being (Barr *et al.*, 2003). Informal actions such as relationships with neighbours, which offer social support to members of the community, can have a positive impact on health. Formal community actions can be organized through different groups able to express the needs they have observed in the community to the appropriate authorities and advocate for the allocation of public resources for specific issues, or attenuate a lack of service by creating social economy enterprises, support groups, peer services for people experiencing similar difficulties, etc. In this context, the linguistic vitality[4] of OLMCs can play an important role in providing access to linguistically appropriate services.

Service Trajectory

Productive interaction in the trajectory of care and services involves collaboration among the person seeking services, that person's caregivers, and service providers, as well as coordination between various service organizations to promote access to services in the chosen official language throughout the continuum. This interaction will be positive if the following conditions are met:

- First, the service provider is proactive, open to networking and to a multifaceted, multistrategy approach, able to actively offer services in both official languages by personally providing service in the user's language or directing the user to an appropriate resource. In addition, clinical tools available to the provider facilitate the process of active offer and coordination of services. It should be remembered here that the interaction between a professional and the person seeking services often takes place in a private space and is not observed by others. This implies that education is needed so that the professional has integrated the value of active offer. Some think that this cannot be achieved through coercion.
- Second, the person and the family or close caregivers are well informed and equipped to manage the patient's chronic health condition, and are also informed of the importance of good communication to quality and safety of care and services. These people will be, as a result, proactive in the decisions that affect them, and capable of understanding and following the recommendations to help them improve their health and living conditions, but also capable of affirming their need for certain procedures to take place in their own language.

These two groups do not operate in a vacuum. People supported by a strong community are more likely to make their needs known (Forgues & Landry, 2014). Service providers supported by their organization or facility will find it easier to actively offer services (Chapter 12). Additionally, knowing that chronic diseases are becoming more prevalent, the likelihood that an individual will need to consult and be treated by several different professionals working in more than one organization in the institutional and community network is very high. In order for the trajectory of care and service to be seamless and uninterrupted, collaborative measures among service providers, and methods to coordinate them, need to be developed—including referral mechanisms that take the language variable into account. In this sense, a single person cannot be responsible for active offer along the entire continuum of care and services. The political and regulatory structure, as well as the organizational structure, must facilitate the coordination of services.

Strategies Promoting Active Offer

In this volume, the authors emphasize the importance of using various strategies to facilitate progress in the active offer of services in both official languages. Therefore, we have outlined their main ideas according to six strategies: legal and political levers; education and engagement of future professionals; organizational culture oriented toward active offer; the leadership of social actors and the community; measures to attract and retain service providers; and mobilization and collaboration among the actors (see Figure 2).

Legal and Political Levers

In the past, representatives of Francophone minority communities primarily relied on legal measures to protect their interests. Indeed, important advances made in one province, such as the favourable court decision at the end of the struggle to save the Hôpital Montfort in Ontario, have served to encourage Francophone communities in other provinces to assert their rights. By rallying actors around language issues, FMCs have succeeded in making concrete progress, and can be expected to advocate and organize to have the right to health[5] fully recognized at the national and provincial levels; language rights in health and social services will then be able to be grafted to the laws and policies that stem from this right. Legal resources (*Canadian Charter of Rights and Freedoms*, Acts, policies, etc.) thus represent an essential lever for OLMCs as they determine their strategies.

414

Figure 2. Six Strategies to Foster Active Offer

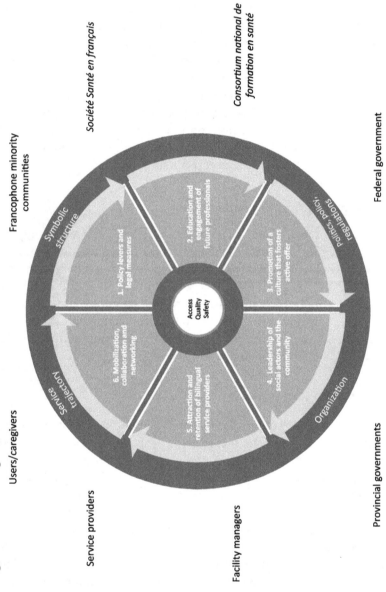

Users/caregivers

Francophone minority communities

Société Santé en français

Service providers

Symbolic structure

1. Policy levers and legal measures

2. Education and engagement of future professionals

3. Promotion of a culture that fosters active offer

Access Quality Safety

Politics, policy, regulations

Consortium national de formation en santé

Federal government

6. Mobilization, collaboration and networking

5. Attraction and retention of bilingual service providers

4. Leadership of social actors and the community

Service trajectory

Organization

Facility managers

Provincial governments

More specifically, actors have designed and proposed different ways to improve French-language services (plans for the development thereof, position of French-language services Commissioner, representation on boards of directors in organizations, lines of accountability, etc.). As Foucher (Chapter 3) points out, despite this progress, we are still a long way from a situation in which citizens in a minority context can "be born, live, be cared for, and die" in their own official language.

In other words, the existence of a favourable legal framework is not enough. It has to be accompanied by political will and a true engagement of actors if the respect for language rights and the active offer of services in the language of the minority population is to actually become a reality. In Chapter 7, Forgues shows that applying language rights remains a complex process involving multiple factors: social, economic, cultural, and political. Organizations operating in a minority context are more effective to the extent that they are able to mobilize and build power relationships, bargaining power, and influence that work in their favour.

Similarly, we have noted that active offer is not a neutral principle and cannot be reduced to a management technique. As Cardinal *et al.* (Chapter 4) observed in the justice sector, active offer has a political dimension since it is subject to a continuing debate between community and governmental actors. Active offer is a principle that informs approaches to management, justice, and development. It relies on policies and directives, service planning, and accountability. On the whole, these observations confirm that the rules of the game shape and condition the strategies of actors who, in turn, are shaped and conditioned by these strategies (Crozier & Friedberg, 1977, p. 212).

Strategies to Educate and Engage Future Professionals

Bouchard *et al.* (Chapter 2) described the way strategic analysis acted as a source of inspiration throughout their project to prepare and equip students in professional programs. They presented a strategy based on this model to educate future professionals; the strategy has been used by the CNFS since 2008 to integrate the values and principles of active offer into post-secondary professional programs. Its long-term objectives are for future professionals to have a greater influence on the setting where they will be working after they graduate, and to play a leadership role, as change makers, to improve the quality of French-language services in every region of the country. The strategy could be summarized as follows: Improving French-language health services necessarily involves the mobilization and engagement of future professionals. At the outset, the educational project sought to document the issues and challenges of active offer and potential solutions to develop practices to improve the active offer of French-language services in minority language settings. Along the way, the project generated a profile of competencies (knowledge, skills, attitudes) suitable for preparing students to take up the challenges of organizing and delivering French-language health care and social services. Among the strategies and solutions identified are engagement and mobilization, identity construction, and the development of learning resources.

This action research project also allowed us to identify a number of zones of uncertainty, in particular those where managers can exercise their power to create a culture oriented towards active offer, by introducing measures ranging from schedules planned in a way that takes language needs into consideration to incentives such as bilingualism bonuses. The research shows that new professionals educated about active offer need to be able to count on organizational support if they are to integrate it into their practice.

New initiatives, such as a developing a reference framework and designing an online tool box to contribute to education on active offer have been undertaken by the CNFS. This information and expertise are becoming sources of power to assist future Francophone, bilingual, and other supportive professionals to protect the interests of FMCs, and thus to reinforce their power within the system of action. Inspired by Crozier's studies, the process for developing these initiatives respected the need to listen attentively to citizens and communities.[6] The process laid the foundation for an educational strategy aligned with one of the goals of the national secretariat of the CNFS, which was to bring the perspectives of different actors from the system into the classroom (for instance by sharing the testimonials of patients and people who have benefited from services), an element facilitated by the creation of the online tool box for the active offer (http://www.offreactive.com/).

We should also mention that actors continue to refine their strategies as they proceed and as they become more aware of the symbolic structure—whether or not they labelled it this way—within which they operate. Analyzing their discourse demonstrates that, over the last few years, many actors have focused on the quality and safety of services rather than on language rights. This allows them to benefit from recent reforms in health care and social service that are person-centred and place the concerns and needs of users at the centre of the system. In this regard, it is interesting to note that during a forum on the quality and safety of health care services in New Brunswick (Bouchard, March 2015), managers were eager to share the efforts they have been making to create a patient-centred culture. Such an approach includes promoting active offer practices and responding to the needs of people in the official language minority group.

Dubouloz *et al.* (Chapter 11) are exploring the needs of professors who play a key role in the education of future professionals. It is important to provide appropriate and useful education and training to professors so they can then prepare and equip their students for professional practice and action in their workplace. The authors propose a conceptual framework for active offer, based on theoretical perspectives defining three types of knowledge (knowledge, skills, and attitudes/people skills) intrinsic to professional competency. Following this line of thinking, structuring the education of professors and instructors who teach in professional programs in a way that integrates the three types of knowledge, and also gives professors a full understanding of active offer, will make it possible for them to help their students learn this content. What results is the knowledge to act: the capacity of the professional to put active offer into practice, to demonstrate leadership skills, and to play a more active role as a change maker in the workplace.

The research of Savard *et al.* (Chapter 12) is also interesting in this respect. Their studies propose tools to evaluate education and training, by assessing active offer behaviours. The authors outline indicators of behaviours associated with the active offer of French-language health care and social services in minority language settings, and discuss tools to measure active offer. By comparing measurements of active offer behaviours among students and professionals to results obtained from other questionnaires, they were able to outline some of the determinants of active offer in official language minority settings.

Of note was the authors' observation that service providers adopted behaviours favourable to active offer that seemed to depend largely on environmental factors (legislative provisions and organizational cultures), as well as on personal factors such as the affirmation of their identity and their proficiency in French. More familiarity with these factors should contribute to awareness and educational strategies that are better adapted to the needs of different target groups (legislators, managers, service providers). In future studies, it will be possible to refine the questionnaires used to define the factors that promote and encourage a commitment to active offer. Development of a tool is planned that will guide learners towards the specific education, training, and targeted awareness activities that are most appropriate for individual needs and circumstances.

In short, several authors in this volume concur with the idea that in order to design a more linguistically and culturally appropriate system, the first step is to address future graduates of health and social service programs by giving them, during their studies, the information and resources they will need. The educational strategy must include new course content; this means developing new knowledge and expertise among future professionals and managers who will be called upon to be ambassadors of active offer in the field. If knowledge is power, as the model of strategic analysis suggests, we have every reason to believe that future graduates will be playing a decisive role in actively offering and promoting linguistically appropriate services. In fact, as Crozier and Friedberg have illustrated with a well-known case of a state-owned tobacco monopoly, the fact that someone possesses expertise (that is competency) that is hard to replace within an organization can be a great source of power. Moreover, the expert is "the only person who has the skills, the knowledge, and the experience in that particular context to be able to resolve certain crucial problems in the organization" (Crozier & Friedberg, 1977, p. 72).

Promoting an Organizational Culture Oriented Toward Active Offer

The analysis of the symbolic structure demonstrated that the value of bilingualism founded on two official languages is not shared equally within the Canadian population. If we are to make significant progress, it would be strategic to appeal to values shared by the majority when we are determining actions that can be taken to help OLMCs. Among the shared values discovered by researchers are: protecting vulnerable people, providing culturally appropriate services, and protecting patient safety; ensuring quality of care and services; fostering collaboration between the person, the person's caregivers, and service providers; and empowering individuals and increasing their capacity to improve their living conditions.

This is what Vézina (Chapter 10) proposes when he examines active offer under the lens of organizational culture, considered a construct in and of itself, just as are the organizational rules of the game. The author believes the idea of a culture centred on bilingualism should be abandoned and replaced by a culture oriented toward active offer. This sort of culture could be positive for OLMCs in that it integrates the values of safety and quality of services in both official languages. In this context, bilingualism becomes a tool among others. The author feels that this shift will foster the support, and perhaps even the engagement and collaboration, of unilingual individuals. Furthermore, adopting values associated with active offer, notably the value of safety, will motivate managers to take the measures required to organize services to promote active offer and to encourage their staff to actively offer these services.

Making actors in the majority language group more aware of the fact that language barriers can represent a major deterrent to health and health care and that they are contradictory to patient-centred practices could, then, be an important lever for action in OLMCs. The language barrier could cause a medical error or make the user more passive when receiving psychological and social treatments. Awareness about language issues can be raised through key messages on quality and safety, which are shared and repeated, using government vocabulary (engaging the population, patient-centred care, putting the patient at the centre of the health system, etc.). The fact that linguistically sensitive services tend to result in greater satisfaction with the care received (Tremblay & Prata, 2012, p. 38) could also be mentioned.

The studies discussed by Savard *et al.* (Chapter 12) show that organizational support influences active offer behaviour. Their research illustrates the importance of making managers and administrators of facilities more aware of new practices in active offer so they can transform organizational culture accordingly. In fact, several authors in this volume argue the commitment of the administration and managers is a key element in progress toward linguistically responsive services. Savard *et al.* (Chapter 12) offer a self-assessment tool that actors interested in the subject can use to improve their practices.

When this new organizational culture affects a greater number of actors, it will be possible to reach not only the organizations that deliver services, but also regional and provincial organizations responsible for the distribution of resources and those that exert influence on political, regulatory, and policy structures. OLMCs may then be able to benefit from new management trends such as reforms centring on the needs of patients. If putting the patient (the person, family, and/ or close caregivers) at the centre of care and services involves policy and administrative restructuring, would this not be an opportune time to propose reforms that recognize the linguistic needs of people, to implement measures to meet these needs in innovative ways, and (especially) to eliminate systemic barriers that negatively affect access to and coordination of services in one's own language along the full continuum of care? For example, we could re-examine the obligation to consult the community and the parameters of designation. When users reside in a certain geographical area where they do not have access to service in both official languages, for instance, services may be available in a neighbouring area; in urban settings, the neighbouring area might be only a few blocks away.

Leadership of Social Actors and Communities

In discussing strategies to improve services, Drolet *et al.* (Chapter 6) recommend developing leadership on two levels. The first level is the leadership of social actors and the community in stimulating the demand for French-language services. The second is the leadership of facilities and decision-makers in organizing services in a way that introduces practices of active offer of French-language services along the entire continuum of care and services. An interesting change appears to be taking place within organizations in terms of the interaction between two partners (the service provider and the person receiving services). From a paradigm of urgent or short-term care characterized by a relationship between an "expert service provider" and a "passive client," there seems to be a shift towards a paradigm of cooperation engaging the person concerned, the person's caregivers, and health and social services providers. In this new context, the professional serves the person and his or her caregivers, who are at the centre of the system; of interest to us here, this includes actively offering services. Once service providers are better educated, prepared, and proactive, it will be easier to envisage changes in their behaviour that contribute to the promotion of active offer and improvements in the living conditions of the people who consult them.

The person who is seeking services is also an important actor in this relationship. In a sense, when an individual or a dyad—an individual and a family member or caregiver—has a better understanding of the importance of receiving services in one's own language, they will also exert influence on the dynamics of this relationship by affirming the need with the service provider. The vitality of the OLMC also facilitates the expression of this need. Indeed, a person living in a minority community is more likely to affirm a need if the environment allows him or her to feel comfortable speaking the chosen language and has a sense that the situation can change and improve (Giles, Bourhis, & Taylor, 1977, in Forgues & Landry, 2014, p. 98). In other words, several new ideas and initiatives have been designed to improve the effectiveness of care and services; they are founded on an egalitarian and dynamic model of the relationship between the service provider and the person and/or caregiver. Therefore, the work of a number of authors in this volume gives us reason to believe we are currently witnessing an important transformation in the system of action. The strategies suggested highlight the importance of focusing efforts on the four dimensions described in *Preventing and Managing Chronic Disease: Ontario's Framework*. They are: strong leadership, aligned resources and incentives, commitment to quality improvement, and accountability for outcomes.

Recruiting and Retaining Bilingual Social Service and Health Care Providers in Minority Communities

The authors of Chapter 9 (Savard *et al.*) argue that the difficulty of recruiting professionals is one of the primary barriers to the linguistic minority population's access to services in their own language. Their study explored the important elements that characterize the conditions of bilingual professionals working in the field of health and social service with members of OLMCs. They also examined factors that facilitated recruitment and retention in a bilingual workplace. Complementing the studies presented by de Moissac *et al.* (Chapter 8), their research was designed to capture information about the expectations and perspectives of bilingual professionals working in two minority language settings.

Due to the predominance of one of the official languages, the reality of work in a bilingual environment poses a number of challenges. Thus, bilingualism can be difficult to put into practice. The authors formulate recommendations for strategies that should be considered by the primary groups of actors involved in improving the recruitment and retention of bilingual staff in bilingual facilities in minority context. Here is a summary of the recommendations for each of the primary groups of actors:

- For bilingual employees, creating informal networks among colleagues in the minority language group may encourage them to use their language. This kind of network may also contribute to enhancing their sense of belonging to their OLMC.
- Employers should be proactive in ensuring that services are actually available in the language of the minority. They must take concrete action to: (1) hire a larger number of bilingual professionals, supervisors, and managers; (2) offer language training for employees to learn both official languages and monitor progress and use, and offer professional development in both official languages to professionals in the facility; (3) adopt measures to promote their employees' sense of belonging to their language community and their awareness of cultural diversity; and (4) recognize and motivate employees who participate in the active offer of bilingual services with incentives (for example, a bilingualism bonus).
- Government departments and agencies should provide adequate funding to support the development and delivery of health care and social services in both official languages. Provincial and national advocacy and community organizations such as the *Société Santé en français* (SSF), the *Consortium national de formation en santé* (CNFS), and the Quebec *Community Health and Social Services Network* (CHSSN) need to continue advocating for the rights of OLMCs and strive to have government bodies adopt legislative and policy provisions to protect official language services in all Canadian provinces and territories. Organizations can also suggest policies to establish incentives for designating bilingual positions, operating rules in designated facilities to encourage bilingualism, and the implementation of other incentives such as a bilingualism bonus, and so on. In other words, the strategies of organizations such as the SSF, the CNFS, and the CHSSN could identify rules of the game that might well

be used to the benefit of OLMCs, by increasing their influence on the system.

Thus, on an organizational level, strategies to recruit health and social services professionals should address the values, needs, and expectations of professionals who want to serve clients in minority language communities. Furthermore, the authors explain that the capacity to recruit bilingual staff who will later offer services to OLMCs in their own language depends on the involvement of the entire community—members of the majority as well as the minority.

Within political, policy, and regulatory structures, certain people are responsible for exploring the best ways to distribute health and social service resources to facilitate access to bilingual resources. If considering the linguistic needs of the population is a recognized part of regional or provincial structures, it would be possible to make any necessary adjustments to the distribution of resources, perhaps through agreements or other means of coordinating delivery. For example, even if provincial directives exist to provide for geographical triage mechanisms, regional managers could decide to introduce procedures for exceptions and for cooperation between two organizations in neighbouring areas for the purpose of improving access to linguistically appropriate services.

Another measure to assist in planning human resources in a way that responds to the needs of OLMCs would be the compilation of an inventory of bilingual service providers within an organization, a region, or a province.

Mobilization, Collaboration, and Networking

As Forgues (Chapter 7) points out, in the years to come, Francophone organizations (CNFS, SSF) will have to meet many challenges. One is to adopt strategies that can move French-language services forward in minority settings through the legal and political framework; this framework differs according to the region and concentration of the Francophone population. It would be valuable to develop mobilization strategies to get actors on board and to introduce measures to coordinate efforts to build their capacity to influence the system. Issues deemed to be essential could be dealt with in a way that is in line with the interests of OLMCs. Research by Savard *et al.* (Chapter 9) suggests that creating an informal network of Francophone colleagues and

Francophile co-workers who are supportive could stimulate the use of French within facilities as well as in the wider community. This would, accordingly, enhance the sense of belonging to the Francophone minority community and contribute to the social capital of Francophones and those who support the use of French.

Research has a role to play as well. Interdisciplinary and collaborative approaches are particularly valuable. In recent years, a growing number of scholars in different fields have adopted new approaches to research.[7] Given the numerous issues arising from active offer, we can understand that models allowing us to gain a better understanding of the subject, in all its complexity, need to be developed. Alliances could be formed among diverse actors and groups of actors, allowing them to reposition themselves to have a greater impact on the concrete system of action.[8]

Synthesis of Recommendations to Promote the Active Offer of Services in Both Official Languages

As we reach the end of this volume, building on the different strategies we have presented, we are able to formulate six recommendations intended to accelerate the shift to the active offer of services in both official languages:

Recommendations to Promote the Active Offer of Services in Both Official Languages

1. Present legal arguments and use policy levers.
2. Pursue efforts dedicated to developing education on active offer to stimulate the commitment of future professionals and the different actors involved in the health care and social services environment.
3. Promote an organizational culture oriented toward active offer.
4. Strengthen the leadership capacity of social actors and communities.
5. Design a strategy to attract and retain bilingual service providers wherever there are members of OLMCs.
6. Rally and engage OLMC advocacy organizations and adopt approaches to increase opportunities for cooperation and networking.

In closing, we would like to put forward the idea that governments have an increasing tendency to emphasize the performance
and accountability of systems. In this kind of context, it is appropriate
to act in ways informed by best practices in active offer. In this regard,
it is also interesting to note the recent link made between Canadian
researchers and their colleagues in Wales,[9] which has allowed us to
compare strategies and to discuss their effectiveness. It is important
to seize every opportunity of this nature in order to better understand the challenges related to active offer and to exchange ideas and
information about innovative practices that could help us respond
better to members of minority communities.

Notes

1. To briefly review the meaning of the four primary concepts of strategic
   analysis presented in the first chapter: **Issues**: what each person hopes
   to gain or runs the risk of losing by putting his or her resources into
   play in a power relationship (Crozier & Friedberg, 1977, p. 68); **Actors**:
   individuals and groups who protect given interests and attempt to
   influence the system of action (Crozier & Friedberg, 1977, p. 397);
   System: a symbolic structure, a political, policy and regulatory structure, and an organizational structure (Champagne *et al.*, 2005);
   Strategies: actions which an actor uses to seize opportunities for the
   purpose of improving her or his own situation and reinforcing her or
   his ability to act. The behaviour of an actor always has meaning, and
   is the result of rational choices based on opportunities available and
   the behaviour of other actors (Crozier & Friedberg, 1977, pp. 47–48).
2. A somewhat more detailed description of these models is presented in
   Chapter 6 (Drolet *et al.*).
3. To learn more about these ideas, we invite the reader to consult research
   on person- or patient-centred care (Canadian Medical Association &
   Canadian Nurses Association [CMA & CNA], 2011; Lévesque *et al.*, 2013),
   user satisfaction (Canadian Foundation for Healthcare Improvement,
   2012), access to care for vulnerable persons and patient safety (Canadian
   Patient Safety Institute, n.d.; Organisation mondiale de la santé, 2009),
   culturally appropriate care (Campinha-Bacote, 2002; Canadian Nurses
   Association [CNA], 2010; Office of Minority Health, 2001).
4. On this topic, see the research of Johnson and Doucet (2006).
5. On this topic, see the *International Covenant on Economic, Social and
   Cultural Rights*, in which every individual's right to "the highest attainable standard of physical and mental health" is included. See also Saint-
   Gal (2016).

6. On this topic, see Crozier (1987) and Pavé (1994).
7. On this subject, see Farrah (2015), p.10.
8. For a deeper understanding of this issue, consult the research of Vincent Lemieux on public policy and actor alliances (Lemieux *et al.*, 2003, pp. 119–144).
9. On this topic, see van Kemenade & Forest (2015).

References

Canadian Medical Association & Canadian Nurses Association (CMA & CNA). (2011). *Principles to Guide Health Care Transformation in Canada*. Retrieved from https://www.cma.ca/Assets/assets-library/document/en/advocacy/HCT-Principlese.pdf#search=soins%20centr%C3% A9s%20 sur%20le%20patien

Canadian Nurses Association (CNA). (2010). *Position Paper: Promoting Cultural Competence in Nursing. CNA Position*. Retrieved from https://www.cna-aiic.ca/~/media/cna/page-content/pdf-en/ps114_cultural_competence_2010_e.pdf?la=en. Accessed March 22, 2017.

Barr, V. J., Robinson, S., Marin-Link, B., Underhill, L., Dotts, A., Ravensdale, D., & Salivaras, S. (2003). The expanded chronic care model: An integration of concepts and strategies from population health promotion and the chronic care model. *Healthcare Quarterly, 7*(1), 73–82. doi:10.12927/hcq.2003.16763.

Bodenheimer, T., Wagner, E. H., & Grumbach, K. (2002). Improving primary care for patients with chronic illness: The chronic care model, part 2. *JAMA, 288*(15), 1909–1914. doi:10.1001/jama.288.15.1909.

Bouchard, P. (under the direction of). (March 2015). *Forum de discussion sur la Qualité, la sécurité et les langues officielles dans l'univers de la santé*. Initiative organized in partnership with:: Département d'administration publique de l'Université de Moncton, Société santé et mieux-être en français du Nouveau-Brunswick and Consortium national de formation en santé— National Secretariat and Université de Moncton section. Discussion forum, Université de Moncton, Moncton, NB.

Campinha-Bacote, J. (2002). The process of cultural competence in the delivery of healthcare services: A model of care. *Journal of Transcultural Nursing, 13*(3), 181–184.

Canadian Foundation for Healthcare Improvement. (2012). Myth: High patient satisfaction means high quality care. Retrieved from http://www.fcass-cfhi.ca/sf-docs/default-source/mythbusters/Myth-Patient-Satisfaction-E.pdf?sfvrsn=0

Canadian Heritage. (2013). *Roadmap for Canada's official languages 2013–2018: Education, Immigration, Communities*. Ottawa, ON: Government of Canada. Retrieved from http://pch.gc.ca/DAMAssetPub/

DAM-secLo-olSec/STAGING/texte-text/road-
map2013-2018_1364313629232_eng.pdf?WT.contentAuthority=11.0

Canadian Patient Safety Institute. (n.d.). *About CSPI.* Retrieved from http://
www.patientsafetyinstitute.ca/en/about/pages/default.aspx

Champagne, F., Contandriopoulos, A., Picot-Touché, J., Béland, F., & Nguyen,
H. (2005). *Un cadre d'évaluation globale de la performance des systèmes de
services de santé: Le modèle EGIPSS.* Montréal, QC: Groupe de recherche
interdisciplinaire en santé de l'Université de Montréal.

Couturier, Y., Gagnon, D., Belzile, L., & Salles, M. (2013). *La coordination en
gérontologie.* Montréal, QC: Presses de l'Université de Montréal.
Retrieved from http://www.pum.umontreal.ca/catalogue/la-coordination-en-
gerontologie/couverture

Crozier, M. (1987). *État modeste, État moderne: stratégie pour un autre changement.* Paris, France: Fayard.

Crozier, M., & Friedberg, E. (1977). *L'acteur et le système.* Paris, France: Seuil.

Farrah, J. (2015). Se positionner pour avoir le plus grand impact: l'inter-
disciplinarité et les collaborations. *Bulletin: La recherche en environnement à l'Université de Moncton, 124,* p. 10. Retrieved from http://www.
umoncton.ca/publications_docs/bulletin/124/files/ assets/basic-html/
page10.html

Forgues, É., & Landry, R. (2014). *L'accès aux services de santé en français et leur
utilisation en contexte francophone minoritaire: Rapport final.* Moncton,
NB: La Société santé en français. Retrieved from http://www.icrml.ca/
fr/recherches-et-publications/publications-de-licrml/item/8709-acces-
aux-services-de-sante-en-francais-et-leur-utilisation-en-contexte-
francophone-minoritaire

Gaudron, P. (2007). Quelle analyse stratégique les directeurs d'Hôpitaux en
France doivent-ils réaliser face aux modifications des règles économiques et financières de leur secteur? *HEC Montréal,* cahier de recherche
no. 07-01-07. Retrieved from http://neumann.hec.ca/chairemsi/pdfca-
hiersrech/07_01_07.pdf

Giles, H., Bourhis, R.Y., & Taylor, D.M. (1977). Toward a theory of ethnic
group relations. In H. Giles (Ed.), *Language, ethnicity and intergroup
relations,* London: Academic Press.

Johnson, M. L., & Doucet, P. (2006). *Une vue plus claire: Évaluer la vitalité des
communautés de langue officielle en situation minoritaire.* Ottawa, ON:
Commissariat aux langues officielles du Canada.

LeBlanc, P. (2008). *Rapport de l'évaluation sommative du projet de formation et de
recherche du Consortium national de formation en santé.* Conseillers en
gestion PRAXIS.

Lemieux, V., Bergeron, P., Bégin, C., & Bélanger, G. (2003). *Le système de santé
au Québec. Organisations, acteurs et enjeux.* Québec, QC: Les Presses de
l'Université Laval.

Levesque, J.-F., Harris, M. F., & Russell, G. (2013). Patient-centred access to health care: Conceptualising access at the interface of health systems and populations. *International Journal for Equity in Health, 12*(1). doi:org/10.1186/1475-9276-12-18

McCurdy, B., MacKay, C., Badley, E., Veinot, P., & Cott, C. (2008). *A proposed evaluation framework for chronic disease prevention and management initiatives in Ontario.* Toronto, ON: Arthritis Community Research & Evaluation (ACREU).

Ontario Ministry of Health and Long-Term Care. (2012). *French language health planning entities under the* Local Health System Integration Act, 2006 *and Regulation 515/09. Retrieved from* http://www.health.gov.on.ca/en/public/programs/flhs/planning.aspx. Accessed March 22, 2017.

Office of Minority Health. (2001). *National standards for culturally and linguistically appropriate services in health care: final report.* Washington, D.C. Retrieved from http://minorityhealth.hhs.gov/assets/pdf/checked/finalreport.pdf

Organisation mondiale de la santé. (2009). *Sécurité des patients.* Retrieved from http://www.who.int/patientsafety/fr/

Pavé, F. (1994). *L'analyse stratégique: Sa genèse, ses applications et ses problèmes actuels, autour de Michel Crozier.* Paris, France: Seuil.

Saint-Gal, A. (2016). *Application du pacte international relatif aux droits économiques, sociaux et culturels.* Paris, France. Retrieved from http://aadh.fr/wp-content/uploads/2016/02/ACTES-formation-au-PIDESC.pdf

Savard, J., Savard, S., Drolet, M., de Moissac, D., Kubina, L.A., van Kemenade, S., Benoit, J.,& Couturier, Y. (2017). *Cadre d'analyse des leviers d'action pour l'accès et l'intégration des services sociaux et de santé pour les francophones en situation minoritaire.* Ottawa, ON. Retrieved from http://www.grefops.ca/ressources-et-outils.html

Tremblay, S., Angus, D., & Hubert, B. (2012). *Étude exploratoire en matière de services de santé intégrés pour les communautés francophones: Rapport présenté au Réseau des services de santé en français de l'Est de l'Ontario.* Ottawa, ON: PGF Consultants Inc. Retrieved from http://www.rssfe.on.ca/files/uploads/rssfefiles/etude9nov12.pdf. Accessed 13 Nov. 2016.

Tremblay, S., & Prata, G. (2012). *Pour des services de santé linguistiquement et culturellement adaptés: l'accessibilité linguistique est un déterminant de la qualité et de la sécurité des services de santé.* Retrieved from http://sante-francais.ca/wp content/uploads/Normes-portrait-canadien-FR.pdf

van Kemenade, S., & Forest, M. (2015). Revue de la littérature: Enjeux des services sociaux et de santé en contexte bilingue ou multilingue national. Ottawa, ON: Association des collèges et universités de la francophonie Canadienne (ACUFC) / Consortium national de formation en santé (CNFS). Retrieved from https://cnfs.net/wp-content/uploads/2015/06/revue-litt--rature-sant---et-bilinguisme-FINAL.pdf

Wagner, E. H., Austin, B. T., & Korff, M. V. (1996). Organizing care for patients with chronic illness. *The Milbank Quarterly, 74*(4), 511–544.

Contributors

Isabelle Arcand has a PhD in Education and was a Research Assistant with the *Groupe de recherche sur la formation professionnelle en santé et en service social en contexte francophone minoritaire* (GReFoPS) at the time the study discussed in this book was taking place. She now works for the Student Academic Success Service at the University of Ottawa (SASS). Both her research and practice are in the areas of positive development in young people in Francophone minority communities, student retention, and support for students experiencing difficulties.

Halimatou Ba, PhD, is an Associate Professor of Social Work at Université de Saint-Boniface in Winnipeg. Her research interests lie in the areas of the social and collective participation of women, the social integration of Francophone immigrants, and the health of Francophone seniors in minority communities.

Boniface Bahi is an Adjunct Professor at the University of Alberta's Campus Saint-Jean. He holds a PhD in Medical Anthropology and has completed graduate studies in Bioethics at Université de Montréal. A graduate of all levels in Sociology and of a Master's in Public Health program (Université Nationale de Côte d'Ivoire) as well as an author, Dr. Bahi has been doing research in the area of health and migration issues in Francophone communities outside Québec since 2007. The phenomena of young people in urban settings are an additional research interest. He was previously an instructor of Anthropology at Université de Montréal (2002-2006).

Josée Benoît is the Senior Research Associate at the *Groupe de recherche sur la formation professionnelle en santé et en service social en contexte francophone minoritaire* (GReFoPS), at the University of Ottawa. During her doctoral studies, she studied the role of music in the identity construction of young Francophones in minority communities. While working with the GReFoPS, she has developed a solid knowledge of the situation in which Francophones in minority communities find themselves when seeking social services and health care.

Kate Bigney has an interdisciplinary doctorate (PhD) and specializes in community engagement as part of policy-making. At the time the study discussed in this book was taking place, she was a Postdoctoral Fellow at the University of Ottawa (with the GreFoPS) and Hôpital Montfort and is currently a policy analyst at Agriculture and Agri-Food Canada. Her own research focuses on the policy discourse surrounding the implementation of the active offer of French language social services and health services in the minority language.

Louise Bouchard, PhD, is a Full Professor in the School of Sociological and Anthropological Studies and in the doctoral program in Population Health at the University of Ottawa. An interdisciplinary researcher in health, her research examines social inequalities of health, health care, human resources, and health services in the minority official language. She is the co-author, with Martin Desmeules, of the book *Minorités de langue officielle du Canada: Égales devant la santé?* (PUQ, 2011).

Pier Bouchard, PhD, is a Full Professor and teaches in the Master's programs in Public Administration and in Health Care Management at Université de Moncton and is a member of the *Groupe de recherche et d'innovation sur l'organisation des services de santé* (GRIOSS). Her fields of expertise are human resources management, governance, and public policy. Her recent research has explored the issues of the accessibility and active offer of French language services in minority contexts.

Richard Bourhis is an Emeritus Professor in the Department of Psychology at the Université du Québec à Montréal. He holds a PhD in Social Psychology from the University of Bristol, UK. Dr. Bourhis published in English and French on immigration and acculturation, cross-cultural communication, discrimination and intergroup relations, and language planning. He received the Robert C. Gardner Award for his research in bilingualism from the International Association of Language and Social Psychology. In 2010 he was awarded a doctorate "honoris causa" at Université de Lorraine in France and was elected Fellow of the Royal Society of Canada in 2012.

Linda Cardinal, PhD, is a Full Professor in the School of Political Studies and holds the Research Chair in Canadian Francophonie and

Public Policies at the University of Ottawa. Among her recent studies is *Le Québec et l'Irlande. Culture, histoire et identité* (Septentrion, 2014), which she co-edited, *Gouvernance et innovation au sein des francophonies néobrunswickoise et ontarienne* (PUL, 2015) and *State Traditions and Language Regimes* (MQUP, 2015). In 2013, she became a Fellow of the Royal Society of Canada. In 2014, she was named Knight of the Ordre des Palmes académiques de la République française, and has been invested as member of the Order of Canada in 2016.

Lynn Casimiro, PhD, is Vice-President responsible for teaching and academic success at La Cité college, and a researcher at the Institut du savoir Montfort - Research in Ottawa, Ontario. Her main research interests are in the active offer of social services and health care in Ontario and in interdisciplinary collaboration in health care.

Manon Cormier is a Research Officer with the *Groupe de recherche et d'innovation sur l'organisation des services de santé* (GRIOSS), part of the Université de Moncton's Public Administration department. She has contributed to various research projects, in particular to studies on active offer. She was actively involved in the development of the Tool Box for the Active Offer, produced and published on line by the *Consortium national de formation en santé* (CNFS) in 2013, as well as the development of online education on active offer. She also contributes to efforts to integrate information about active offer into educational programs for both future health and social service professionals and those already working in the field.

Danielle de Moissac, PhD, is a Full Professor in the Faculty of Science at Université de Saint-Boniface. Her research deals primarily with the health of Francophones living in minority communities in Manitoba, and on their access to French language social services and health care.

Martin Desmeules, MA in History (UQAM, 2009) / DESS in Teaching (UQAM, 2012) and doctoral candidate in History (UQAM, 2015), has been a professional researcher in history since 2009 and in health sciences since 2010. He has completed studies on the history of social regulations, the health of Canadian linguistic minorities, social science research methodology, and the history of mental health.

Marie Drolet holds a PhD in Social Work. She is a Full Professor in the School of Social Work, Faculty of Social Sciences, at the University of Ottawa and a founding member of the *Groupe de recherche sur la formation professionnelle en santé et en service social en contexte francophone minoritaire* (GReFoPS). Actively involved in the Franco-Ontarian community, her expertise lies in the area of access to French language social services and health care in minority language settings, social issues in health, and the practice of social work with children, adolescents, seniors, and their families.

Claire-Jehanne Dubouloz, PhD, is a Full Professor in the School of Rehabilitation Sciences in University of Ottawa's Faculty of Health Sciences. Her research looks at change in occupational therapy clients, and she has recently developed a Meaning Perspectives Transformation model, which is currently in the validation phase. She directs research on the active offer of health services and offers education in the same area to various actors involved in professional development. Dr. Dubouloz is a founding member of the *Groupe de recherche sur la formation professionnelle en santé et en service social en contexte francophone minoritaire* (GReFoPS). In 2014, she received the Muriel Driver Lectureship Award from the Canadian Association of Occupational Therapists for her contribution to the profession, teaching and research development in the discipline.

Éric Forgues, PhD, has an academic background in Sociology. Since 2012, he has served as the Executive Director of the Canadian Institute for Research on Linguistic Minorities (CIRLM). From 2003 to 2012, he was Assistant Director and Researcher at the same institute. His work focuses on the development of minority language communities, in particular with regard to governance, community organization, and the organization of services directed to the Francophone population.

Pierre Foucher is a Full Professor in the Faculty of Law at the University of Ottawa, and works in both common law and civil law. He is the current director of the Centre for Research on French Canadian Culture (Centre de recherche en civilisation canadienne-française (CRCCF)) at the University of Ottawa. His particular expertise is in the language rights of Francophone minorities in Canada. In 2016, he received the Ordre de la Pléiade from the Ontario branch of the Assemblée parlementaire de la Francophonie (APF) and in 2017, the Ordre des francophones d'Amérique by the Conseil supérieur de la langue française.

Florette Giasson is a Professor at Université de Saint-Boniface's School of Social Work, Director of the school, and its field placement coordinator. Her field of research is the health of Francophones living in minority communities.

Paulette Guitard, PhD, is an Associate Professor in the School of Rehabilitation Sciences in University of Ottawa's Faculty of Health Sciences, where she teaches in the Occupational Therapy program. Her research interests and expertise lie in the areas of French language services, playfulness in adults, the occupational therapist's role in sex reorientation, and technical aids and the environment.

Lucy-Ann Kubina has a Master's in Health Sciences and is a Research Associate with the *Groupe de recherche sur la formation professionnelle en santé et en service social en contexte francophone minoritaire* (GReFoPS). Since 2004, she has developed a solid expertise in qualitative research, and has contributed to several research projects on participation in meaningful activities after a stroke and on social services and health care for Francophones in minority communities.

Marie-Josée Laforge is a Research Officer with the *Groupe de recherche et d'innovation sur l'organisation des services de santé* (GRIOSS) in Université de Moncton's Public Administration department. Since 2014, she has contributed to a number of research projects on active offer, by supporting professors and researchers, conducting research, and delivering educational programs to future health professionals.

Josée Lagacé is an Audiologist with a doctorate in Clinical Sciences. She is an Associate Professor at the University of Ottawa's School of Rehabilitation Sciences and a member of the GReFoPS. Her primary research interest is difficulties in speech perception, particularly in Francophone or bilingual children with academic learning difficulties.

Pascal Lefebvre, PhD, is a speech-language pathologist and an Associate Professor in the Faculty of Health at Laurentian University in Sudbury, Ontario. His research is on speech, language and literacy in children and on the application of knowledge in these fields by professionals working in health and education.

Jacques Michaud, PhD, has been an independent researcher, educator, and community worker for several decades. His research focuses on the French language services provided to Francophone minority communities in Canada. He has worked with the Canadian Institute for Research on Linguistic Minorities (CIRLM) and the Institut franco-ontarien (IFO) at Laurentian University, among other institutions, in order to advance knowledge in the areas of education, community development, and the health and wellness of seniors in linguistic minority settings.

Martin Normand completed his PhD in Political Science at Université de Montréal. His thesis dealt with linguistic mobilization in Ontario, New Brunswick, and Wales. He is currently pursuing a postdoctoral internship at the Institut du savoir Montfort - Research as part of a fellowship in conjunction with the CNFS, University of Ottawa component. Dr. Normand is also a member of the Centre de recherche sur les politiques et le développement social de l'Université de Montréal and an Associate Researcher affiliated with University of Ottawa's Chair in Canadian Francophonie and Public Policies.

Nathalie Plante has been the Coordinator and Senior Analyst at the University of Ottawa's Chair in Canadian Francophonie and Public Policies since 2004. She has also been responsible for knowledge transfer and mobilization with the *Alliance de recherche: Les savoirs de la gouvernance communautaire* since 2010.

Jacinthe Savard is an Occupational Therapist and has a PhD in Public Health. She is an Associate Professor at the School of Rehabilitation Sciences at the University of Ottawa, and a member of the Groupe de recherche sur la formation professionnelle en santé et en service social en contexte francophone minoritaire (GReFoPS). Her particular expertise is in the organization of health services for seniors, in active offer and the education of professionals in practice using an inter-professional co-operation approach.

Sébastien Savard, PhD, is an Associate Professor in the School of Social Work, University of Ottawa. He is particularly interested in the practice of community organization in social work and in social services management. His current research deals with partnerships between community organizations and public institutions, the development of vulnerable communities, and the active offer of social services and health care to Francophones living in minority communities in Ontario. He is a member of the *Groupe de recherche sur la formation des professionnels en santé et service social en contexte francophone minoritaire* (GReFoPS).

Solange van Kemenade has a doctorate in Sociology. She is a Research Associate with the *Groupe de recherche sur la formation professionnelle en santé et en service social en contexte francophone minoritaire* (GReFoPS) at the University of Ottawa and an Instructor at Université du Québec en Outaouais and Université de Montréal. In the past, she worked as the Senior Research Analyst at the Public Health Agency of Canada and Health Canada. Since 2013, she has been working in the field of population health in linguistic minority settings.

Sylvain Vézina is a Full Professor in the Department of Public Administration, Université de Moncton. He is particularly interested in the areas of organizational theory, public policy, and health services management. His most recent studies, as a member of the *Groupe de recherche et d'innovation sur l'organisation des services de santé* (GRIOSS), examine access by members of Francophone minority communities to high-quality and safe health services, and in particular with the concept of active offer.

Faiçal Zellama is an Associate Professor of Economics and Management, and the Director of the School of Business Administration at Université de Saint-Boniface. His particular interests are in economic policy, public policy and social programs, and organizational practices in the area of human resources management.

Health and Society

Series editor: Sanni Yaya

The *Health and Society* series provides a space for dialogue where different fields of expertise (sociology, psychology, political science, biology, nutrition, medicine, nursing, human kinetics, and rehabilitation sciences) generate new insights into health matters from the individual as well as the global perspectives on population health.

Previous titles in this collection

Martin Rovers, Judith Malette and Manal Guirguis-Younger (editors), *Therapeutic Touch: Research, Practice and Ethics*, 2017

Manal Guirguis-Younger, Ryan McNeil and Stephen W. Hwang (editors), *Homelessness & Health in Canada*, 2014

www.press.uottawa.ca

Printed in the USA
CPSIA information can be obtained
at www.ICGtesting.com
JSHW011520221024
72172JS00015B/124